Carbohydrates: Role in Health and Disease

Carbohydrates: Role in Health and Disease

Editor: Clark Turner

AMERICAN
MEDICAL PUBLISHERS
www.americanmedicalpublishers.com

AMERICAN
MEDICAL PUBLISHERS
www.americanmedicalpublishers.com

Cataloging-in-Publication Data

Carbohydrates : role in health and disease / edited by Clark Turner.
p. cm.
Includes bibliographical references and index.
ISBN 978-1-63927-621-9
1. Carbohydrates. 2. Carbohydrates in the body. 3. Carbohydrates in human nutrition.
4. Carbohydrates--Metabolism. 5. Carbohydrates--Metabolism--Disorders.
6. Food--Carbohydrate content. 7. Diet in disease. 8. Nutrition. I. Turner, Clark.
QP701 .C373 2023
612.396--dc23

American Medical Publishers,
41 Flatbush Avenue,
1st Floor, New York,
NY 11217, USA

ISBN 978-1-63927-621-9 (Hardback)

Contents

Preface

Carbohydrates are referred to as the sugar molecules that provide energy to the body. The natural sources of carbohydrates include fruits and vegetables, while some carbohydrates are processed and refined. The most abundant and common types of carbohydrates include fiber, starch or complex carbs, and sugars or simple carbs. Legumes, whole grains, beans and potatoes are some good sources of complex carbohydrates. They play a key role in the prevention of diseases and maintenance of weight. Higher intake of carbohydrates is associated with complications like obesity and associated conditions like heart diseases and diabetes. The breakdown of carbohydrates into glucose causes an increase in the blood sugar levels. This may lead to insulin resistance and the risk of developing metabolic syndrome. Healthy carbohydrates that contain essential vitamins, nutrients and fiber can help prevent insulin resistance. The topics included in this book on carbohydrates and their role in health and disease are of utmost significance and bound to provide incredible insights to readers. It will serve as a reference to a broad spectrum of readers.

Significant researches are present in this book. Intensive efforts have been employed by authors to make this book an outstanding discourse. This book contains the enlightening chapters which have been written on the basis of significant researches done by the experts.

Finally, I would also like to thank all the members involved in this book for being a team and meeting all the deadlines for the submission of their respective works. I would also like to thank my friends and family for being supportive in my efforts.

Editor

1

Quantity and Quality of Carbohydrate Intake during Pregnancy, Newborn Body Fatness and Cardiac Autonomic Control: Conferred Cardiovascular Risk?

Kirsty M. Mckenzie [1,2], Hasthi U. Dissanayake [1,2], Rowena McMullan [1,2,3], Ian D. Caterson [1], David S. Celermajer [2,3], Adrienne Gordon [2,3], Jonathan Hyett [2], Alice Meroni [1], Melinda Phang [1], Camille Raynes-Greenow [4], Jaimie W. Polson [2,5] and Michael R. Skilton [1,2,*]

1 Boden Institute of Obesity, Nutrition, Exercise & Eating Disorders, D17-Charles Perkins Centre, University of Sydney, Camperdown, NSW 2006, Australia; kirstymacknz@gmail.com (K.M.M.); hdis1775@uni.sydney.edu.au (H.U.D.); rowenamcm@gmail.com (R.M.); ian.caterson@sydney.edu.au (I.D.C.); alice.meroni@sydney.edu.au (A.M.); melinda.phang@sydney.edu.au (M.P.)

2 Sydney Medical School, D17-Charles Perkins Centre, University of Sydney, Camperdown, NSW 2006, Australia; David.Celermajer@health.nsw.gov.au (D.S.C.); adrienne.gordon@sydney.edu.au (A.G.); Jon.Hyett@sswahs.nsw.gov.au (J.H.); jaimie.polson@sydney.edu.au (J.W.P.)

3 Royal Prince Alfred Hospital, Missenden Road, Camperdown, NSW 2050, Australia

4 Sydney School of Public Health, Edward Ford Building, Fisher Road, University of Sydney, Sydney, NSW 2006, Australia; camille.raynes-greenow@sydney.edu.au

5 School of Medical Science & Bosch Institute, Anderson Stuart Building (F13), University of Sydney, Sydney, NSW 2006, Australia

* Correspondence: michael.skilton@sydney.edu.au

Abstract: The fetal environment has an important influence on health and disease over the life course. Maternal nutritional status during pregnancy is potentially a powerful contributor to the intrauterine environment, and may alter offspring physiology and later life cardio-metabolic risk. Putative early life markers of cardio-metabolic risk include newborn body fatness and cardiac autonomic control. We sought to determine whether maternal dietary carbohydrate quantity and/or quality during pregnancy are associated with newborn body composition and cardiac autonomic function. Maternal diet during pregnancy was assessed in 142 mother-infant pairs using a validated food frequency questionnaire. Infant adiposity and body composition were assessed at birth using air-displacement plethysmography. Cardiac autonomic function was assessed as heart rate variability. The quantity of carbohydrates consumed during pregnancy, as a percentage of total energy intake, was not associated with meaningful differences in offspring birth weight, adiposity or heart rate variability ($p > 0.05$). There was some evidence that maternal carbohydrate quality, specifically higher fibre and lower glycemic index, is associated with higher heart rate variability in the newborn offspring ($p = 0.06$). This suggests that poor maternal carbohydrate quality may be an important population-level inter-generational risk factor for later cardiac and hemodynamic risk of their offspring.

Keywords: carbohydrate; maternal diet; fibre; glycaemic index; glycaemic load; autonomic function; body composition; heart rate variability; infant; adiposity

---

1. Introduction

Cardiovascular disease (CVD) remains the leading cause of morbidity and mortality worldwide. The World Health Organization estimates that 17.5 million people die each year from CVD, an estimated 31% of all deaths worldwide [1]. Both human and animal studies have provided strong evidence to suggest that the fetal environment impacts the risk of cardio-metabolic diseases in later life.

Impaired fetal growth is recognized as an important early life risk factor for CVD [2–4]. Fetal growth is affected by a range of genetic, environmental and maternal factors, and impaired fetal growth is associated with higher blood pressure and markers of poorer vascular health from early childhood through adulthood [5,6], which likely mediate at least part of the association with CVD. High birth weight is also an important risk factor for obesity in adulthood [7], and therefore also poses a risk for CVD. A proportion of the association between obesity and CVD may relate to autonomic dysfunction [8], an important factor in the early aetiology and ongoing pathophysiology of hypertensive and cardiovascular disorders [9–13]. Indeed, there is evidence that newborns with high body fatness, putatively a better marker of risk than birth weight, have altered autonomic control [14].

Maternal nutritional status is a powerful contributor to the overall intrauterine environment to which the fetus is exposed, with considerable evidence linking dietary restrictions to adverse offspring outcomes. For example, the offspring of women exposed to extreme famines while pregnant, such as the Dutch Hunger Winter, have reduced birth weights [15], subsequently linked to CVD and increased mortality in later life [16]. However, severe dietary restriction is uncommon in developed nations, in which dietary composition is likely to be of greater relevance. Both maternal dietary protein and fat intake have been shown to influence offspring cardiometabolic function, playing an integral role in the modification of genetic programming of fetal physiology and morphology in experimental models [17]. However, as glucose is the main energy substrate for fetal growth, maternal dietary carbohydrate intake is an important fetal exposure. Both dietary glycaemic index (GI) and glycaemic load (GL) are markers of dietary carbohydrate quality, and are strong determinants of circulating glucose levels throughout the day during pregnancy [18]. In turn, blood glucose levels are associated with increased risk of adverse outcomes in the offspring, including being born large-for-gestational age, in a linear dose-dependent manner [19].

Nonetheless, there is limited evidence directly linking maternal dietary carbohydrate quantity and quality with offspring body fatness and cardiac autonomic control during the perinatal period.

Therefore, we sought to determine whether maternal dietary carbohydrate intake, and GI and fibre as markers of the quality thereof, are associated with newborn anthropometric measures including body fatness, and cardiac autonomic function. We predicted that maternal intake of higher quality carbohydrates during pregnancy would be correlated with reduced body fatness and improved markers of infant autonomic control.

2. Materials and Methods

2.1. Participants

Mothers and their newborn babies were recruited (n = 224; between April 2015 and September 2016) from the maternity wards of RPA Women & Babies, Royal Prince Alfred Hospital, Sydney, Australia as part of a broader study examining the associations of body fatness, diet and late preterm birth with cardiovascular risk in the offspring. Participants were eligible if they met all of the following criteria: singleton born at the RPA Women & Babies, infants had body fatness assessed by air-displacement plethysmography within 24 h of birth, and gestational age $\geq$ 34 weeks. Exclusion criteria included infants with major congenital abnormalities or who required respiratory support, and those from a multiple birth pregnancy. For this manuscript, mothers with gestational diabetes mellitus (GDM) (n = 36), preeclampsia (n = 8), and neonates born pre-term (gestational age $\leq$ 36 weeks, n = 8), were excluded prior to analysis, ultimately leaving 142 participants for analysis.

The study was conducted in accordance with ethical standards and approved by the Sydney Local Health District (HREC/14/RPAH/478). Participation was voluntary and informed written consent was obtained from the participating mothers before taking part in the study.

2.2. *Maternal Characteristics and Dietary Intake*

A self-administered questionnaire recorded maternal demographic characteristics and perinatal outcomes, with confirmation from health records.

Dietary data and intakes during pregnancy were collected using a validated electronic food frequency questionnaire (FFQ) which includes the foods and drinks typically consumed in Australia [20]. Women were requested by the study investigators to specifically think about their dietary consumption during the entirety of their pregnancy when completing the FFQ. Food specific nutrient values were derived from AUSNUT 2007, and GI and GL values from NUTTAB 2010.

2.3. *Infant Anthropometry and Autonomic Function*

Birth weight, length and head circumference were collected clinically as part of the newborn early assessment program (RPAH_GL2013_019) and obtained from medical records. Infant body fat percentage, lean body mass and body composition were assessed by air-displacement plethysmography (PEA POD, COSMED, Italy) as part of routine clinical practice [21]. Gestational age was estimated from the date of last menstrual period and early pregnancy ultrasound [22].

Autonomic function was assessed as heart rate variability (HRV) derived from electrocardiogram (ECG) recordings. ECG was recorded continuously for 15 min using a standard neonatal 3-lead configuration (Powerlab, ADInstruments, Australia) in infants sleeping in a supine position. Analog output was digitized at 500 Hz. During recordings, the infants' behavior were closely monitored, noting any occasions when the infant woke up, which were subsequently removed from analysis. Frequency domain analysis of HRV was performed using LabChart (HRV 1 module, version 7, ADInstruments, Australia) from 3 R-R interval epochs of exactly 4 min. Peak detection on the ECG signal was used to create RR interval sequences. A fast Fourier transformation (256 point, Hanning window) with 50% overlap was used to analyze the frequency domain. A range of 0–1.1 Hz was used to investigate the spectral bands for HRV that incorporated the respiratory frequency of the infant [23]. High frequency (HF) was defined at 0.15 to 1.1 Hz and low frequency (LF) at 0.04 to 0.15. The very low frequency band was not analyzed because of probable non-harmonic components and trend removal artifacts [24]. Of the 142 participants who met the inclusion criteria for analysis, successful cardiac autonomic function assessments were available for 101 infants. The primary reasons for unsuccessful cardiac autonomic function assessment were infants failing to settle during the recordings, early discharge prior to assessment and equipment related issues.

2.4. *Statistical Analysis*

Descriptive data are presented as mean (SD) for continuous variables and n (%) for categorical variables, unless otherwise stated. Data were visually assessed for normality and confirmed using the Kolmogorov-Smirnov test. Non-normally distributed data were transformed using an appropriate transformation. Associations between maternal dietary factors, newborn autonomic functions, and body composition measures were determined by multivariable linear regression models, adjusting for maternal total energy intake during pregnancy, maternal age and newborn gender as covariates. Our sample size of $n = 142$ mother-child pairs provides us with 85% power to detect a correlation coefficient of 0.25 at $2p < 0.05$.

Maternal carbohydrate intake during pregnancy was derived from the FFQ as crude intake (g/day), and subsequently converted to proportion of daily energy intake (%) for statistical analysis using a conversion factor of 17 kJ per gram of carbohydrate [25]. Maternal dietary intakes, specifically carbohydrate intake, GI, GL and fibre were analyzed as continuous variables and as categorical variables derived from quartiles. Cut-offs for quartiles were: Carbohydrate: Min 28.6% of total energy intake; 25th percentile 37.0; 50th percentile 40.9; 75th percentile 43.3; max 59.1. GI: Min 41.7% of total energy intake; 25th percentile 47.0; 50th percentile 49.8; 75th percentile 52.1; max 59.8. Quartiles for fibre (g/day) and GL were derived using the residual method [26]. For the four groups stratified by carbohydrate intake, the mean macronutrient proportions (Carbohydrate:Fat:Protein) were: Q1 34:42:22; Q2 39:40:19; Q3 42:37:19; Q4 47:33:18. All statistical analysis was undertaken with IBM SPSS Statistics (version 22.0; IBM Corp., Somers, NY, USA), and statistical significance inferred at $2p < 0.05$.

3. Results

3.1. Demographics

Characteristics of the 142 mother-child pairs are shown in Table 1. Mothers who participated in the study were, on average, in their early thirties (33 years (SD 4.4)) and with pre-pregnancy BMI (22.0 (IQR 3.6) kg/m^2). On average, women obtained 41% of their daily energy intake from carbohydrate, GI was relatively low and fibre intake was slightly lower than the recommended adequate intake for pregnant women in Australia [27] (Table 1).

Table 1. Maternal characteristics, including diet, and neonatal anthropometry.

Characteristic		
Maternal characteristics		*Cardiac autonomic function subgroup*
Maternal age, years	33.3 ± 4.4	33.2 ± 4.6
Maternal height, m	165.3 ± 6.5	165.0 ± 6.6
Pre-pregnancy BMI, kg/m^2	22.0 ± 3.6	22.1 ± 4.1
Total energy intake, kJ/day	7854 ± 3756	7478 ± 3464
Total fat intake, % energy	37.7 ± 4.6	37.9 ± 4.3
Protein intake, % energy	19.4 ± 2.8	19.0 ± 3.3
Carbohydrate, % energy	41.0 ± 5.0	41.0 ± 4.8
Fibre, g/day	22.8 ± 9.8	21.9 ± 8.7
Glycaemic Index	49.8 ± 5.1	49.4 ± 0.
Glycaemic Load	89.3 ± 44.8	96.3 ± 5.3
Newborn characteristics		
Female, n%	83 (58%)	58 (57%)
Gestation, week	39.3 ± 1.2	39.2 ± 1.1
Birth Weight, g	3426 ± 521	3436 ± 558
Birth length, cm	49.9 ± 2.3	49.9 ± 2.5
Head circumference, cm	34.8 ± 1.4	34.8 ± 1.4
Body Fatness, %	11.1 ± 5.1	11.3 ± 5.4
Fat Free Mass, %	88.9 ± 5.1	88.7 ± 5.4
HRV – TP, ms^2	-	1124 ± 1113
HRV – LF, ms^2	-	285 ± 286
HRV – HF, ms^2	-	122 ± 168

Values are mean ± SD for continuous variables and n (%) for categorical variables. n = 131 for maternal height, n = 134 for pre-pregnancy BMI, n = 147 for gestational age, birth weight, birth length, head circumference, body fatness and fat free mass. For the autonomic function subgroup, n = 91 for pre-pregnancy BMI, n = 104 for TP, LF & HF, n = 142 for all other variables and n = 101 for all other cardiac autonomic function variables. Pre-pregnancy BMI, GI, GL, TP, LF and HF were not normally distributed, and are expressed as median ± interquartile range (IQR).

3.2. Body Composition and Maternal Carbohydrate Intake

There was no association of carbohydrate intake, either quantity or quality, with infant birth weight or body fatness (Table 2). Results were similar when dietary exposures were treated as continuous or categorical variables. Further adjustment for carbohydrate intake did not modify the association of maternal dietary fibre intake with newborn body fat or birth weight.

Table 2. Associations between maternal carbohydrate intake, both quantity and quality, with newborn body composition (n = 142).

	Birth Weight (g)		Body Fatness (%)	
	β (95% CI)	**p Value**	**β (95% CI)**	**p Value**
Carbohydrate (%)	43 (−23, 108)	0.20	0.01 (−0.18, 0.16)	0.90
Q_1	*Reference*		*Reference*	
Q_2	222 (−33, 478)	0.09	2.18 (−0.30, 4.67)	0.09
Q_3	143 (−109, 396)	0.26	0.35 (−2.11, 2.80)	0.78
Q_4	124 (−124, 372)	0.33	1.44 (−0.98, 3.85)	0.24
Glycaemic Index	291 (−970, 1553)	0.65	1.73 (−10.59, 14.04)	0.78
Q_1	*Reference*		*Reference*	
Q_2	−13 (−259, 233)	0.91	−0.58 (−3.00, 1.83)	0.63
Q_3	122 (−129, 372)	0.34	0.37 (−2.08, 2.82)	0.77
Q_4	32 (−218, 282)	0.80	0.26 (−2.19, 2.71)	0.83
Glycaemic Load	265 (−138, 667)	0.20	0.88 (−3.07, 4.83)	0.66
Q_1	*Reference*		*Reference*	
Q_2	−236 (−478, 6)	0.06	−1.79 (−4.20, 0.61)	0.14
Q_3	125 (−114, 363)	0.30	0.55 (−1.82, 2.93)	0.65
Q_4	−56 (−294, 181)	0.64	−0.28 (−2.64, 2.08)	0.81
Fibre (g)	45 (−51, 141)	0.36	0.01 (−0.15, 0.16)	0.95
Q_1	*Reference*		*Reference*	
Q_2	−98 (−340, 144)	0.43	−0.11 (−2.42, 2.20)	0.93
Q_3	97 (−147, 341)	0.43	2.56 (0.23, 4.90)	0.03
Q_4	−30 (−273, 214)	0.81	−0.39 (−2.72, 1.94)	0.75

Values are unstandardized β-regression coefficients (95% CI) from multivariable regression analyses, and represent the differences in newborn birth weight (g) and body fatness (%) per unit increase in the independent variable (maternal dietary characteristic), adjusted for maternal age, newborn gender and total energy intake. Glycaemic Index and glycaemic load were log transformed (ln) for analysis.

3.3. Infant Autonomic Function and Maternal Carbohydrate Intake

In the 101 infants in whom cardiac autonomic control was assessed, maternal carbohydrate intake as a proportion of energy was not associated with measures of cardiac autonomic control (total power, LF, HF and LF:HF). There was weak evidence of an association of better carbohydrate quality (higher fibre, lower GI) with higher LF band of heart rate variability, considered to be a marker of sympathetic modulation. This was similar for analysis of GI as either a continuous variable or as a categorical variable (Table 3), and for fibre (Table 3; Figure 1). These associations were slightly strengthened by adjustment for pre-pregnancy weight, e.g., LF: −2.17 [−4.36, 0.03] per unit GI (p = 0.05) and 0.66 (0.08, 1.24) per unit fibre (p = 0.03) and were only slightly weakened by adjustment for newborn body fatness, e.g., LF: (−1.8 [−4.0, 0.4]) per unit GI (p = 0.12), adjusted for body fatness (%).

Table 3. Associations between maternal carbohydrate content and quality with newborn heart rate variability (autonomic cardiac control).

	TP *, ms^2		LF *, ms^2		HF *, ms^2		LF:HF *	
	β (95% CI)	p Value	β (95% CI)	p Value	β (95% CI)	p Value	β (95% CI)	p Value
Carbohydrate, %	0.01 (−0.04, 0.03)	0.75	0.00 (−0.03, 0.03)	0.97	0.00 (−0.04, 0.05)	0.96	0.00 (−0.03, 0.03)	0.85
Q_1	*Reference*		*Reference*		*Reference*		*Reference*	
Q_2	−0.03 (−0.50, 0.44)	0.90	−0.20 (−0.70, 0.30)	0.42	−0.32 (−0.96, 0.32)	0.32	0.23 (−0.22, 0.68)	0.31
Q_3	0.17 (0.26, 0.60)	0.44	−0.11 (−0.34, 0.57)	0.62	0.22 (−0.37, 0.81)	0.46	−0.01 (−0.42, 0.40)	0.96
Q_4	−0.03 (−0.46, 0.41)	0.91	−0.01 (−0.47, 0.45)	0.97	−0.09 (−0.67, 0.50)	0.76	0.12 (−0.29, 0.53)	0.57
Glycaemic Index *	−1.37 (−3.43, 0.70)	0.19	−1.94 (−4.12, 0.24)	0.08	−1.59 (−4.46, 1.27)	0.27	−0.10 (−2.09, 1.89)	0.92
Q_1	*Reference*		*Reference*		*Reference*		*Reference*	
Q_2	−0.11 (−0.51, 0.30)	0.61	−0.21 (−0.64, 0.21)	0.32	−0.28 (−0.84, 0.27)	0.32	0.10 (−0.29, 0.49)	0.60
Q_3	0.00 (−0.46, 0.46)	0.99	−0.13 (−0.62, 0.35)	0.58	0.00 (−0.64, 0.63)	1.00	0.07 (−0.37, 0.51)	0.76
Q_4	−0.31 (−0.73, 0.12)	0.16	−0.44 (−0.89, 0.01)	0.05	−0.42 (−1.01, 0.17)	0.16	0.06 (−0.35, 0.47)	0.77
Glycaemic load *	0.38 (−0.34, 1.09)	0.30	0.19 (−0.57, 0.95)	0.62	0.34 (−0.65, 1.33)	0.49	−0.15 (−0.83, 0.54)	0.67
Q_1	*Reference*		*Reference*		*Reference*		*Reference*	
Q_2	0.19 (−0.32, 0.62)	0.39	0.20 (−0.25, 0.65)	0.38	0.22 (−0.37, 0.82)	0.46	0.08 (−0.34, 0.49)	0.71
Q_3	−0.05 (−0.48, 0.37)	0.80	−0.21 (−0.66, 0.23)	0.34	−0.11 (−0.69, 0.47)	0.71	0.05 (−0.36, 0.45)	0.82
Q_4	−0.02 (−0.46, 0.42)	0.92	0.00 (−0.47, 0.46)	1.00	−0.15 (−0.76, 0.46)	0.62	0.14 (−0.29, 0.56)	0.52
Fibre, g	0.02 (−0.01, 0.05)	0.14	0.03 (−0.00, 0.06)	0.06	0.01 (−0.04, 0.05)	0.79	0.03 (−0.00, 0.06)	0.06
Q_1	*Reference*		*Reference*		*Reference*		*Reference*	
Q_2	0.23 (−0.19, 0.65)	0.29	0.45 (−0.01, 0.89)	0.05	0.28 (−0.31, 0.86)	0.35	0.19 (−0.21, 0.59)	0.34
Q_3	0.24 (−0.19, 0.66)	0.28	0.21 (−0.24, 0.65)	0.36	0.09 (−0.51, 0.68)	0.78	0.26 (−0.15, 0.66)	0.22
Q_4	0.27 (−0.16, 0.70)	0.22	0.40 (−0.05, 0.85)	0.08	0.15 (−0.45, 0.75)	0.62	0.26 (−0.15, 0.67)	0.21

Values are unstandardized β-regression coefficients (95% CI) from multivariable models (n = 101). Results shown are differences in newborn cardiac autonomic control per unit increase in maternal GI (glycaemic index), GL (glycaemic load) and carbohydrate intake (%), adjusted for maternal age, newborn gender and total energy intake. * Log transformed for analysis. TP, total power; LF, low frequency; HF, high frequency; LF:HF, ratio of low frequency to high frequency.

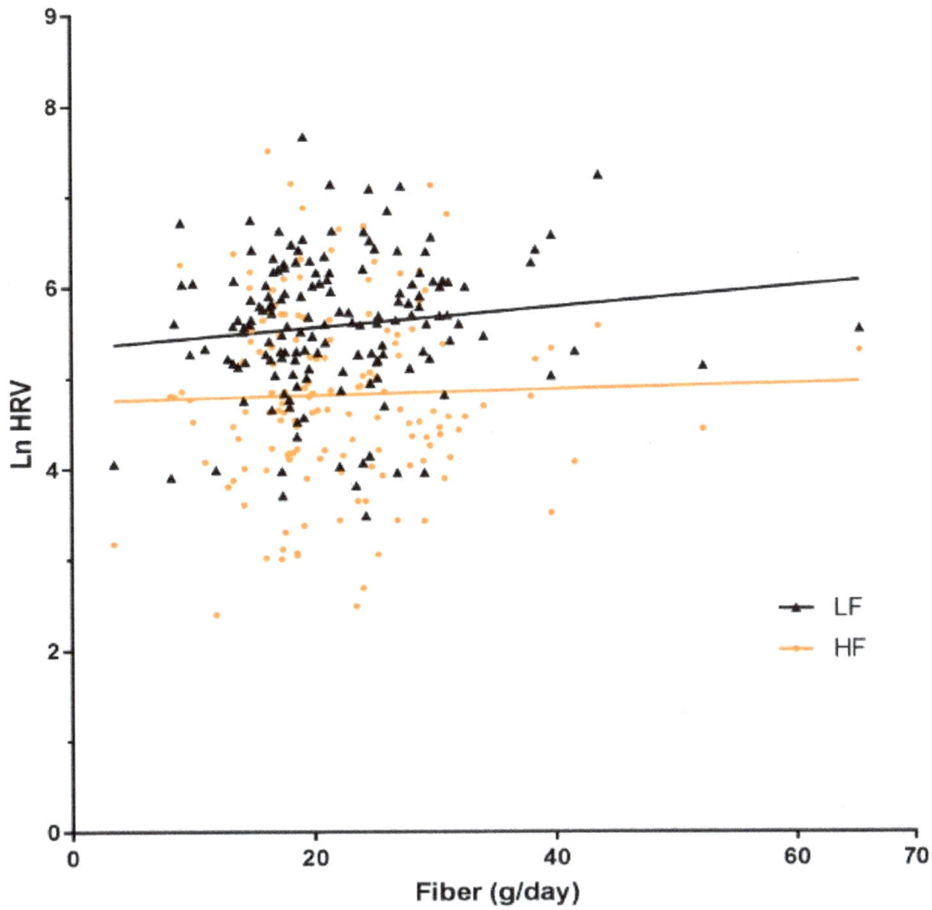

Figure 1. Correlation between maternal fibre (g/day) intake for the duration of pregnancy and newborn autonomic function (HRV).

4. Discussion

Our findings indicate maternal carbohydrate quality, as measured by GI and fibre intake, are weakly associated with physiological differences in infant cardiac autonomic function. In contrast, the quantity of maternal carbohydrate intake during pregnancy was not associated with meaningful differences in offspring body composition or autonomic control, including amongst those who consumed the highest proportion of energy as carbohydrate. Autonomic nervous system activity predicts future risk of cardiovascular disease [24,28] and plays a role in the development and etiology of adult hypertension [29,30]. HRV is a non-invasive marker of autonomic modulation of heart rate and is categorised into three main spectral components; the frequency domain measures of very low frequency (VLF), low frequency (LF) and high frequency (HF). Both the distribution of the measure of total power, as well as the power within the LF and HF bands may vary in relation to changes in autonomic modulations of heart rate [31,32]. The HF band is associated with respiratory sinus arrhythmia and is largely influenced by vagal nerve activity, while the interpretation of the LF band is more complex [24]. The LF component is believed to reflect both vagal and sympathetic activity [33,34], or alternatively as a quantitative marker of sympathetic modulations [35,36]. Accordingly our finding that carbohydrate quality was weakly associated with the LF band of heart rate variability, suggests that higher quality maternal carbohydrate intake may be linked with improved sympathetic modulation in their newborn offspring. Conversely, the offspring of women who consumed poorer quality carbohydrates during pregnancy may have worse cardiac autonomic control, which may mechanistically predispose these infants to later hemodynamic and cardiovascular disorders. Future studies may determine whether this is indeed the case, and if so, seek to quantify the effectiveness of interventions that seek to improve maternal carbohydrate quality during pregnancy [22].

The quality of maternal carbohydrate intake during pregnancy influences fetal glucose supply and consequently fetal growth [19,37,38]. The adverse newborn cardio-metabolic profile associated with higher maternal glucose levels may therefore result from a complex interaction between fetal growth, body fatness, vascular changes and cardiac autonomic modulation, which is consistent with the association between autonomic function and maternal carbohydrate quality being weakened by adjustment for newborn birth weight or body fatness.

Carbohydrates represent the largest individual macronutrient component of most diets [39], and both their quantity and quality has been independently associated with maternal blood glucose concentrations and pregnancy outcomes [40]. In this study we used GI and fibre as measures of carbohydrate quality. Both are components of healthy dietary patterns and are associated with improved cardio-metabolic profiles in adults [41–43]. While strong continuous associations have been found between maternal glucose levels and the incidence of infant macrosomia [19,40], low GI dietary interventions in pregnant women have not been clearly demonstrated to affect the incidence of macrosomia, and have little influence on birth weight [40,44,45] or body composition in infancy [46]. We saw no clear or consistent evidence for an association between maternal dietary carbohydrate quality and newborn birth weight or body fatness. This may be explained by the robust physiological transfer of nutrients from mothers to the developing fetus, within the normal range of dietary intakes of women with uncomplicated pregnancies living in developed nations. Indeed, the body fatness and fat free mass of newborns in our study were similar to healthy values from normative data [47]. However, our findings differ from those of a previous small study which showed an inverse association between dietary GI and infant fat free mass in a group of women at risk of GDM [48]. These differences may relate to the risk nature of the participants or timing of dietary assessment.

In contrast, there is evidence that interventions that target GI may be associated with improved vascular health outcomes in the offspring during infancy [22]. This complements our finding that carbohydrate quality may be weakly associated with cardiac autonomic control in newborns. Our results expand upon the etiology of early vascular disease and haemodynamic risk, and inform on age-appropriate cardiovascular risk markers that may identify risk relating to maternal dietary intake. It remains to be determined whether the effect size of the observed association of carbohydrate quality with cardiac autonomic control would be more marked in pregnancies at high risk of poorer cardio-metabolic outcomes.

The main strength of this study lies in the use of air-displacement plethysmography to assess newborn body fatness and fat free mass [49]. There are relatively few studies of body fatness in newborns using air displacement plethysmography, which is the gold-standard non-invasive methodology. Newborn body fatness is potentially a more appropriate marker of the net effect of the intrauterine environment and the maternal nutritional state on fetal growth. Accordingly, it has been proposed that infant body fatness may be a more accurate predictor for later life CVD and metabolic disease, in comparison to newborn birth weight and lean body mass, which are known to be more greatly influenced by genetic factors [50]. Additionally, the intensive newborn measures collected, combined with the assessment of maternal [51] dietary intake, provide unique data regarding the potential associations between maternal dietary carbohydrate intake, infant autonomic function, and adiposity.

All dietary assessment methods have limitations, with FFQs being prone to mis- or under-reporting of exact quantities of nutrient intakes [52]. Accordingly, we have used measures that are proportionate to total energy intake (e.g., carbohydrate intake as percentage energy), and/or adjusted for total energy intake in our statistical analyses. The advantage of utilising a FFQ is that it removes the incentive for study participants to prospectively alter dietary intake, is less burdensome on the subjects [53], and provides a validated measure of habitual dietary intake. Assessment of dietary intake at multiple times during pregnancy, specifically during each trimester and also during the peri-conception period, would provide a clearer and more definitive indication of any critical timings of dietary intake during pregnancy. Blood pressure changes markedly during the early neonatal period, and is logistically difficult to obtain reproducible measures. Accordingly, we did not measure blood pressure in these participants, although it would have informed the cardiac autonomic function results. We excluded pregnancies affected by GDM and preeclampsia to avoid reverse causation, and as such our results should be taken within the context of healthy pregnancies. Future studies that prospectively assess diet in early pregnancy, prior to the development of GDM or preeclampsia, will inform further on whether these complications of pregnancy alter the observed associations. Our sample size is similar to other papers in the field detailing cardiac autonomic control in infants [54], but made sub-analysis of low birth weight babies unfeasible. Family history of cardiovascular disease and gestational weight gain also influence early life markers of cardiometabolic disease [55,56], although were not assessed in the current study. Our sample size also restricts our ability to study the interaction between maternal dietary intake and the genetic programming of cardiometabolic disease [17]. The role of these factors as putative confounders or mediators of the observed associations should be the focus of future studies with a larger sample size.

Weight trajectory during infancy and early childhood may also be an important predictor of later life cardiometabolic disease [5,6]. Future longitudinal studies taking into account the distinct associations of maternal carbohydrate quality and childhood growth trajectories with autonomic activity, would further inform on the independence and potential interaction between these early life exposures.

5. Conclusions

Our findings suggest that quality, but not quantity, of carbohydrates consumed during pregnancy is weakly associated with cardiac autonomic control in the newborn offspring, highlighting a novel putative link between maternal dietary intake and offspring cardiovascular and haemodynamic risk. Whether these associations with cardiac autonomic control have potential long-term implications for disease outcomes, or in risk stratification, remains to be determined. Furthermore, our findings are consistent with a proportionally high carbohydrate diet having neither beneficial nor detrimental effects on newborn cardiovascular risk, birth weight and body fatness, in this otherwise healthy population.

Acknowledgments: The authors thank Professor Graham Giles of the Cancer Epidemiology Centre, Cancer Council Victoria, for permission to use the Dietary Questionnaire for Epidemiological Studies (Version 2), Melbourne: Cancer Council Victoria, 1996. M.R.S. is supported by a Future Leader fellowship from the National Heart Foundation of Australia (#100419).

Author Contributions: K.M.M., H.U.D., A.G., A.M., R.M., M.P., J.W.P. and M.R.S. contributed to the conception and design of the study, and data collection. K.M.M. was responsible for statistical analysis and interpretation, and drafted the manuscript. I.D.C., D.S.C., H.U.D., A.G., J.H., A.M., R.M., M.P., J.W.P., C.R.-G. and M.R.S. read, critically reviewed for meaningful intellectual insight and approved the final manuscript.

References

1. WHO. Cardiovascular Diseases (CVD's). Available online: http://www.who.int/mediacentre/factsheets/fs317/en/ (accessed on 27 August 2017).
2. Reynolds, C.M.; Gray, C.; Li, M.; Segovia, S.A.; Vickers, M.H. Early life nutrition and energy balance disorders in offspring in later life. *Nutrients* **2015**, *7*, 8090–8111. [CrossRef] [PubMed]
3. Barker, D.J.; Osmond, C.; Forsen, T.J.; Kajantie, E.; Eriksson, J.G. Trajectories of growth among children who have coronary events as adults. *N. Engl. J. Med.* **2005**, *353*, 1802–1809. [CrossRef] [PubMed]
4. Visentin, S.; Grumolato, F.; Nardelli, G.B.; Di Camillo, B.; Grisan, E.; Cosmi, E. Early origins of adult disease: Low birth weight and vascular remodeling. *Atherosclerosis* **2014**, *237*, 391–399. [CrossRef] [PubMed]
5. Sehgal, A.; Skilton, M.R.; Crispi, F. Human fetal growth restriction: A cardiovascular journey through to adolescence. *J. Dev. Orig. Health Dis.* **2016**, *7*, 626–635. [CrossRef] [PubMed]

6. Whincup, P.H.; Bredow, M.; Payne, F.; Sadler, S.; Golding, J. Size at birth and blood pressure at 3 years of age. The avon longitudinal study of pregnancy and childhood (ALSPAC). *Am. J. Epidemiol.* **1999**, *149*, 730–739. [CrossRef] [PubMed]
7. Schellong, K.; Schulz, S.; Harder, T.; Plagemann, A. Birth weight and long-term overweight risk: Systematic review and a meta-analysis including 643,902 persons from 66 studies and 26 countries globally. *PLoS ONE* **2012**, *7*, e47776. [CrossRef] [PubMed]
8. Yadav, R.L.; Yadav, P.K.; Yadav, L.K.; Agrawal, K.; Sah, S.K.; Islam, M.N. Association between obesity and heart rate variability indices: An intuition toward cardiac autonomic alteration—A risk of CVD. *Diabetes Metab. Syndr.* **2017**, *10*, 57–64. [CrossRef] [PubMed]
9. Judy, W.V.; Farrell, S.K. Arterial baroreceptor reflex control of sympathetic nerve activity in the spontaneously hypertensive rat. *Hypertension* **1979**, *1*, 605–614. [CrossRef] [PubMed]
10. Judy, W.V.; Watanabe, A.M.; Henry, D.P.; Besch, H.R., Jr.; Murphy, W.R.; Hockel, G.M. Sympathetic nerve activity: Role in regulation of blood pressure in the spontaenously hypertensive rat. *Circ. Res.* **1976**, *38*, 21–29. [CrossRef] [PubMed]
11. Grassi, G. Sympathetic neural activity in hypertension and related diseases. *Am. J. Hypertens.* **2010**, *23*, 1052–1060. [CrossRef] [PubMed]
12. Grassi, G.; Seravalle, G.; Quarti-Trevano, F. The 'neuroadrenergic hypothesis' in hypertension: Current evidence. *Exp. Physiol.* **2010**, *95*, 581–586. [CrossRef] [PubMed]
13. Esler, M.; Straznicky, N.; Eikelis, N.; Masuo, K.; Lambert, G.; Lambert, E. Mechanisms of sympathetic activation in obesity-related hypertension. *Hypertension* **2006**, *48*, 787–796. [CrossRef] [PubMed]
14. Dissanayake, H.; McMullan, R.; Phang, M.; Gordon, A.; Hyatt, J.; Rains-Greenow, C.; Celermajer, D.; Polson, J.; Skilton, M. Newborn body fatness and autonomic function: Identification of infants at risk of later cardiovascular disease. *FASEB J.* **2017**, *31*, 1071–1078.
15. Schulz, L.C. The Dutch Hunger Winter and the developmental origins of health and disease. *Proc. Natl. Acad. Sci. USA* **2010**, *107*, 16757–16758. [CrossRef] [PubMed]
16. Roseboom, T.; de Rooij, S.; Painter, R. The Dutch famine and its long-term consequences for adult health. *Early Hum. Dev.* **2006**, *82*, 485–491. [CrossRef] [PubMed]
17. Costa-Silva, J.H.; Simoes-Alves, A.C.; Fernandes, M.P. Developmental origins of cardiometabolic diseases: Role of the maternal diet. *Front. Physiol.* **2016**, *7*, 504. [CrossRef] [PubMed]
18. Kizirian, N.V.; Goletzke, J.; Brodie, S.; Atkinson, F.S.; Markovic, T.P.; Ross, G.P.; Buyken, A.; Brand-Miller, J.P. Lower glycemic load meals reduce diurnal glycemic oscillations in women with risk factors for gestational diabetes. *BMJ Open Diabetes Res. Care* **2017**, *5*, e000351. [CrossRef] [PubMed]
19. HAPO Study Cooperative Research Group; Metzger, B.E.; Lowe, L.P.; Dyer, A.R.; Trimble, E.R.; Chaovarindr, U.; Coustan, D.R.; Hadden, D.R.; McCance, D.R.; Hod, M.; et al. Hyperglycemia and adverse pregnancy outcomes. *N. Engl. J. Med.* **2008**, *358*, 1991–2002. [CrossRef] [PubMed]
20. Giles, G.G.; Ireland, P.D. *Dietary Questionnaire for Epidemiological Studies*; Version 2; Victorian Cancer Council: Melbourne, Australia, 1996.
21. Breij, L.M.; Steegers-Theunissen, R.P.; Briceno, D.; Hokken-Koelega, A.C. Maternal and fetal determinants of neonatal body composition. *Horm. Res. Paediatr.* **2015**, *84*, 388–395. [CrossRef] [PubMed]
22. Kizirian, N.V.; Kong, Y.; Muirhead, R.; Brodie, S.; Garnett, S.P.; Petocz, P.; Sim, K.A.; Celermajer, D.S.; Louie, J.C.; Markovic, T.P.; et al. Effects of a low-glycemic index diet during pregnancy on offspring growth, body composition, and vascular health: A pilot randomized controlled trial. *Am. J. Clin. Nutr.* **2016**, *103*, 1073–1082. [CrossRef] [PubMed]
23. Polson, J.W.; McCallion, N.; Waki, H.; Thorne, G.; Tooley, M.A.; Paton, J.F.; Wolf, A.R. Evidence for cardiovascular autonomic dysfunction in neonates with coarctation of the aorta. *Circulation* **2006**, *113*, 2844–2850. [CrossRef] [PubMed]
24. Task Force of the European Society of Cardiology. Heart rate variability: Standards of measurement, physiological interpretation and clinical use. *Circulation* **1996**, *93*, 1043–1065.
25. NHMRC. *Nutrient Reference Values for Australia and New Zealand*; Australian Government Department of Health and Ageing, New Zealand Ministry of Health: Canberra, Australia, 2006.
26. Willett, K.; Stampfer, M. *Implications of Total Energy Intake for Epidemiologic Analyses*; Oxford University Press: New York, NY, USA, 1998; pp. 1273–1301.

27. Australian Government. *Healthy Eating During Your Pregnancy*; Health, D.O., Ed.; National Medical Health and Medical Research Council: Canberra, Australia, 2013.
28. Lown, B.; Verrier, R.L. Neural activity and ventricular fibrillation. *N. Engl. J. Med.* **1976**, *294*, 1165–1170. [PubMed]
29. Thayer, J.F.; Lane, R.D. The role of vagal function in the risk for cardiovascular disease and mortality. *Biol. Psychol.* **2007**, *74*, 224–242. [CrossRef] [PubMed]
30. Seravalle, G.; Mancia, G.; Grassi, G. Role of the sympathetic nervous system in hypertension and hypertension-related cardiovascular disease. *High Blood Press. Cardiovasc. Prev.* **2014**, *21*, 89–105. [CrossRef] [PubMed]
31. Malliani, A.; Pagani, M.; Lombardi, F.; Cerutti, S. Cardiovascular neural regulation explored in the frequency domain. *Circulation* **1991**, *84*, 482–492. [CrossRef] [PubMed]
32. Pagani, M.; Lombardi, F.; Guzzetti, S.; Rimoldi, O.; Furlan, R.; Pizzinelli, P.; Sandrone, G.; Malfatto, G.; Dell'Orto, S.; Piccaluga, E.; et al. Power spectral analysis of heart rate and arterial pressure variabilities as a marker of sympatho-vagal interaction in man and conscious dog. *Circ. Res.* **1986**, *59*, 178–193. [CrossRef] [PubMed]
33. Wolf, M.M.; Varigos, G.A.; Hunt, D.; Sloman, J.G. Sinus arrhythmia in acute myocardial infarction. *Med. J. Aust.* **1978**, *2*, 52–53. [PubMed]
34. Appel, M.L.; Berger, R.D.; Saul, J.P.; Smith, J.M.; Cohen, R.J. Beat to beat variability in cardiovascular variables: Noise or music? *J. Am. Coll. Cardiol.* **1989**, *14*, 1139–1148. [CrossRef]
35. Montano, N.; Ruscone, T.G.; Porta, A.; Lombardi, F.; Pagani, M.; Malliani, A. Power spectrum analysis of heart rate variability to assess the changes in sympathovagal balance during graded orthostatic tilt. *Circulation* **1994**, *90*, 1826–1831. [CrossRef] [PubMed]
36. Kamath, M.V.; Fallen, E.L. Power spectral analysis of heart rate variability: A noninvasive signature of cardiac autonomic function. *Crit. Rev. Biomed. Eng.* **1993**, *21*, 245–311. [PubMed]
37. Catalano, P.M.; McIntyre, H.D.; Cruickshank, J.K.; McCance, D.R.; Dyer, A.R.; Metzger, B.E.; Lowe, L.P.; Trimble, E.R.; Coustan, D.R.; Hadden, D.R.; et al. The hyperglycemia and adverse pregnancy outcome study: Associations of GDM and obesity with pregnancy outcomes. *Diabetes Care* **2012**, *35*, 780–786. [CrossRef] [PubMed]
38. Tzanetakou, I.P.; Mikhailidis, D.P.; Perrea, D.N. Nutrition during pregnancy and the effect of carbohydrates on the offspring's metabolic profile: In search of the "Perfect Maternal Diet". *Open Cardiovasc. Med. J.* **2011**, *5*, 103–109. [CrossRef] [PubMed]
39. Australian Bereau of Statistics. Australian Health Survey. Available online: http://www.abs.gov.au/ausstats/abs@.nsf/Lookup/by%20Subject/4364.0.55.007~2011-12~Main%20Features~Carbohydrate~705 (accessed on 16 November 2017).
40. Walsh, J.M.; McAuliffe, F.M. Impact of maternal nutrition on pregnancy outcome—Does it matter what pregnant women eat? *Best Pract. Res. Clin. Obstet. Gynaecol.* **2015**, *29*, 63–78. [CrossRef] [PubMed]
41. Pereira, M.A.; Swain, J.; Goldfine, A.B.; Rifai, N.; Ludwig, D.S. Effects of a low-glycemic load diet on resting energy expenditure and heart disease risk factors during weight loss. *JAMA* **2004**, *292*, 2482–2490. [CrossRef] [PubMed]
42. Ebbeling, C.B.; Leidig, M.M.; Feldman, H.A.; Lovesky, M.M.; Ludwig, D.S. Effects of a low-glycemic load vs low-fat diet in obese young adults: A randomized trial. *JAMA* **2007**, *297*, 2092–2102. [CrossRef] [PubMed]
43. Liyanage, T.; Ninomiya, T.; Wang, A.; Neal, B.; Jun, M.; Wong, M.G.; Jardine, M.; Hillis, G.S.; Perkovic, V. Effects of the mediterranean diet on cardiovascular outcomes—A systematic review and meta-analysis. *PLoS ONE* **2016**, *11*, e0159252. [CrossRef] [PubMed]
44. Walsh, J.M.; McGowan, C.A.; Mahony, R.; Foley, M.E.; McAuliffe, F.M. Low glycaemic index diet in pregnancy to prevent macrosomia (ROLO study): Randomised control trial. *BMJ* **2012**, *345*, e5605. [CrossRef] [PubMed]
45. Horan, M.K.; McGowan, C.A.; Gibney, E.R.; Donnelly, J.M.; McAuliffe, F.M. Maternal low glycaemic index diet, fat intake and postprandial glucose influences neonatal adiposity—Secondary analysis from the ROLO study. *Nutr. J.* **2014**, *13*, 78. [CrossRef] [PubMed]
46. Louie, J.C.; Markovic, T.P.; Perera, N.; Foote, D.; Petocz, P.; Ross, G.P.; Brand-Miller, J.C. A randomized controlled trial investigating the effects of a low-glycemic index diet on pregnancy outcomes in gestational diabetes mellitus. *Diabetes Care* **2011**, *34*, 2341–2346. [CrossRef] [PubMed]
47. Hawkes, C.P.; Hourihane, J.O.; Kenny, L.C.; Irvine, A.D.; Kiely, M.; Murray, D.M. Gender- and gestational age-specific body fat percentage at birth. *Pediatrics* **2011**, *128*, E645–E651. [CrossRef] [PubMed]

48. Kizirian, N.V.; Markovic, T.P.; Muirhead, R.; Brodie, S.; Garnett, S.P.; Louie, J.C.; Petocz, P.; Ross, G.P.; Brand-Miller, J.C. Macronutrient balance and dietary glycemic index in pregnancy predict neonatal body composition. *Nutrients* **2016**, *8*, 270. [CrossRef] [PubMed]
49. Kuhle, S.; Maguire, B.; Ata, N.; MacInnis, N.; Dodds, L. Birth weight for gestational age, anthropometric measures, and cardiovascular disease markers in children. *J. Pediatr.* **2017**, *182*, 99–106. [CrossRef] [PubMed]
50. Skilton, M.R.; Marks, G.B.; Ayer, J.G.; Garden, F.L.; Garnett, S.P.; Harmer, J.A.; Leeder, S.R.; Toelle, B.G.; Webb, K.; Baur, L.A.; et al. Weight gain in infancy and vascular risk factors in later childhood. *Pediatrics* **2013**, *131*, e1821–e1828. [CrossRef] [PubMed]
51. Hull, H.R.; Dinger, M.K.; Knehans, A.W.; Thompson, D.M.; Fields, D.A. Impact of maternal body mass index on neonate birthweight and body composition. *Am. J. Obstet. Gynecol.* **2008**, *198*, e411–e416. [CrossRef] [PubMed]
52. Cade, J.; Thompson, R.; Burley, V.; Warm, D. Development, validation and utilisation of food-frequency questionnaires—A review. *Public Health Nutr.* **2002**, *5*, 567–587. [CrossRef] [PubMed]
53. Subar, A.F.; Ziegler, R.G.; Thompson, F.E.; Johnson, C.C.; Weissfeld, J.L.; Reding, D.; Kavounis, K.H.; Hayes, R.B.; Colorectal and Ovarian Cancer Screening Trial Investigators. Is shorter always better? Relative importance of questionnaire length and cognitive ease on response rates and data quality for two dietary questionnaires. *Am. J. Epidemiol.* **2001**, *153*, 404–409. [CrossRef] [PubMed]
54. Yiallourou, S.R.; Sands, S.A.; Walker, A.M.; Horne, R.S.C. Maturation of heart rate and blood pressure variability during sleep in term-born infants. *Sleep* **2012**, *35*, 177–186. [CrossRef] [PubMed]
55. Oken, E.; Kleinman, K.P.; Belfort, M.B.; Hammitt, J.K.; Gillman, M.W. Associations of gestational weight gain with short- and longer-term maternal and child health outcomes. *Am. J. Epidemiol.* **2009**, *170*, 173–180. [CrossRef] [PubMed]
56. Stotland, N.E.; Cheng, Y.W.; Hopkins, L.M.; Caughey, A.B. Gestational weight gain and adverse neonatal outcome among term infants. *Obstet. Gynecol.* **2006**, *108*, 635–643. [CrossRef] [PubMed]

2

Glucose-6 Phosphate: A Central Hub for Liver Carbohydrate Metabolism

Fabienne Rajas [1,2,3,*], Amandine Gautier-Stein [1,2,3] and Gilles Mithieux [1,2,3]

1 Institut National de la Santé et de la Recherche Médicale, U1213, F-69008 Lyon, France; amandine.gautier-stein@univ-lyon1.fr (A.G.-S.); gilles.mithieux@univ-lyon1.fr (G.M.)
2 Université de Lyon, F-69008 Lyon, France
3 Université Lyon 1, F-69622 Villeurbanne, France
* Correspondence: fabienne.rajas@univ-lyon1.fr

Abstract: Cells efficiently adjust their metabolism according to the abundance of nutrients and energy. The ability to switch cellular metabolism between anabolic and catabolic processes is critical for cell growth. Glucose-6 phosphate is the first intermediate of glucose metabolism and plays a central role in the energy metabolism of the liver. It acts as a hub to metabolically connect glycolysis, the pentose phosphate pathway, glycogen synthesis, de novo lipogenesis, and the hexosamine pathway. In this review, we describe the metabolic fate of glucose-6 phosphate in a healthy liver and the metabolic reprogramming occurring in two pathologies characterized by a deregulation of glucose homeostasis, namely type 2 diabetes, which is characterized by fasting hyperglycemia; and glycogen storage disease type I, where patients develop severe hypoglycemia during short fasting periods. In these two conditions, dysfunction of glucose metabolism results in non-alcoholic fatty liver disease, which may possibly lead to the development of hepatic tumors. Moreover, we also emphasize the role of the transcription factor carbohydrate response element-binding protein (ChREBP), known to link glucose and lipid metabolisms. In this regard, comparing these two metabolic diseases is a fruitful approach to better understand the key role of glucose-6 phosphate in liver metabolism in health and disease.

Keywords: de novo lipogenesis; carbohydrate response element-binding protein; ChREBP; diabetes; glucose production; glycogen; glycolysis; glycogen storage disease type I; hexosamine; nonalcoholic fatty liver disease; NAFLD; pentose phosphate pathway; steatosis

---

1. Introduction

The liver plays a crucial role in the maintenance of glucose homeostasis by extracting glucose from the blood and then storing it after a meal, and also by producing glucose in post-absorptive state. When its concentration increases in the bloodstream, glucose enters the hepatocytes mainly through the glucose transporter 2 (GLUT2). Within the cells, free glucose is immediately phosphorylated on the sixth carbon by glucokinase (also named hexokinase IV), producing glucose-6 phosphate (G6P) and consuming one molecule of ATP. Contrary to the other hexokinases, glucokinase has relatively low affinity for glucose and is not inhibited by G6P [1]. Glucokinase expression is transcriptionally regulated by hormones [induced by insulin through the transcription factor SREBP1c (Sterol Response Element-Binding Protein 1c) and inhibited by glucagon] and metabolites of glucose and glucokinase activity is dependent on its binding to a specific inhibitor named glucokinase regulatory protein (GKRP) (see [2] for a review of glucokinase regulation). Other binding proteins such as 6-phosphofructo-2-kinase/fructose 2,6 biphosphatase (PFK2/FBP2) are also able to activate glucokinase by direct interaction with this enzyme [3].

The phosphorylation of glucose by glucokinase adds a charged phosphate group to this molecule. Consequently, G6P cannot cross the cell membrane, preventing the diffusion of free glucose out of the cells. Thanks to this phosphorylation step, glucokinase enables hepatocytes to trap glucose. During fasting periods, G6P is also produced after isomerization of glucose-1 phosphate during the breakdown of glycogen and by gluconeogenesis in the hepatocyte. It should be noted that a limited amount of free glucose can be directly released from glycogen through the action of the debranching enzyme α-1,6-glucosidase (AGL) and/or the lysosomal acid α-1,4 glucosidase (also known as acid maltase) [4].

Within the cells, G6P has many possible fates and therefore it represents a central hub for carbohydrate metabolism (Figure 1). After isomerization, it initiates major metabolic pathways, i.e., glycolysis, pentose phosphate pathway (PPP), glycogen synthesis, hexosamine pathway, and glucose production according to the nutritional or hormonal states. This review is focused on the key metabolic roles of G6P in cell signaling in the healthy or pathological liver. Here, we will highlight the metabolic reprogramming taking place in two metabolic diseases characterized by a dysfunction of glucose metabolism, namely type 2 diabetes and glycogen storage disease type I (GSDI). Interestingly, type 2 diabetes is an epidemic disease characterized by hyperglycemia, while GSDI is a rare genetic disease due to a loss of endogenous glucose production leading to severe hypoglycemia during short fasting. In type 2 diabetes, hyperglycemia is responsible for an increase in metabolic pathways downstream of G6P, while in GSDI the blockage of glucose production leads to the accumulation of G6P in the hepatocytes, which also increases all the metabolic pathways downstream of G6P (Figure 2). These two diseases are characterized by an accumulation of ectopic lipids in the liver, which leads to the development of hepatic steatosis and promotes hepatic tumorigenesis over time [5]. In this review, we will also consider the well-established role of the Carbohydrate-Responsive Element-Binding Protein (ChREBP) as the carbohydrate sensor that coordinates glucose and lipid metabolism in the liver according to nutritional states.

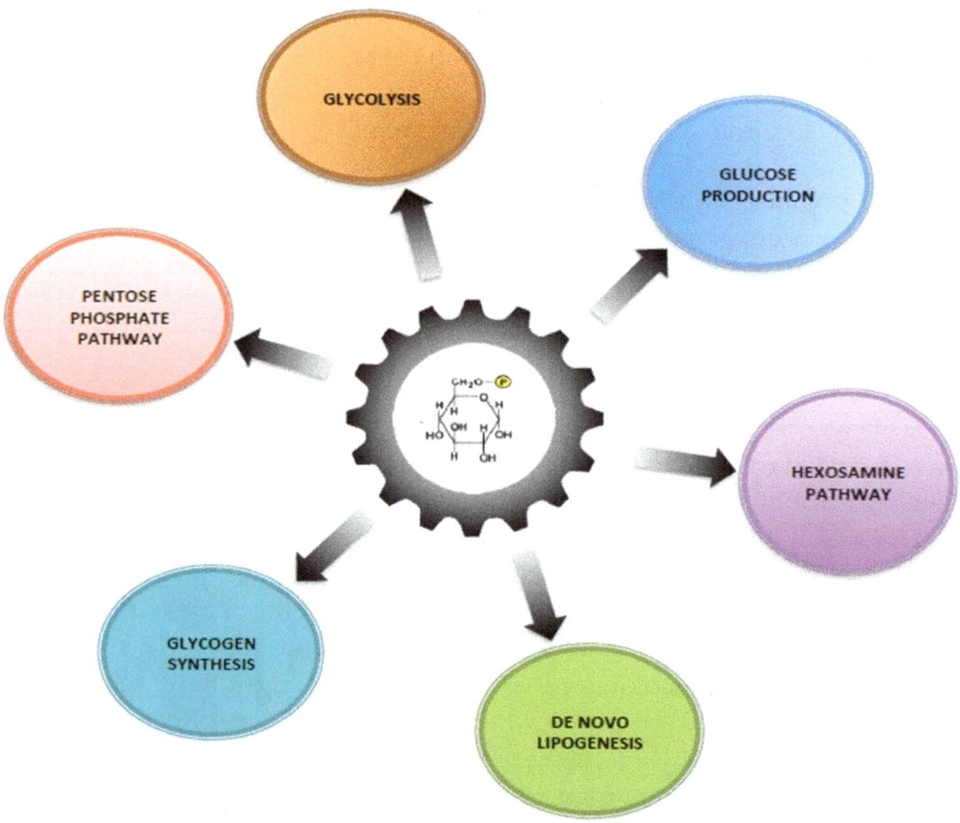

Figure 1. Glucose-6 phosphate, a central hub for liver carbohydrate metabolism. The increase of flux through G6P is responsible for increasing glycogen synthesis, glycolysis, pentose phosphate pathway (PPP), hexosamine pathway and de novo lipogenesis.

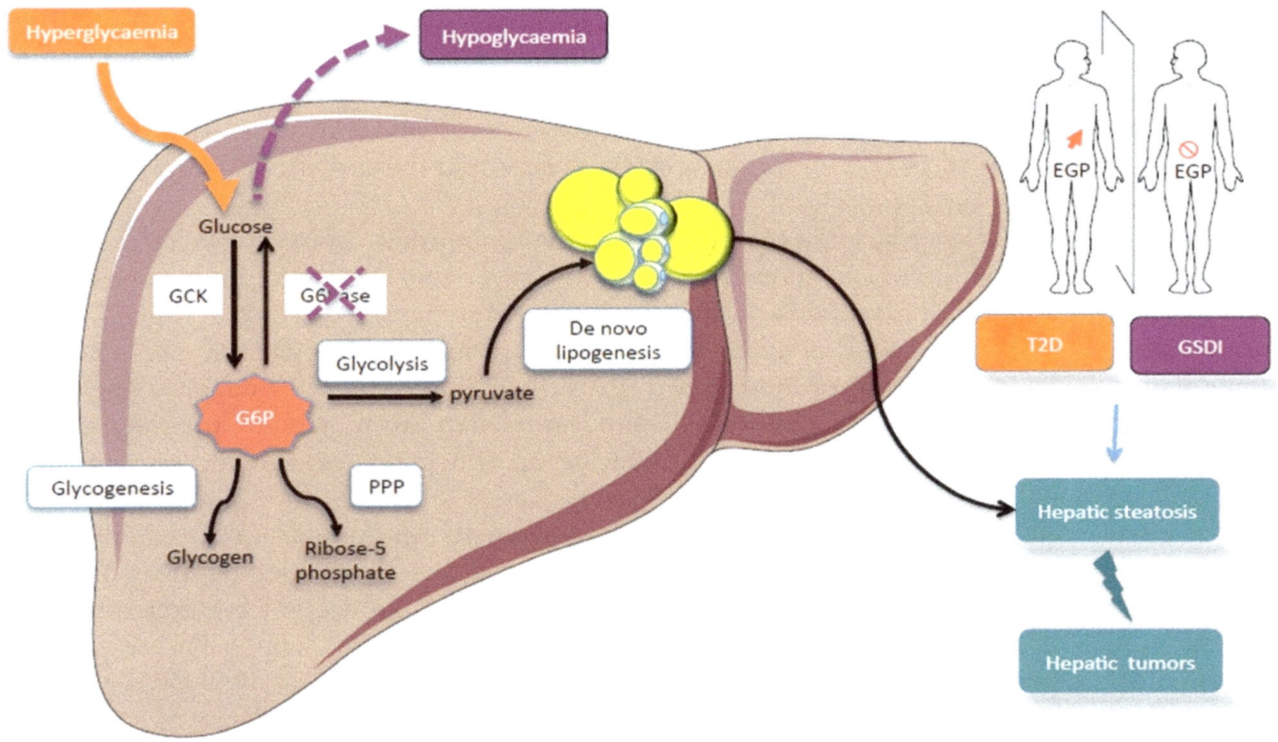

Figure 2. Comparison of hepatic glucose metabolism in glycogen storage disease type I (GSDI) or type 2 diabetes. Type 2 diabetes is characterized by an increase in endogenous glucose production (EGP) while GSDI is due to an absence of EGP. In GSDI, the absence of G6Pase activity is responsible for G6P accumulation in the hepatocyte. In diabetes, hyperglycemia is responsible for the increase flux through G6P. In both cases, this leads to a metabolic reprogramming characterized by the activation of glycolysis, PPP, and de novo lipogenesis. This metabolic reprogramming promotes hepatic steatosis in type 2 diabetes and GSDI, in which the risk of liver tumorigenesis is increased. Figures were drawn using Sevier Medical Art images.

2. Metabolic Fate of Glucose-6 Phosphate in the Healthy Liver

In order to control cell metabolism and proliferation, G6P enters different metabolic pathways to provide energy and/or precursors for biomolecule synthesis needed to sustain these processes. First, glucose concentrations fluctuate between the fed state and fasting periods. The liver plays a crucial role in maintaining blood glucose levels by its capacity to produce glucose during fasting periods. Moreover, in the case of overnutrition, excessive G6P is converted into fatty acids via de novo lipogenesis in the liver. Secondly, during fasting periods, glucose should be preserved to supply precursors for maintaining biomass, especially for cell renewal. Ketone bodies then become a major energy source for most tissues. Thus, the liver plays a central role by coordinating the storage and synthesis of glucose and the redistribution of nutrients, through the G6P metabolism.

2.1. Glucose and Lipid Storage

After a meal, a large portion of the excess carbohydrates (approximately 30–40% of the glucose ingested) is stored as glycogen in the liver, inside the hepatocytes, and in muscles (glycogenesis). In healthy individuals, hepatic glycogen represents around 5% of the liver weight. Glycogen is a polymer of glucose residues linked by α-(1,4) and α-(1,6)-glycosidic bonds. To synthesize glycogen, G6P is isomerized into glucose-1 phosphate and then converted into UDP-glucose. For de novo glycogen synthesis, UDP-glucose molecules are attached to a protein known as glycogenin. Once a linear chain of 10–20 glucose moieties is formed, glycogen synthase extends the glycogen chain, forming α-1-4 glycosidic links, and a branching enzyme introduces a branch point. The branching enzyme transfers a glycosyl chain of 6 to 8 units to the glycogen thread forming an α-1-6 linkage [6]. G6P is a precursor for glycogen synthesis but it also plays a huge role in regulating the activities of glycogen synthase and glycogen phosphorylase. Indeed, G6P is an allosteric inhibitor of glycogen phosphorylase and an allosteric activator of glycogen synthase, thus favoring hepatic glycogen increase [7]. In addition, glycogen synthesis/degradation is tightly regulated by hormones and nutritional states, which has been extensively described (see [7] for a review). It is of note that the presence of high insulin level after a meal favors glycogen synthesis.

Importantly, the capacity to store glycogen in the liver is limited. In case of excessive feeding of carbohydrates or in pathological states such as GSDI, glycogen turnover allows to continually breakdown glycogen to limit glycogen accumulation [4,8]. Moreover, the excess of dietary glucose that cannot be stored as glycogen is converted into fat by de novo lipogenesis (see below) [9]. A deregulation of glycogen storage or metabolic dysfunctions leading to abnormal glycogen storage in the liver results in hepatic glycogen storage diseases, which are metabolic inherited diseases characterized by hypoglycemia. GSDI belongs to this group of hepatic diseases, representing about 30% of GSD cases [10].

In the liver, triglycerides can be packed into very low density lipoproteins (VLDL) and secreted into the circulation, stored as lipid droplets, or be metabolized by the β-oxidation pathway. Excessive G6P is converted into fatty acids via de novo lipogenesis using the acetyl-CoA generated from glycolysis-driven pyruvate and NADPH derived from PPP. After glucose load, lipogenesis is markedly increased at the expense of glycogen synthesis; conversely, low carbohydrate diets reduce de novo lipogenesis [9]. Interestingly, insulin secreted in response to elevated blood glucose levels and glucose can induce hepatic lipogenesis through the synergistically activation of SREBP-1c and ChREBP, respectively [11]. Thus, increased consumption of simple sugars leads to the ectopic accumulation of lipids in the liver and increases the risk of metabolic diseases such as obesity, type 2 diabetes and nonalcoholic fatty liver disease (NAFLD).

2.2. Maintenance of Glycaemia and Endogenous Glucose Production

The liver plays a key role in the maintenance of blood glucose, particularly during the beginning of fasting periods. Just after the intestinal glucose absorption from food is completed, hepatic G6P is mainly derived from glycogen breakdown, while gluconeogenesis becomes the major source of G6P after more prolonged fasting. Indeed, hepatic glycogen stores are depleted after a 12h-fasting in mice and an overnight fasting period in Humans [12,13]. Glycogenolysis requires the intervention of two different enzymes: glycogen phosphorylase that degrades the glycogen chain down to a chain length of 4 units into glucose-1 phosphate, and glycogen debranching enzyme (GDE) that first transfers 3 glucose units to the terminal end of another chain and then cleaves off the final glucose unit, releasing it as free glucose. Glucose-1-phosphate must further be converted by phosphoglucomutase into G6P to enter the metabolism mainstream. During a longer fast or starvation, the liver synthetizes glucose de novo mainly from lactate, alanine, and glycerol while glutamine is a predominant gluconeogenic substrate in the kidney and intestine [14,15]. Interestingly, the contribution of hepatic glucose production decreases during fasting [16]. This decrease is compensated by glucose production from the kidneys and intestine, which are especially capable of producing glucose thanks to gluconeogenesis and to participate in the maintenance of blood glucose when fasting is prolonged [17–20]. The significance of the renal and intestinal gluconeogenesis has been firmly demonstrated in mice that are incapable to produce glucose by the liver (Liver-specific *G6pc* knockout mice- L.G6pc$^{-/-}$) [21]. Indeed, despite a drop in blood sugar levels in the post-prandial period, L.G6pc$^{-/-}$ mice regulate their blood sugar similarly to control mice after several hours of fasting thanks to an induction of gluconeogenic genes in the kidney and the intestine [13,22].

To be released as glucose into the bloodstream, G6P has to be dephosphorylated into glucose by glucose-6 phosphatase (G6Pase), which is expressed only in the liver, kidneys, and intestine. G6P is first translocated into the endoplasmic reticulum by the G6Pase transporter subunit (G6PT) and subsequently hydrolyzed into free glucose and inorganic phosphate by the G6Pase catalytic subunit

(G6PC). Glucose is finally released from the cytosol into the bloodstream through GLUT2. Thus, the liver, kidneys, and intestine play a central role in maintaining blood glucose levels at around 1 g/L (5 mM) since most mammals, including Humans, are incapable of tolerating hypoglycemia for more than a few minutes. Failure to activate these physiological pathways results in severe hypoglycemia that can be fatal, especially in GSDI or in diabetic patients treated with inappropriate doses of insulin.

2.3. Glucose-6 Phosphate: A Source of Energy and Carbon Skeletons

In feeding periods, glucose can be oxidized to CO_2 through a series of metabolic pathways, namely glycolysis in the cytosol, followed by the tricarboxylic acid cycle and the respiratory chain in the mitochondria. The first step of glycolysis is the isomerization of G6P into fructose-6 phosphate to produce triose-phosphate, then resulting in the generation of 2 pyruvate molecules and a small amount of ATP (net gain of 2 ATP molecules). The oxidation of pyruvate then generates the bulk of ATP under aerobic conditions in quiescent differentiated cells (Figure 3).

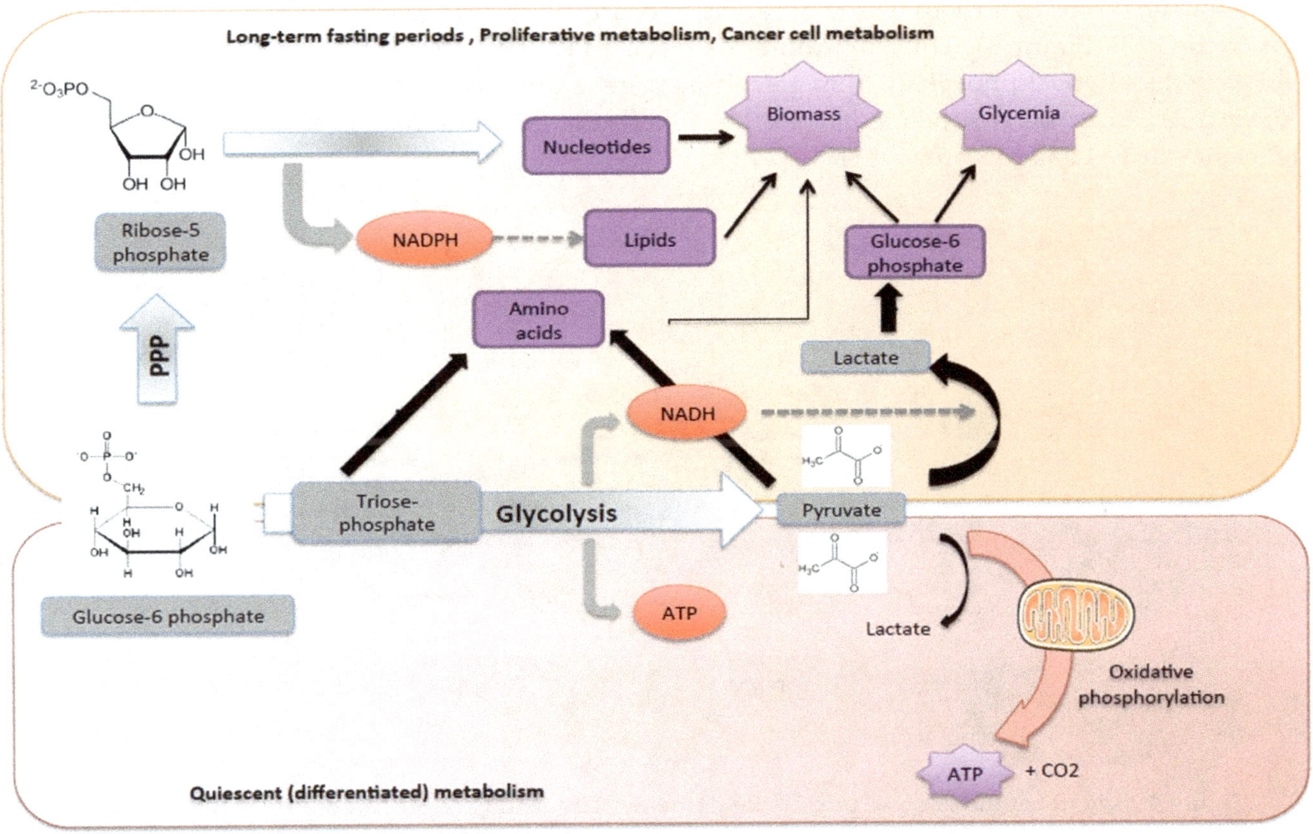

Figure 3. Glucose-6 phosphate: a source of energy and carbon skeletons. The G6P is metabolized either through the glycolytic pathway or PPP, which are tightly connected, depending on metabolic demands. Non-dividing normal differentiated cells mainly depend on mitochondrial oxidative phosphorylation of pyruvate, which is produced from glycolysis, to generate ATP. During cell proliferation or starvation periods, G6P is preferentially metabolized via PPP to maintain carbon homeostasis and produce biomass. In this case, glycolysis produces pyruvate and lactate as final metabolites and becomes inefficient in producing ATP. Indeed, G6P is preferentially metabolized via PPP to provide precursors for nucleotide and amino acid biosynthesis and to provide reducing molecules in the form of NADPH used in reductive biosynthesis reactions within cells (e.g., fatty acid synthesis). Lactate is also used by the hepatocyte to produce glucose and maintain glycaemia.

While glucose is generally considered to be the main source of cell energy, it is above all a major provider of carbon skeletons for cell growth and survival [16]. Indeed, glucose oxidation to CO_2 to produce energy should be avoided to permit to supply essential functions in some situations, in particular during long-term fasting or during cell proliferation. Glycolysis supplies 3 carbon-compounds, such as triose-phosphate, pyruvate and lactate that can be used to maintain cellular homeostasis and produce biomass (Figure 3). Hence, global glucose turnover decreases and glucose is used to supply PPP that provides the carbon skeletons needed for the synthesis of nucleotides, chromosomal duplication and cell proliferation (Figure 3). PPP is an important metabolic pathway known to provide reducing equivalents (NADPH) for anabolism and it plays a pivotal role in counteracting oxidative stress. Indeed, during oxidative stress, NADPH is needed for the generation of reduced glutathione. In the first step of PPP, G6P is oxidized into gluconolactone and carbon dioxide by glucose-6 phosphate dehydrogenase and 6-phosphogluconic dehydrogenase (oxidative branch). Ribulose-5 phosphate yielded is then isomerized to ribose-5 phosphate, which is the critical precursor for de novo ribonucleotide synthesis or epimerized into xylulose-5 phosphate. Additionally, a series of reversible reactions that recruit additional glycolytic intermediates, such as fructose-6 phosphate and glyceraldehyde-3-phosphate, can be converted into pentose phosphates and vice versa (non-oxidative branch). Transketolase (TKT) and transaldolase (TALDO) are the two major reversible enzymes that mediate the non-oxidative PPP and determine the diversion of metabolite flux in the PPP (Figure 4). Thus, in proliferative cells, TKT and TALDO divert fructose-6 phosphate and glyceraldehyde-3-phosphate from glycolysis to generate additional ribonucleotides. Interestingly, cancer cells can accelerate non-oxidative PPP by elevating the expression of these enzymes [23], while deficiency in TALDO can prevent HCC [24].

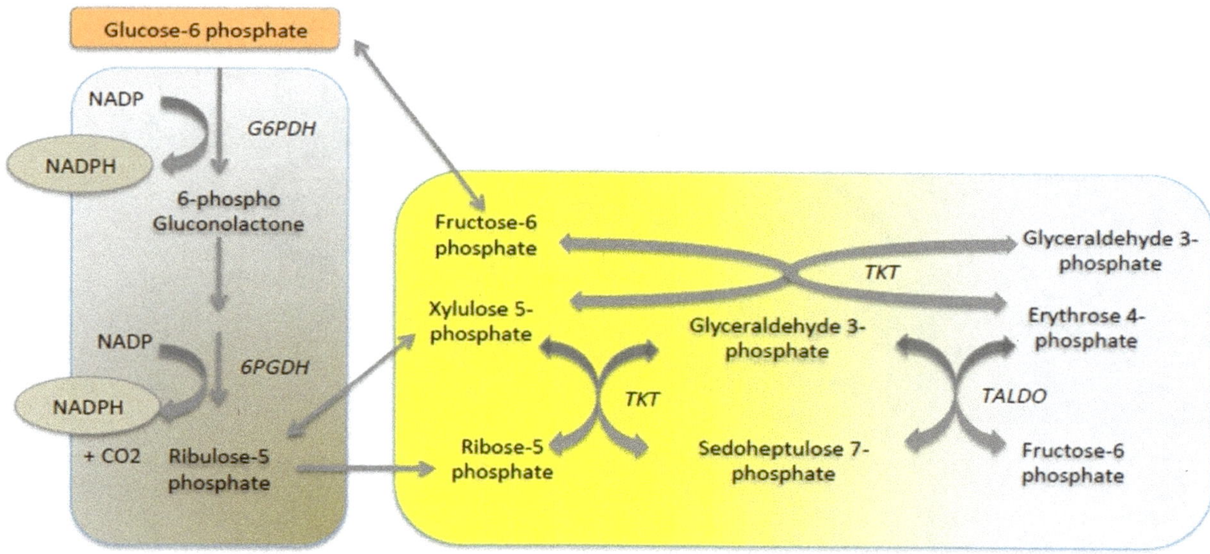

Figure 4. Scheme of the pentose phosphate pathway. The oxidative branch of PPP is highlighted in the brown part and the non-oxidative branch is represented in the yellow part of the figure. G6PDH: glucose-6 phosphate dehydrogenase; 6PGDH: 6-phosphogluconic dehydrogenase; TKT: Transketolase; TALDO: transaldolase.

Thus, the ability to switch the glucose metabolism from a catabolic to an anabolic process is critical for cells to thrive, especially during long fasting periods. This capacity is also an advantage for cancer cells that can grow and multiply by using glucose as a carbon source to build proteins and nucleotides rather than as an energy source, thanks to the Warburg effect [25].

2.4. Hexosamine Pathway

When G6P is increased, the hexosamine pathway produces carbohydrate units for glycosylation of proteins and contributes to the synthesis of complex molecules such as glycolipids, proteoglycans and glycosylphosphatidylinositol anchors. First, G6P is converted into fructose-6 phosphate, which may either enter the hexosamine pathway in combination with glutamine to produce

UDP-Nacetylglucosamine or it can follow the glycolytic pathway. The hexosamine pathway usually accounts for only 2–5% of total glucose metabolism. Interestingly, O-GlcNAcylation of different key transcription factors involved in energy metabolism, including ChREBP and the nuclear receptor Farnesoid X receptor (FXR), requires the hexosamine pathway [26].

3. ChREBP: A Glucose Sensor

In the hepatocyte, the transcriptional effects of glucose on gene expression are mediated by the transcription factor ChREBP, which in interaction with Max-like protein (Mlx) binds conserved consensus sequences (Carbohydrate Response Element, ChoRE). Indeed, in response to increased glucose concentration, ChREBP is translocated to the nucleus and it activates several genes involved in glucose and lipid metabolism [such as liver-Pyruvate kinase (L-PK), Fatty Acid Synthase (FAS) acetyl-CoA carboxylase (ACC), and stearoyl-CoA desaturase (SCD1)], but also genes involved in insulin signaling [27–29]. Recently, ChREBP was pointed out as a potential regulator of VLDL secretion in the liver [30]. Thus, it is assumed that ChREBP has important roles in the development of liver diseases including NAFLD [31]. In consequence, inactivation of ChREBP or liver-specific inhibition of ChREBP led to a decrease in glycolytic and lipogenic gene expression and a decrease in hepatic steatosis in mice [29,32,33]. On the contrary, the overexpression of ChREBP led to the development of hepatic steatosis without concomitant insulin resistance [27]. More recently, a key regulatory role for ChREBP in hepatic tumorigenesis was also suggested, since ChREBP expression was found to be increased in non-tumorous surrounding tissue in liver samples and further increased in HCC in Humans [34]. In addition, a recent study reported the importance of ChREBP in HCC [35]. The genetic deletion of ChREBP in mice impaired hepatocarcinogenesis driven by protein kinase B/Akt overexpression [36]. Furthermore, in vitro studies of ChREBP silencing in hepatoma cells resulted in a metabolic switch from aerobic glycolysis to mitochondrial oxidative phosphorylation, concomitantly with a reduction of cell proliferation [37]. In GSDI, the overexpression of ChREBP has been linked to glucose and lipid metabolism reprogramming [38,39]. In this context, enhanced ChREBP could partly account for increased proliferation of hepatocytes by favoring cancer cell-like metabolism. Further investigation is required to unravel the exact role of ChREBP in hepatocarcinogenesis in the context of NAFLD.

Two isoforms of ChREBP have been recently described originating from an alternative first exon promoter - ChREBP α and β [40]. The presence of a ChoRE sequence in the exon promoter 1β suggests that ChREBPα directly regulates the expression of ChREBPβ, considered as a constitutively active isoform (due to the loss of a regulatory inhibitory domain). Consequently, the response to glucose under hyperglycemic conditions could be exacerbated. The regulation of ChREBP activity by glucose is complex and the relative role of xylulose-5 phosphate, G6P or other glucose metabolites on the triggering of ChREBP activation is still discussed [41]. It was shown that xylulose-5 phosphate activates PP2A promoting dephosphorylation of ChREBP and its nuclear translocation and activation [42]. However, G6P seems to have a central role for the increase in ChREBP activity, especially by favoring ChREBP translocation to the nucleus and transactivation [28]. The key role of G6P was supported by the identification of a putative G6P recognition motif in the transactivation domain, called glucose-activation conserved element (GRACE), suggesting the possibility of an allosteric regulation of ChREBP by G6P [43]. High glucose also stimulates ChREBP activity and affinity to ChoRE sequences through acetylation and/or O-GlcNacetylation [44,45]. Finally, during fasting periods, phosphorylation of ChREBP by AMPK, in response to glucagon or to an increase in cellular AMP, is responsible for its cytoplasmic retention and/or for its decreased binding to target promoters [46,47].

In conclusion, ChREBP is a carbohydrate-signaling transcription factor, which masters, in the liver, the storage of lipids in feeding response. Recent studies have also supported the importance of ChREBP in the regulation of fructose metabolism [48,49].

4. Imbalance of Glucose-6 Phosphate Metabolism Leads to Metabolic Diseases and Promotes Hepatocarcinogenesis

In this review, we have chosen to illustrate two different pathological states characterized by impaired glucose metabolism. Firstly, type 2 diabetes is a chronic disease with the status of a global pandemic that is closely linked to overnutrition and obesity [50,51]. The main hallmark of diabetes is hyperglycemia due to insulin resistance and an overproduction of glucose by the body [52]. Hyperglycemia results in non-enzymatic glycosylation (glycation) and thus loss of function of proteins, glucose-induced oxidative damage and other adverse effects such as macrovascular and microvascular complications [53]. The second metabolic disease characterized by carbohydrate metabolism disruption is GSDI. This is a rare genetic disease (1 birth over 100,000) due to mutations in *G6PC* (that cause GSDIa) or *G6PT* (that cause GSDIb) leading to a loss of G6Pase activity and endogenous glucose production. In consequence, patients develop severe hypoglycemia during short fasting periods [54]. Thus, although type 2 diabetes and GSDI appear to be opposite diseases in terms of glucose production and insulin sensitivity, the liver is chronically exposed to either hyperglycemia or G6P accumulation, respectively, leading the same metabolic consequences, in particular hepatic steatosis (Figure 2). Comparing type 2 diabetes and GSDI will allow us to highlight metabolic perturbations that promote tumour development in relation to the ectopic accumulation of lipids in the liver.

In both type 2 diabetes and GSDI, liver metabolism is characterized by an increased metabolic flux downstream of G6P (Figure 2). Even if glucose uptake is impaired in obese and/or diabetic mice or patients, high blood glucose levels are responsible for the activation of all G6P-dependent pathways previously described [7]. Subsequently, one major metabolic consequence is an increase in triglyceride synthesis by the liver leading to hepatic steatosis [55,56]. Indeed, up to 70% of diabetic subjects may present NAFLD [56,57] and all GSDI develop a NAFLD-like pathology [54]. In insulin-resistant states, hyperglycemia and hyperinsulinemia are in part responsible for enhancing de novo lipogenesis through the activation of both ChREBP and SREBP1c. Interestingly, both transcription factors are also induced in the context of a high carbohydrate feeding independently of insulin signaling [58]. As previously mentioned, it has been shown that the global or liver-specific inhibition of ChREBP protected mice against carbohydrate-induced hepatic steatosis [29,33]. However, the effects of ChREBP inhibition on hepatic insulin sensitivity are still controversial. In GSDI, the absence of G6Pase activity leads to the accumulation of G6P in the liver and consequently the accumulation of glycogen and lipids, responsible for hepatomegaly and hepatic steatosis. Contrarily to diabetes, lipid synthesis is activated by ChREBP but independently of liver X receptor (LXR) and SREBP-1c [59]. The lack of SREBP-1c activation is probably due to a low intensity of insulin signaling in GSDI [37]. De novo lipogenesis is not the only process contributing to fatty liver. Indeed, the accumulation of lipid is also caused by an unbalanced diet, elevated non-esterified fatty acid due to a decreased inhibition of adipose tissue lipolysis, and reduced hepatic VLDL export [60,61]. All these disturbances contribute to hypertriglyceridemia and hypercholesteridemia observed in diabetes and GSDI. In conclusion, the liver metabolism of diabetes and GSDI is very similar, albeit exacerbated in GSDI, with G6P being at the metabolic crossroad as a main responsible for metabolic reprogramming [39,62].

Interestingly, both diabetes and GSDI patients are prone to the development of hepatic tumors. In diabetes, NAFLD can progress to liver fibrosis associated with inflammation i.e., non-alcoholic steatohepatitis NASH, cirrhosis and finally to the development of HCC. However, an important fraction of obese/diabetic patients develop HCC in the absence of liver cirrhosis [63,64]. Interestingly, GSDI subjects develop simple hepatic steatosis, which was long considered as a benign reversible condition. Nonetheless, lipid accumulation in the liver is a fertile ground for the development of hepatic tumors and most of patients with GSDI develop hepatocellular adenomas (HCA) that can later progress into HCC [54]. Despite the important accumulation of glycogen and lipids, GSDI patients present only low-grade hepatic inflammation and no hepatic injuries (namely normal hepatic transaminase levels and absence of liver failure). It is noteworthy that in obese/diabetic patients a part of HCA arises at the state of NAFLD characterized by a low-grade inflammation and may progress to HCC [65].

The comparison of HCC occurrence in NAFLD and GSDI livers argues for a dominant role of metabolic reprogramming in the molecular induction of tumor development.

Interestingly, tumor cells are metabolically reprogrammed to fuel cell proliferation, mostly by increasing glucose uptake and flux through aerobic glycolysis (Warburg effect) and anabolic pathways (PPP and de novo lipogenesis). The Warburg effect is characterized by high rates of glycolysis and lactic acid fermentation that occur in the cytosol regardless of the oxygen level. This provides essential bioenergetic substrates for cell growth and replication, i.e., components needed for cellular membrane biogenesis and amino acids and nucleotide synthesis for cell division. Recently, we showed that GSDI hepatocytes exhibit the main characteristics of cancer cell metabolism, with a Warburg-like metabolic reprogramming that predisposes GSDIa livers to tumor development [15]. Indeed, we observed a hyperactivation of the glycolysis pathway notably characterized by an overexpression of the M2 isoform of pyruvate kinase in the tumors and an increase in lactate production. Moreover, OXPHOS analyses revealed a decrease in mitochondrial respiration with a reduction of pyruvate oxidation [39].

A rational therapeutic approach for the treatment of NAFLD is to increase hepatic energy expenditure and thereby increase hepatic fat oxidation. Recently, we showed that the use of PPAR-α agonists, in particular fenofibrate, prevented NAFLD and hepatic injuries in GSDI, as previously described in diabetes [66–68]. Interestingly, the activation of β-oxidation by fenofibrate promoted the utilization of G6P through lipid metabolism, avoiding the accumulation of glycogen [66]. In diabetes, thyroid hormone receptor-β agonist combined with glucagon treatment, or glucacon like peptide 1 agonist-gastric inhibitory peptide-glucagon tri-conjugate [69], or liver targeted mitochondrial protonophores [70,71] were shown to reverse NAFLD in preclinical studies. Interestingly, glucose-lowering medications such as metformin also reduce the risk of HCC in diabetes, suggesting that better control of hepatic glucose metabolism should permit prevention of carcinogenesis.

To conclude, the activation of G6P-mediated metabolism is a hallmark of both GSDI and diabetes that causes hepatic steatosis and may promote cell proliferation and liver cancer. Thus, an optimal metabolic control, thanks to a strict diet with a reduced consumption of simple carbohydrates, should prevent tumor occurrence in GSDI [54]. In diabetes, better control of hyperglycemia should also permit better control of glucose/G6P metabolism and its possible consequences in hepatocytes. Thus, comparing these two metabolic diseases is a useful approach to better understand the key role of G6P in the liver both in health and pathological conditions.

Author Contributions: Wrote, reviewed and edited the manuscript, F.R.; Reviewed the manuscript, A.G.-S. and G.M.

Acknowledgments: The authors thank all past and current colleagues in the laboratory who contributed to the work reviewed. We would particularly like to thank Monika Gjorgjieva for her kind contribution to the manuscript.

References

1. Van Schaftingen, E.; Detheux, M.; Veiga da Cunha, M. Short-term control of glucokinase activity: Role of a regulatory protein. *FASEB J.* **1994**, *8*, 414–419. [CrossRef] [PubMed]
2. Agius, L. Hormonal and Metabolite Regulation of Hepatic Glucokinase. *Annu. Rev. Nutr.* **2016**, *36*, 389–415. [CrossRef] [PubMed]
3. Baltrusch, S.; Lenzen, S.; Okar, D.A.; Lange, A.J.; Tiedge, M. Characterization of glucokinase-binding protein epitopes by a phage-displayed peptide library identification of 6-phosphofructo-2-kinase/fructose-2,6-bisphosphatase as a novel interaction partner. *J. Biol. Chem.* **2001**, *276*, 43915–43923. [CrossRef] [PubMed]
4. Hijmans, B.S.; Boss, A.; van Dijk, T.H.; Soty, M.; Wolters, H.; Mutel, E.; Groen, A.K.; Derks, T.G.J.; Mithieux, G.; Heerschap, A.; et al. Hepatocytes contribute to residual glucose production in a mouse model for glycogen storage disease type Ia. *Hepatology* **2017**, *66*, 2042–2054. [CrossRef]
5. Rajas, F.; Labrune, P.; Mithieux, G. Glycogen storage disease type 1 and diabetes: Learning by comparing and contrasting the two disorders. *Diabetes Metab.* **2013**, *39*, 377–387. [CrossRef]

6. Adeva-Andany, M.M.; González-Lucán, M.; Donapetry-García, C.; Fernández-Fernández, C.; Ameneiros-Rodríguez, E. Glycogen metabolism in humans. *BBA Clin.* **2016**, *5*, 85–100. [CrossRef]
7. Petersen, M.C.; Vatner, D.F.; Shulman, G.I. Regulation of hepatic glucose metabolism in health and disease. *Nat. Rev. Endocrinol.* **2017**, *13*, 572–587. [CrossRef]
8. Magnusson, I.; Rothman, D.L.; Jucker, B.; Cline, G.W.; Shulman, R.G.; Shulman, G.I. Liver glycogen turnover in fed and fasted humans. *Am. J. Physiol.* **1994**, *266*, E796–E803. [CrossRef]
9. McDevitt, R.M.; Bott, S.J.; Harding, M.; Coward, W.A.; Bluck, L.J.; Prentice, A.M. De novo lipogenesis during controlled overfeeding with sucrose or glucose in lean and obese women. *Am. J. Clin. Nutr.* **2001**, *74*, 737–746. [CrossRef]
10. Ozen, H. Glycogen storage diseases: New perspectives. *World J. Gastroenterol.* **2007**, *13*, 2541–2553. [CrossRef]
11. Linden, A.G.; Li, S.; Choi, H.Y.; Fang, F.; Fukasawa, M.; Uyeda, K.; Hammer, R.E.; Horton, J.D.; Engelking, L.J.; Liang, G. Interplay between ChREBP and SREBP-1c coordinates postprandial glycolysis and lipogenesis in livers of mice. *J. Lipid Res.* **2018**, *59*, 475–487. [CrossRef]
12. Xu, K.; Morgan, K.T.; Todd Gehris, A.; Elston, T.C.; Gomez, S.M. A Whole-Body Model for Glycogen Regulation Reveals a Critical Role for Substrate Cycling in Maintaining Blood Glucose Homeostasis. *PLoS Comput. Biol.* **2011**, *7*, e1002272. [CrossRef] [PubMed]
13. Mutel, E.; Gautier-Stein, A.; Abdul-Wahed, A.; Amigó-Correig, M.; Zitoun, C.; Stefanutti, A.; Houberdon, I.; Tourette, J.A.; Mithieux, G.; Rajas, F. Control of Blood Glucose in the Absence of Hepatic Glucose Production During Prolonged Fasting in Mice. *Diabetes* **2011**, *60*, 3121–3131. [CrossRef] [PubMed]
14. Mithieux, G. New data and concepts on glutamine and glucose metabolism in the gut. *Curr. Opin. Clin. Nutr. Metab. Care* **2001**, *4*, 267–271. [CrossRef] [PubMed]
15. Mithieux, G.; Rajas, F.; Gautier-Stein, A. A novel role for glucose 6-phosphatase in the small intestine in the control of glucose homeostasis. *J. Biol. Chem.* **2004**, *279*, 44231–44234. [CrossRef] [PubMed]
16. Soty, M.; Gautier-Stein, A.; Rajas, F.; Mithieux, G. Gut-Brain Glucose Signaling in Energy Homeostasis. *Cell Metab.* **2017**, *25*, 1231–1242. [CrossRef]
17. Pillot, B.; Soty, M.; Gautier-Stein, A.; Zitoun, C.; Mithieux, G. Protein feeding promotes redistribution of endogenous glucose production to the kidney and potentiates its suppression by insulin. *Endocrinology* **2009**, *150*, 616–624. [CrossRef]
18. Gerich, J.E.; Meyer, C.; Woerle, H.J.; Stumvoll, M. Renal gluconeogenesis: Its importance in human glucose homeostasis. *Diabetes Care* **2001**, *24*, 382–391. [CrossRef]
19. Croset, M.; Rajas, F.; Zitoun, C.; Hurot, J.M.; Montano, S.; Mithieux, G. Rat small intestine is an insulin-sensitive gluconeogenic organ. *Diabetes* **2001**, *50*, 740–746. [CrossRef]
20. Mithieux, G.; Gautier-Stein, A.; Rajas, F.; Zitoun, C. Contribution of intestine and kidney to glucose fluxes in different nutritional states in rat. *Comp. Biochem. Physiol. B Biochem. Mol. Biol.* **2006**, *143*, 195–200. [CrossRef]
21. Mutel, E.; Abdul-Wahed, A.; Ramamonjisoa, N.; Stefanutti, A.; Houberdon, I.; Cavassila, S.; Pilleul, F.; Beuf, O.; Gautier-Stein, A.; Penhoat, A.; et al. Targeted deletion of liver glucose-6 phosphatase mimics glycogen storage disease type 1a including development of multiple adenomas. *J. Hepatol.* **2011**, *54*, 529–537. [CrossRef] [PubMed]
22. Penhoat, A.; Fayard, L.; Stefanutti, A.; Mithieux, G.; Rajas, F. Intestinal gluconeogenesis is crucial to maintain a physiological fasting glycemia in the absence of hepatic glucose production in mice. *Metab. Clin. Exp.* **2014**, *63*, 104–111. [CrossRef] [PubMed]
23. Heinrich, P.C.; Morris, H.P.; Weber, G. Behavior of transaldolase (EC 2.2.1.2) and transketolase (EC 2.2.1.1) Activities in normal, neoplastic, differentiating, and regenerating liver. *Cancer Res.* **1976**, *36*, 3189–3197. [PubMed]
24. Hanczko, R.; Fernandez, D.R.; Doherty, E.; Qian, Y.; Vas, G.; Niland, B.; Telarico, T.; Garba, A.; Banerjee, S.; Middleton, F.A.; et al. Prevention of hepatocarcinogenesis and increased susceptibility to acetaminophen-induced liver failure in transaldolase-deficient mice by N-acetylcysteine. *J. Clin. Investig.* **2009**, *119*, 1546–1557. [CrossRef]
25. Koppenol, W.H.; Bounds, P.L.; Dang, C.V. Otto Warburg's contributions to current concepts of cancer metabolism. *Nat. Rev. Cancer* **2011**, *11*, 325–337. [CrossRef]
26. Benhamed, F.; Filhoulaud, G.; Caron, S.; Lefebvre, P.; Staels, B.; Postic, C. O-GlcNAcylation Links ChREBP and FXR to Glucose-Sensing. *Front. Endocrinol.* **2015**, *5*, 230. [CrossRef]

27. Benhamed, F.; Denechaud, P.D.; Lemoine, M.; Robichon, C.; Moldes, M.; Bertrand-Michel, J.; Ratziu, V.; Serfaty, L.; Housset, C.; Capeau, J.; et al. The lipogenic transcription factor ChREBP dissociates hepatic steatosis from insulin resistance in mice and humans. *J. Clin. Investig.* **2012**, *122*, 2176–2194. [CrossRef]
28. Dentin, R.; Tomas-Cobos, L.; Foufelle, F.; Leopold, J.; Girard, J.; Postic, C.; Ferré, P. Glucose 6-phosphate, rather than xylulose 5-phosphate, is required for the activation of ChREBP in response to glucose in the liver. *J. Hepatol.* **2012**, *56*, 199–209. [CrossRef]
29. Iizuka, K.; Miller, B.; Uyeda, K. Deficiency of carbohydrate-activated transcription factor ChREBP prevents obesity and improves plasma glucose control in leptin-deficient (ob/ob) mice. *Am. J. Physiol. Endocrinol. Metab.* **2006**, *291*, E358–E364. [CrossRef]
30. Niwa, H.; Iizuka, K.; Kato, T.; Wu, W.; Tsuchida, H.; Takao, K.; Horikawa, Y.; Takeda, J. ChREBP Rather Than SHP Regulates Hepatic VLDL Secretion. *Nutrients* **2018**, *10*, 321. [CrossRef]
31. Poungvarin, N.; Chang, B.; Imamura, M.; Chen, J.; Moolsuwan, K.; Sae-Lee, C.; Li, W.; Chan, L. Genome-Wide Analysis of ChREBP Binding Sites on Male Mouse Liver and White Adipose Chromatin. *Endocrinology* **2015**, *156*, 1982–1994. [CrossRef] [PubMed]
32. Dentin, R.; Benhamed, F.; Hainault, I.; Fauveau, V.; Foufelle, F.; Dyck, J.R.B.; Girard, J.; Postic, C. Liver-specific inhibition of ChREBP improves hepatic steatosis and insulin resistance in ob/ob mice. *Diabetes* **2006**, *55*, 2159–2170. [CrossRef] [PubMed]
33. Jois, T.; Chen, W.; Howard, V.; Harvey, R.; Youngs, K.; Thalmann, C.; Saha, P.; Chan, L.; Cowley, M.A.; Sleeman, M.W. Deletion of hepatic carbohydrate response element binding protein (ChREBP) impairs glucose homeostasis and hepatic insulin sensitivity in mice. *Mol. Metab.* **2017**, *6*, 1381–1394. [CrossRef] [PubMed]
34. Calvisi, D.F.; Wang, C.; Ho, C.; Ladu, S.; Lee, S.A.; Mattu, S.; Destefanis, G.; Delogu, S.; Zimmermann, A.; Ericsson, J.; et al. Increased lipogenesis, induced by AKT-mTORC1-RPS6 signaling, promotes development of human hepatocellular carcinoma. *Gastroenterology* **2011**, *140*, 1071–1083. [CrossRef] [PubMed]
35. Ribback, S.; Sonke, J.; Lohr, A.; Frohme, J.; Peters, K.; Holm, J.; Peters, M.; Cigliano, A.; Calvisi, D.F.; Dombrowski, F. Hepatocellular glycogenotic foci after combined intraportal pancreatic islet transplantation and knockout of the carbohydrate responsive element binding protein in diabetic mice. *Oncotarget* **2017**, *8*, 104315–104329. [CrossRef] [PubMed]
36. Ribback, S.; Che, L.; Pilo, M.G.; Cigliano, A.; Latte, G.; Pes, G.M.; Porcu, A.; Pascale, R.M.; Li, L.; Qiao, Y.; et al. Oncogene-dependent addiction to carbohydrate-responsive element binding protein in hepatocellular carcinoma. *Cell Cycle* **2018**, *17*, 1496–1512. [CrossRef]
37. Tong, X.; Zhao, F.; Mancuso, A.; Gruber, J.J.; Thompson, C.B. The glucose-responsive transcription factor ChREBP contributes to glucose-dependent anabolic synthesis and cell proliferation. *Proc. Natl. Acad. Sci. USA* **2009**, *106*, 21660–21665. [CrossRef]
38. Abdul-Wahed, A.; Gautier-Stein, A.; Casteras, S.; Soty, M.; Roussel, D.; Romestaing, C.; Guillou, H.; Tourette, J.A.; Pleche, N.; Zitoun, C.; et al. A link between hepatic glucose production and peripheral energy metabolism via hepatokines. *Mol. Metab.* **2014**, *3*, 531–543. [CrossRef]
39. Gjorgjieva, M.; Calderaro, J.; Monteillet, L.; Silva, M.; Raffin, M.; Brevet, M.; Romestaing, C.; Roussel, D.; Zucman-Rossi, J.; Mithieux, G.; et al. Dietary exacerbation of metabolic stress leads to accelerated hepatic carcinogenesis in glycogen storage disease type Ia. *J. Hepatol.* **2018**, *69*, 1074–1087. [CrossRef]
40. Eissing, L.; Scherer, T.; Tödter, K.; Knippschild, U.; Greve, J.W.; Buurman, W.A.; Pinnschmidt, H.O.; Rensen, S.S.; Wolf, A.M.; Bartelt, A.; et al. De novo lipogenesis in human fat and liver is linked to ChREBP-β and metabolic health. *Nat. Commun.* **2013**, *4*, 1528. [CrossRef]
41. Filhoulaud, G.; Guilmeau, S.; Dentin, R.; Girard, J.; Postic, C. Novel insights into ChREBP regulation and function. *Trends Endocrinol. Metab.* **2013**, *24*, 257–268. [CrossRef] [PubMed]
42. Kabashima, T.; Kawaguchi, T.; Wadzinski, B.E.; Uyeda, K. Xylulose 5-phosphate mediates glucose-induced lipogenesis by xylulose 5-phosphate-activated protein phosphatase in rat liver. *Proc. Natl. Acad. Sci. USA* **2003**, *100*, 5107–5112. [CrossRef] [PubMed]
43. McFerrin, L.G.; Atchley, W.R. A novel N-terminal domain may dictate the glucose response of Mondo proteins. *PLoS ONE* **2012**, *7*, e34803. [CrossRef] [PubMed]
44. Bricambert, J.; Miranda, J.; Benhamed, F.; Girard, J.; Postic, C.; Dentin, R. Salt-inducible kinase 2 links transcriptional coactivator p300 phosphorylation to the prevention of ChREBP-dependent hepatic steatosis in mice. *J. Clin. Investig.* **2010**, *120*, 4316–4331. [CrossRef]

45. Guinez, C.; Filhoulaud, G.; Rayah-Benhamed, F.; Marmier, S.; Dubuquoy, C.; Dentin, R.; Moldes, M.; Burnol, A.F.; Yang, X.; Lefebvre, T.; et al. O-GlcNAcylation Increases ChREBP Protein Content and Transcriptional Activity in the Liver. *Diabetes* **2011**, *60*, 1399–1413. [CrossRef]
46. Davies, M.N.; O'Callaghan, B.L.; Towle, H.C. Glucose activates ChREBP by increasing its rate of nuclear entry and relieving repression of its transcriptional activity. *J. Biol. Chem.* **2008**, *283*, 24029–24038. [CrossRef]
47. Sato, S.; Jung, H.; Nakagawa, T.; Pawlosky, R.; Takeshima, T.; Lee, W.R.; Sakiyama, H.; Laxman, S.; Wynn, R.M.; Tu, B.P.; et al. Metabolite Regulation of Nuclear Localization of Carbohydrate-response Element-binding Protein (ChREBP): ROLE OF AMP AS AN ALLOSTERIC INHIBITOR. *J. Biol. Chem.* **2016**, *291*, 10515–10527. [CrossRef]
48. Ortega-Prieto, P.; Postic, C. Carbohydrate Sensing Through the Transcription Factor ChREBP. *Front. Genet.* **2019**, *10*, 472. [CrossRef]
49. Kim, M.S.; Krawczyk, S.A.; Doridot, L.; Fowler, A.J.; Wang, J.X.; Trauger, S.A.; Noh, H.L.; Kang, H.J.; Meissen, J.K.; Blatnik, M.; et al. ChREBP regulates fructose-induced glucose production independently of insulin signaling. *J. Clin. Investig.* **2016**, *126*, 4372–4386. [CrossRef]
50. Unnikrishnan, R.; Pradeepa, R.; Joshi, S.R.; Mohan, V. Type 2 Diabetes: Demystifying the Global Epidemic. *Diabetes* **2017**, *66*, 1432–1442. [CrossRef]
51. Chen, L.; Magliano, D.J.; Zimmet, P.Z. The worldwide epidemiology of type 2 diabetes mellitus–present and future perspectives. *Nat. Rev. Endocrinol.* **2012**, *8*, 228–236. [CrossRef] [PubMed]
52. Lin, H.V.; Accili, D. Hormonal regulation of hepatic glucose production in health and disease. *Cell Metab.* **2011**, *14*, 9–19. [CrossRef] [PubMed]
53. Brownlee, M. Biochemistry and molecular cell biology of diabetic complications. *Nature* **2001**, *414*, 813–820. [CrossRef] [PubMed]
54. Kishnani, P.S.; Austin, S.L.; Abdenur, J.E.; Arn, P.; Bali, D.S.; Boney, A.; Chung, W.K.; Dagli, A.I.; Dale, D.; Koeberl, D.; et al. Diagnosis and management of glycogen storage disease type I: A practice guideline of the American College of Medical Genetics and Genomics. *Genet. Med.* **2014**, *16*, e1. [CrossRef] [PubMed]
55. Smith, B.W.; Adams, L.A. Non-alcoholic fatty liver disease. *Crit. Rev. Clin. Lab. Sci.* **2011**, *48*, 97–113. [CrossRef]
56. Hazlehurst, J.M.; Woods, C.; Marjot, T.; Cobbold, J.F.; Tomlinson, J.W. Non-alcoholic fatty liver disease and diabetes. *Metab. Clin. Exp.* **2016**, *65*, 1096–1108. [CrossRef]
57. Williamson, R.M.; Price, J.F.; Glancy, S.; Perry, E.; Nee, L.D.; Hayes, P.C.; Frier, B.M.; Van Look, L.A.F.; Johnston, G.I.; Reynolds, R.M.; et al. Prevalence of and risk factors for hepatic steatosis and nonalcoholic Fatty liver disease in people with type 2 diabetes: The Edinburgh Type 2 Diabetes Study. *Diabetes Care* **2011**, *34*, 1139–1144. [CrossRef]
58. Matsuzaka, T.; Shimano, H. Insulin-dependent and -independent regulation of sterol regulatory element-binding protein-1c. *J. Diabetes Investig.* **2013**, *4*, 411–412. [CrossRef]
59. Grefhorst, A.; Schreurs, M.; Oosterveer, M.H.; Cortés, V.A.; Havinga, R.; Herling, A.W.; Reijngoud, D.J.; Groen, A.K.; Kuipers, F. Carbohydrate-response-element-binding protein (ChREBP) and not the liver X receptor α (LXRα) mediates elevated hepatic lipogenic gene expression in a mouse model of glycogen storage disease type 1. *Biochem. J.* **2010**, *432*, 249–254. [CrossRef]
60. Postic, C.; Girard, J. Contribution of de novo fatty acid synthesis to hepatic steatosis and insulin resistance: Lessons from genetically engineered mice. *J. Clin. Investig.* **2008**, *118*, 829–838. [CrossRef]
61. Bandsma, R.H.J.; Prinsen, B.H.; de Sain-van der Velden, M.; Rake, J.P.; Boer, T.; Smit, G.P.A.; Reijngoud, D.J.; Kuipers, F. Increased de novo Lipogenesis and Delayed Conversion of Large VLDL into Intermediate Density Lipoprotein Particles Contribute to Hyperlipidemia in Glycogen Storage Disease Type 1a. *Pediatr. Res.* **2008**, *63*, 702–707. [CrossRef] [PubMed]
62. Gjorgjieva, M.; Oosterveer, M.H.; Mithieux, G.; Rajas, F. Mechanisms by Which Metabolic Reprogramming in GSD1 Liver Generates a Favorable Tumorigenic Environment. *J. Inborn Errors Metab. Screen.* **2016**, *4*. [CrossRef]
63. Calzadilla Bertot, L.; Adams, L.A. The Natural Course of Non-Alcoholic Fatty Liver Disease. *Int. J. Mol. Sci.* **2016**, *17*, 774. [CrossRef] [PubMed]
64. Sanyal, A.; Poklepovic, A.; Moyneur, E.; Barghout, V. Population-based risk factors and resource utilization for HCC: US perspective. *Curr. Med. Res. Opin.* **2010**, *26*, 2183–2191. [CrossRef] [PubMed]

65. Bengtsson, B.; Stål, P.; Wahlin, S.; Björkström, N.K.; Hagström, H. Characteristics and outcome of hepatocellular carcinoma in patients with NAFLD without cirrhosis. *Liver Int.* **2019**, *39*, 1098–1108. [CrossRef] [PubMed]
66. Monteillet, L.; Gjorgjieva, M.; Silva, M.; Verzieux, V.; Imikirene, L.; Duchampt, A.; Guillou, H.; Mithieux, G.; Rajas, F. Intracellular lipids are an independent cause of liver injury and chronic kidney disease in non alcoholic fatty liver disease-like context. *Mol. Metab.* **2018**, *16*, 100–115. [CrossRef]
67. Musso, G.; Cassader, M.; Gambino, R. Non-alcoholic steatohepatitis: Emerging molecular targets and therapeutic strategies. *Nat. Rev. Drug Discov.* **2016**, *15*, 249–274. [CrossRef]
68. Waskowicz, L.R.; Zhou, J.; Landau, D.J.; Brooks, E.D.; Lim, A.; Yavarow, Z.A.; Kudo, T.; Zhang, H.; Wu, Y.; Grant, S.; et al. Bezafibrate induces autophagy and improves hepatic lipid metabolism in glycogen storage disease type Ia. *Hum. Mol. Genet.* **2018**, *28*, 143–154. [CrossRef]
69. Finan, B.; Clemmensen, C.; Zhu, Z.; Stemmer, K.; Gauthier, K.; Müller, L.; De Angelis, M.; Moreth, K.; Neff, F.; Perez-Tilve, D.; et al. Chemical Hybridization of Glucagon and Thyroid Hormone Optimizes Therapeutic Impact for Metabolic Disease. *Cell* **2016**, *167*, 843–857. [CrossRef]
70. Perry, R.J.; Zhang, D.; Zhang, X.M.; Boyer, J.L.; Shulman, G.I. Controlled-release mitochondrial protonophore reverses diabetes and steatohepatitis in rats. *Science* **2015**, *347*, 1253–1256. [CrossRef]
71. Perry, R.J.; Kim, T.; Zhang, X.M.; Lee, H.Y.; Pesta, D.; Popov, V.B.; Zhang, D.; Rahimi, Y.; Jurczak, M.J.; Cline, G.W.; et al. Reversal of hypertriglyceridemia, fatty liver disease, and insulin resistance by a liver-targeted mitochondrial uncoupler. *Cell Metab.* **2013**, *18*, 740–748. [CrossRef] [PubMed]

3

Simple vs. Complex Carbohydrate Dietary Patterns and the Global Overweight and Obesity Pandemic

Fabrizio Ferretti * and Michele Mariani

Department of Communication and Economics, School of Social Sciences, University of Modena and Reggio Emilia, Palazzo Dossetti—Viale Allegri 9, 42121 Reggio Emilia, Italy; michele.mariani@unimore.it
* Correspondence: fabrizio.ferretti@unimore.it

Academic Editor: Stuart Schweitzer

Abstract: Nowadays, obesity and being overweight are among the major global health concerns. Many, diet-related diseases impose high tangible and intangible costs, and threaten the sustainability of health-care systems worldwide. In this study, we model, at the macroeconomic level, the impact of energy intake from different types of carbohydrates on the population's BMI (body mass index). We proceed in three steps. First, we develop a framework to analyse both the consumption choices between simple and complex carbohydrates and the effects of these choices on people health conditions. Second, we collect figures for 185 countries (over the period 2012–2014) regarding the shares of simple (sugar and sweetener) and complex (cereal) carbohydrates in each country's total dietary energy supply. Third, we use regression techniques to: (1) estimate the impact of these shares on the country's prevalence of obesity and being overweight; (2) compute for each country an indicator of dietary pattern based on the ratio between simple and complex carbohydrates, weighted by their estimated effects on the prevalence of obesity and being overweight; and (3) measure the elasticity of the prevalence of obesity and being overweight with respect to changes in both carbohydrate dietary pattern and income per capita. We find that unhealthy eating habits and the associated prevalence of excessive body fat accumulation tend to behave as a 'normal good' in low, medium- and high-HDI (Human Development Index) countries, but as an 'inferior good' in very high-HDI countries.

Keywords: carbohydrates; dietary patterns; human development; overweight and obesity; nutrition transition

1. Introduction

There is increasing emphasis on obesity as a major global public health and economic problem [1]. According to the World Health Organization (WHO), the prevalence of obesity worldwide has more than doubled since 1980 and, today, most of the world's populations live in countries where being overweight and obesity kill more people than being underweight [2]. It is widely acknowledged that obesity and being overweight are important risk factors for a variety of chronic non-communicable diseases (including cardiovascular diseases, diabetes, musculoskeletal disorders, and even some types of cancer) [3].

These diet-related diseases impose high tangible and intangible costs on society and threaten the sustainability of health-care systems worldwide—a problem usually exacerbated by the contemporary rising global trends in population ageing [4]. The so-called 'obesity pandemic' is, indeed, not restricted to advanced economies. The growth of the prevalence of obesity and being overweight is often faster in emerging economies than in the Western countries [5]. In China, for instance, the prevalence of obesity and being overweight has grown significantly during the last two decades, especially among children in urban areas, where overweight and obesity rates have increased more than ten times since 1985 [6].

Obesity and being overweight are complex health issues with a multi-factorial aetiology, involving genetic, behavioral, and environmental (i.e., cultural, economic and social) factors [7]. Despite this, comprehensive epidemiological analysis of world trends in the Body Mass Index (BMI) usually pay little attention to the economic forces that underlies the overweight and obesity pandemic [8,9]. However, research has consistently shown that the increasing prevalence of obesity and being overweight—and especially its spread in rapidly growing economies—reflects structural changes in people's health-related habits and behaviors, which are inextricably linked with improving living standards [10,11].

The main characteristic of the conditions of obesity and being overweight is the abnormal (or excessive) accumulation of body fat resulting from an energy imbalance between two flows: the inflow of calories consumed and the outflow of calories expended [12]. In the vast majority of world cultures and geographic regions, carbohydrates usually serve as the human body's primary source of calories [13]. However, not all carbohydrates 'are created equal' in nutritional sciences. Specifically, complex carbohydrates—derived from whole and unprocessed plant-based foods—are generally considered healthier than simple carbohydrates, especially those derived from high-processed and sugar-added foods and beverages—which usually provide 'empty calories' (i.e., calories without nutrients)—whose increasing consumption is regarded as a major driver of the worldwide spread of obesity and being overweight, notably among children and young adults [14–16].

In this study, we model—at the macroeconomic level—the impact of energy intake from different types of carbohydrates on the population's BMI. To this end, we proceed in three steps. Firstly, we develop a theoretical framework to analyse both the consumption choices between simple and complex carbohydrates and the effects of these choices on consumers' health conditions. Second, we collect figures for 185 countries (over the period 2012–2014) regarding the shares of simple (sugar and sweetener) and complex (cereal) carbohydrates in each country's total dietary energy supply. Third, we use regression techniques to: (1) estimate the impact of these shares on the country's prevalence of obesity and being overweight; (2) compute for each country an indicator of dietary pattern based on the ratio between simple and complex carbohydrates, weighted by their estimated effects on the prevalence of obesity and being overweight; and (3) measure the elasticity of the prevalence of obesity and being overweight with respect to changes in both carbohydrate dietary pattern and income per capita.

The remainder of the paper is structured as follows. In the next section we develop the model of consumer food choice that grounds our quantitative work. Section 3 illustrates the econometric methods and data sources. The results are presented in Section 4. Finally, Section 5 concludes with a discussion and some brief policy recommendations.

2. Theory

After Grossman's seminal model of the demand for health [17], it is usual to model consumers' behavior by combining the utility function (and the budget constraint) with a health production function that indicates the impact of the consumers' health-related choices on their health status (measured in terms of morbidity, mortality, life expectancy, or other health-adjusted indicators of quality of life). From this approach, as shown by Wagstaff [18], a simple macroeconomic model can be derived to empirically study how changes in health-related choices (due, for instance, to changes in consumers' preferences or income) affect individuals' health conditions and, thus, the prevalence of health problems in a given population. In this paper, a generalization of Wagstaff's model, recently provided by Coppola [19], is adapted to the study of the effects on BMI of different carbohydrate dietary patterns.

Let us consider a simplified economy in which there are only two types of foods: (1) low-processed foods, made with whole cereals and vegetables; and (2) high-processed foods, made with refined flours and added sugars. The former are the source of complex carbohydrates with a low glycaemic index, whereas the latter are the source of simple carbohydrates with a high glycaemic index. We assume that people consuming any positive combination of these two kinds of foods in order to meet their daily energy requirements. However, the health effects of low- and high-processed foods are different. A whole-grain- and vegetable-based diet (i.e., a diet based mainly on low-calorie and high-nutrient foods) has 'protective' health effects, helping people to maintain a healthy weight and decreasing their likelihood of developing diet-related chronic non-communicable diseases. Conversely, a refined-flour- and added-sugar-based diet (i.e., a diet based mainly on high-calorie and low-nutrient foods) is one of the leading causes of unhealthy weight gains and is associated with the onset of the Metabolic Syndrome, which tends to raise the risk of developing several diet-related chronic non-communicable diseases [20–22].

In the following, let us denote by H a measure of the individual's health status. Specifically, H is the difference between the actual and the ideal body weight, measured according to the WHO recommended healthy BMI range [23]. Our focus is on obesity and being overweight, thus, H is positive or at least equal to zero (i.e., we do not deal with problems of undernourishment). As a result, the greater the value of H the greater is the unhealthy excess of body weight and, thus, the more severe is the individual's overweight or obesity condition. The health effects of the individual's eating habits are described by the following health production function:

$$H = s^{\rho} \times c^{-\sigma} \tag{1}$$

where s stands for 'sugar' (i.e., the consumption of simple carbohydrates from high-processed foods) and c stands for 'cereal' (i.e., the consumption of complex carbohydrates from low-processed foods). Both, s and c are measured in kcal per capita per day. In Equation (1), the exponents ρ and σ measure the elasticity of H with respect to s and c. Since H measures the excess of body weight compared to set health standards, ρ and σ are, respectively, positive and negative, because the consumption of s worsens health by promoting obesity and being overweight, whereas the consumption of c improves health by protecting against the onset of obesity and being overweight. For these reasons, hereafter, we will refer to c and s simply as healthy and unhealthy food, respectively.

The dimension of ρ and σ is ultimately determined by the functioning of the metabolic processes that underlie the physiology of human nutrition. However, these coefficients may be manipulated by the agro-food industry. Such manipulations are constrained by the available technology and the country's regulatory framework, and may have either positive or negative effects on consumers' health. For instance, in the case of s, the agro-food industry can operate by adding sweeteners, such as the high-fructose corn syrup, so as to increase the food palatability, but worsening its adverse health effects (and, thus, raising the value of ρ).

In this simplified economy, people have preferences regarding food consumption and health conditions [24]. These preferences are described by the following Cobb–Douglas utility function:

$$U = c^{\alpha} \times s^{\beta} \times H^{-\eta} \tag{2}$$

where U is the consumer's utility (i.e., the total satisfaction that results from any given combination of goods and health status). In Equation (2), the parameters α, β, and η are elasticity coefficients that measure the reactivity of U with respect to c, s, and H. The value of these coefficients depends on individual preferences and, thus, it changes from one consumer to another.

Specifically, regarding food consumption, we assume that Equation (2) has the usual property of positive, but diminishing, marginal utility (i.e., c and s are 'goods', whose consumption increases the total utility but at a decreasing rate ($0 < \alpha < 1$ and $0 < \beta < 1$). In the case of health, we assume, instead, that η is negative, because the condition of being overweight or obese is a 'bad' (i.e., something that confers disutility). In other words, if η were equal to zero the consumer would not care about being overweight or obese. On the contrary, $\eta < 0$ implies that we are assuming health-conscious consumers who, at least partially, are concerned about their health conditions. This can be explained by the awareness of the negative effects of obesity and being overweight on future health status (i.e., the increasing risk of developing some overweight and obesity-related diseases) and/or by the cultural and social pressure to conform to a stereotype of an 'ideal body shape' (e.g., the social pressure on girls and young women to be thin).

Equations (2) and (3) define a framework in which the population's health conditions, measured by the number of individuals that are overweight or obese, depend on people choices as consumers. The usual population's eating habits determine a general profile of food consumption—i.e., a dietary pattern—that affects the prevalence of obesity and being overweight. This can be shown by replacing H in the utility function (Equation (2)) with its expression from the health production function (Equation (1)), as follows:

$$U = c^{\alpha + \sigma\eta} \times s^{\beta - \rho\eta} \tag{3}$$

This expression shows that the individuals' eating habits are a function of three fundamental factors: (1) the consumers' tastes and preferences regarding the different kinds of foods available in the market (that is, the elasticity of utility with respect to c and s, measured by the parameters α and β); (2) the role that health plays in the individuals' preferences, captured here by the importance of not being overweight or obese (thus, the elasticity of utility with respect to H, measured by the parameter η); and, finally, (3) the size of the (positive or negative) effects on people's health of the consumption of the healthy and unhealthy foods (that is, the elasticity of H with respect to c and s, measured here by the parameters ρ and σ).

Health-related choices, besides preferences, also depend on the consumer's purchasing power. We describe the set of consumer's feasible consumption bundles by the following standard budget constraint: $p_c c + p_s s = Y$, where p_c and p_s denote the prices of the healthy and unhealthy foods respectively, and Y denotes the amount of money that consumer spends on foods (which we simply indicate as the consumer's disposable income). Thus, each individual is facing a constrained optimization problem: to maximize utility from the consumption of goods s and c subject to the constraint of a given amount of income to spend (Y) and the food prices (p_c and p_s), that is: $max_{C,S}\ U(c, s) = c^{\alpha + \sigma\eta} \times s^{\beta - \rho\eta}$ subject to $p_c c + p_s s = Y$.

By optimally solving this problem, we obtain the consumer's demand functions for the unhealthy and healthy food:

$$Q_S = \frac{\beta - \rho\eta}{\alpha + \beta + \eta(\sigma - \rho)} \times \frac{Y}{p_S} \tag{4}$$

$$Q_C = \frac{\alpha + \sigma\eta}{\alpha + \beta + \eta(\sigma - \rho)} \times \frac{Y}{p_C} \tag{5}$$

where the first term on the right-hand side of each equation is the share of the consumer's income spent on s and c (i.e., $p_c c/Y$ and $p_s s/Y$, respectively). Hence, by denoting these expenditure shares with X_S and X_C, Equations (4) and (5) become $Q_S = X_S \times (Y/p_S)$ and $Q_C = X_C \times (Y/p_c)$, respectively. Finally, if we substitute these last two expressions—which indicate the composition of the optimal consumption bundle (i.e., the quantity demanded of s and c) given the consumer's disposable income and the food market prices—in Equation (1), we obtain the level of overweight or obesity (H) as a function of the variables that drives the demand for the healthy and unhealthy food:

$$H = (X_S \times \frac{Y}{p_S})^{\rho} \times (X_C \times \frac{Y}{p_C})^{-\sigma} \tag{6}$$

which, by factoring out prices and income, we can more usefully rewrite as follows:

$$H = (X_S^{\rho} \times X_C^{-\sigma}) \times (\frac{p_C^{\sigma}}{p_S^{\rho}}) \times Y^{\rho - \sigma} \tag{7}$$

Equation (7) shows that the excess of body fat accumulation depends on four fundamental factors, namely: (1) the share of disposable income that consumers spend on unhealthy and healthy foods (i.e., X_S and X_C, respectively); (2) the food market prices (i.e., p_c and p_s); (3) the consumers' disposable income (Y); and, finally, (4) the elasticity of the body weight accumulation with respect to s and c (i.e., the parameters of the health production function, ρ and σ). It is worth noting that the exponent of the disposable income—the difference between ρ and σ (that hereafter we will denote by $\theta = \rho - \sigma$)—may be either positive ($\rho > \sigma$) or negative ($\rho < \sigma$). This means that, by increasing the average income, the economic development may push people towards a healthier or unhealthier dietary pattern. As a result, in each population the prevalence of health problems due to obesity and being overweight may be mitigated or exacerbated by an increasing living standard. Testing the nature of this relationship is the main purpose of the next section.

3. Methods and Data

The central question in which we are interested is the relationship between unhealthy body fat accumulation, carbohydrate dietary patterns, and living standards. Moreover, given the hierarchical nature of the consumers' nutritional needs and wants, variations in food prices may only anticipate or postpone demand-side structural changes that result from the overcoming of rising income threshold levels, beyond which consumers modify their health-related lifestyles [25,26]. We can therefore simplify Equation (7) by rewriting it as a relationship between three key variables: the condition of being overweight or obese (H), the consumption of healthy and unhealthy food (X_C and X_S), and the disposable income (Y), as follows:

$$H = (X_S^{\rho} \times X_C^{-\sigma}) \times Y^{\rho-\sigma} \tag{8}$$

to emphasize the role of the standard of living—captured here by the level of disposable income—in determining the prevalence of obesity and being overweight. Finally, because in this model consumers spend all income on food, and both s and c are measured in terms of energy (i.e., in kcal/person/day), in Equation (8) the variables X_S and X_C directly measure the shares of the total consumers' energy intake derived from simple and complex carbohydrates, respectively.

Our quantitative analysis is conducted at the macroeconomic level, by using cross-section data for 185 countries worldwide, over the period 2012–2014. Data come from three main sources: the Food and Agriculture Organization (FAO), the WHO, and the United Nations Development Report (UNDR). Specifically, we collected figures from:

- the FAO database [27], about the population mean consumption of simple and complex carbohydrates. These figures measure, in percentage, the shares of sugar and sweeteners (X_S) and cereals (X_C) in each country Dietary Energy Supply—(DES), the DES is an indicator of the total amount of food, usually expressed in kcal/person/day, available in a given country and year for human consumption;
- the WHO database [3], regarding the age-standardized adjusted rates of overweight and obesity prevalence, measured in each country by the percentage of adults (ages 20+) who have a BMI (kg/m^2) greater than 25 (overweight, H_{OW}) or greater than 30 (obese, H_{OB});
- and, finally, the UNDR database [28], concerning the level human development and that of average income, measured in each country respectively by the Human Development Index (HDI) and the Gross National Income per capita (Y, adjusted for purchasing power parity);

Table 1 contains a brief description of each variable, as well as basic summary statistics. The full database is available in the Supplementary material section (Tables S1–S3).

We, thus, proceed in three steps. First, by combining data on X_S and X_C with figures on Y, we estimate Equation (8) in order to measure the values of the parameters ρ and σ. For such a purpose, we use a double-log specification—that is, $\ln H_i = \beta_0 + \beta_1 \ln X_{Si} + \beta_2 \ln X_{Ci} + \beta_3 \ln Y_i + \varepsilon_i$, where the coefficients β_1, β_2, and β_3 measure the parameters ρ, σ, and $\theta = \rho - \sigma$, respectively—by running two regressions, one for the prevalence of overweight (H_{OW}) and the other for that of obesity (H_{OB}). Second, we use the estimated coefficients ρ and σ to compute, for each country, an indicator of the population carbohydrate dietary pattern (that is, a carbohydrates dietary pattern index, *CDP*), based upon the ratio of the shares of simple to complex carbohydrates in the country's DES, in which each share is weighted by the value of its negative or positive impact on health conditions:

$$CDP_i = \frac{\rho X_{S_i}}{\sigma X_{C_i}} \times 100 \quad (9)$$

where i stands for the ith country, and which we use as a basic measure of unhealthy eating habits, since its value increases the greater the share of calories from unhealthy foods (X_S), and the greater the negative impact on health of the unhealthy food (ρ), and vice versa for X_C and σ. Third, and finally, we estimate an equation in which the prevalence of obesity and being overweight in each country is regressed against the population's *CDP* index and the average income per capita, by using a double-log quadratic model—that is, $\ln H_i = \beta_0 + \beta_1 \ln DPI_i + \beta_2 \ln Y_i + \beta_3 \ln Y_i^2 + \varepsilon_i$—which allows for a non-constant income elasticity of H_{OW} and H_{OB} with respect to Y.

Table 1. Summary of statistics.

Variable	Description	Mean	Median	Max	Min	Std. Dev.	*n*
HDI	Human Development Index	0.697	0.727	0.949	0.352	0.155	185
Y	Gross National Income (GNI) per capita 2011, PPP $	16,867.1	10,382.7	129,915.6	587.5	18,521.1	185
H_{OW}	Prevalence of overweight (population aged 18+) Age-standardized rate, both sex	47.7	54.8	79.3	14.5	17.0	185
H_{OB}	Prevalence of obesity (population aged 18+) Age-standardized rate, both sex	19.0	20.1	47.6	2.2	10.2	185
X_C	Cereals Share of dietary energy supply (% DES)	41.8	40.6	98.1	16.6	13.6	185
X_S	Sugar and sweeteners Share of dietary energy supply (% DES)	9.7	10.0	21.8	1.1	4.3	185

4. Results

The regression results are collected in Tables 2 and 3. Table 2 reveals that the shares of simple and complex carbohydrates in the total population's *DES* have a significant impact on the country's prevalence of obesity and being overweight. In both equations, the adjusted R^2 is around 0.5, all coefficients have the expected sign and are statistically significant ($p < 0.001$). Specifically, our model predicts that a 1% increase in the share of sugar and sweeteners, on average, increases the country's overweight rate by 0.3% and the obesity rate by 0.5%. On the contrary, a 1% increase in the share of cereal in the country's *DES*, on average, decreases the overweight rate by 0.2% and the obesity rate by around 0.4%. It is worth noting that the theoretical model finds full empirical support in the results of the econometric analysis. As predicted by Equation (7), the coefficient of disposable income ($\rho - \sigma = \theta$) is indeed almost equal to the algebraic sum of the coefficients of the shares of simple (X_S) and complex (X_C) carbohydrates ($0.30 - 0.21 \approx 0.12$ and $0.53 - 0.38 \approx 0.16$, for H_{OW} and H_{OB}, respectively).

Table 2. Regression results: H_{OW} and H_{OB} regressed on X_S, X_C and Y (double-log model).

Dependent Variable	Constant	Share Sugar	Share Cereal	Income	Adj. R^2	*n*
		X_S	X_C	Y		
Prevalence of Overweight (H_{OW})	2.72	0.30 * 0.05 (6.52)	−0.21 * 0.07 (−2.83)	0.12 * 0.02 (5.45)	0.57	185
Prevalence of Obesity (H_{OB})	1.48	0.53 * 0.08 (6.51)	−0.38 * 0.13 (−2.94)	0.16 * 0.04 (3.96)	0.50	185

Note: t-statistics in brackets, * denote statistical significance at the 1% level ($p < 0.001$).

Table 3. Carbohydrate dietary pattern (CDP) index.

Countries by HDI Group		CDP_{OW}	CDP_{OB}	
Very High	Mean	59.8	57.6	
	Std. Dev.	22.3	21.5	
	Max	117.7	113.3	USA
	Min	28.2	27.1	Slovenia
High	Mean	45.3	43.6	
	Std. Dev.	19.9	19.1	
	Max	101.7	97.9	Barbados
	Min	6.9	6.6	China
Medium	Mean	28.1	27.0	
	Std. Dev.	16.1	15.5	
	Max	77.5	74.6	Kiribati
	Min	3.0	2.9	Nepal
Low	Mean	17.0	16.4	
	Std. Dev.	8.8	8.5	
	Max	35.4	34.1	Swaziland
	Min	4.8	4.6	Benin

Along with each country's values of X_S and X_C, the estimated coefficients ρ and σ were then used to compute the *CDP* index, according to Equation (9). We obtained two indicators: one, CDP_{OW}, for overweight and the other, CDP_{OB}, for obesity, because for a given X_S/X_C ratio, the impact of dietary composition on the prevalence of overweight is slightly different from that on obesity. The results of these calculations are collected in Table 3 where, for ease of exposition, the average value of the *CDP* index in four groups of countries is shown, clustered according to their level of human development (measured by the HDI). The average value of the *DPI* index increases with the country's human development, by varying from a minimum of about 15 in low-HDI countries to a maximum of about 60 in very high-HDI countries. It should be noted, however, that there is great variability within each HDI group (in the very high-HDI countries, for instance, the US index is around four times greater than that of Slovenia).

Table 4 contains the results of the econometric analysis in which H_{OW} and H_{OB} are regressed against *CDP* and *Y*. We can see that the model explains more than a half of the cross-country variation in the age-standardized overweight and obesity rates (here the adjusted R^2 is equal to 0.58 and 0.53, respectively), and all coefficients are statistically significant ($p < 0.001$ for *DPI* and *Y*, and $p < 0.005$ for Y^2). The output elasticity of both obesity and being overweight with respect to the dietary pattern (hereafter, EHD_{OW} and EHD_{OB}) is positive, but less than one (the value of these coefficients is 0.26 and 0.47 for overweight and obesity, respectively). The strong relationship between the *CDP* index and the health outcome is evident from Figure 1, where *CDP* is plotted against the prevalence of obesity, H_{OB}.

Table 4. Regression results: H_{OW} and H_{OB} regressed on CDP index and Y (double-log quadratic model).

	Constant	Carbohydrate Dietary Pattern CDP Index	Income	Income^2	Adj. R^2	n
Dependent Variable			Y	Y^2		
Prevalence of Overweight (H_{OW})	−1.65	0.26 * 0.04 (7.09)	0.88 * 0.24 (3.67)	−0.04 ** 0.01 (−3.15)	0.58	185
Prevalence of Obesity (H_{OB})	−6.00	0.47 * 0.06 (7.14)	1.43 * 0.42 (3.38)	−0.07 ** 0.02 (−3.01)	0.53	185

Note: t-statistics in brackets, * and ** denote statistical significance at the 1% and 5% levels ($p < 0.001$ and $p < 0.005$).

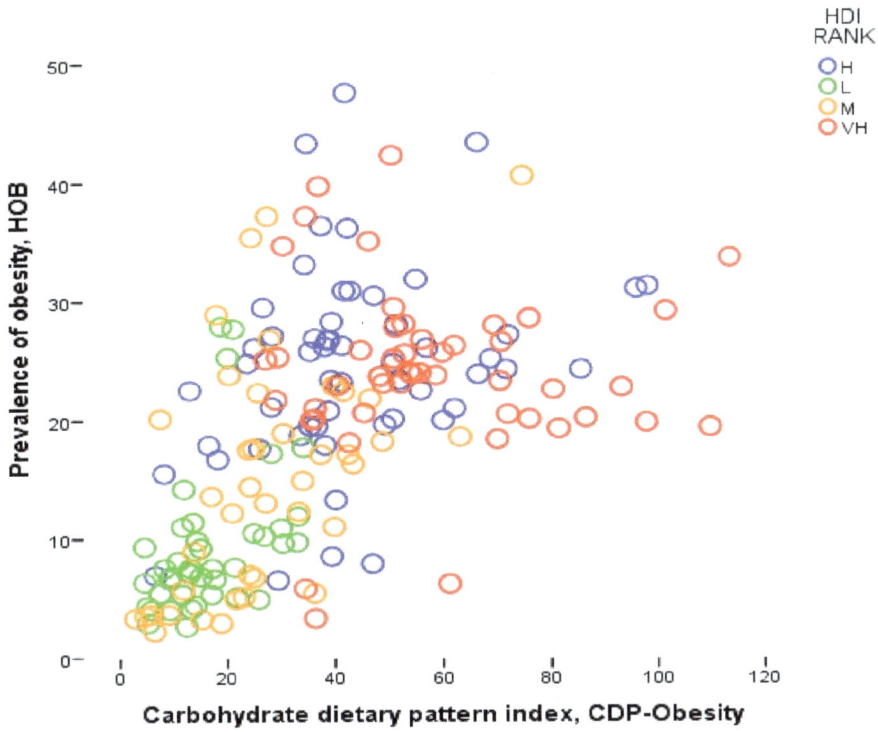

Figure 1. Carbohydrate dietary pattern (CDP) index and the rate of prevalence of obesity.

From the results collected in Table 4, we are also able to compute the income elasticity of H_{OW} and H_{OB}—calculated as $\beta_2 + 2\beta_3\ln(Y)$, and hereafter denoted by EHY_{OW} and EHY_{OB}, respectively. As shown in Table 5, it appears that there is a strong negative relation between these elasticities and the level of human development. Overall, the value of EHY_{OW} and EHY_{OB} is close to zero, or even negative, in very high- and high-HDI countries, and it increases with the decrease of the country's HDI, until becoming equal, on average, at 0.25 and 0.37 in low-HDI countries for overweight and obesity, respectively.

Table 5. Output and Income Elasticities.

Countries by HDI Group		Overweight			Obesity			
		EHY	EHD	EDY	EHY	EHD	EDY	
Very High	Mean	0.003	0.266	0.010	−0.048	0.471	−0.102	
	Std. Dev.	0.036		0.135	0.061		0.128	
	Max	0.076		0.285	0.075		0.159	Montenegro
	Min	−0.103		−0.389	−0.226		−0.480	Qatar
High	Mean	0.091	0.266	0.341	0.100	0.471	0.212	
	Std. Dev.	0.034		0.129	0.057		0.122	
	Max	0.166		0.623	0.226		0.480	Tonga
	Min	0.008		0.031	−0.038		−0.081	Oman
Medium	Mean	0.158	0.266	0.594	0.213	0.471	0.452	
	Std. Dev.	0.048		0.181	0.081		0.172	
	Max	0.234		0.881	0.342		0.725	Nepal
	Min	0.048		0.179	0.028		0.059	Eq. Guinea
Low	Mean	0.255	0.266	0.960	0.377	0.471	0.799	
	Std. Dev.	0.049		0.184	0.082		0.175	
	Max	0.350		1.318	0.537		1.139	C. African Rep.
	Min	0.136		0.512	0.176		0.374	Swaziland

Note: HDI (Human Development Index) rank denotes the level (low, medium, high, and very high) of human development.

In our simplified model, the country's prevalence of obesity and being overweight is determined by the carbohydrate dietary pattern but, at the same time, the country's carbohydrate dietary pattern is determined by the level of income per capita. In our notation, $H = f(CDP)$ and $CDP = g(Y)$. Thus, by substituting the latter equation in the former, we obtain $H = f[g(Y)]$, and by differentiating H with respect to Y—given that $(\partial H/\partial Y)\times(Y/H)$ measure the elasticity of health conditions with respect to income—EHY can be expressed as the product of two elasticities: the elasticity of obesity and being overweight with respect to the dietary pattern (EHD), and the elasticity of the dietary patterns with respect to income per capita (EDY).

In other words, the income elasticity of the population health condition can be decomposed as follows: $EHY = EHD \times EDY$ [29,30]. We use this latter relationship to compute the value of EDY; that is, to measure for each country the reactivity of the carbohydrate dietary pattern to income per capita. Such calculations yield the results collected in the last columns of Table 5. Attention is drawn to the fact that in the low HDI countries the reactivity of the carbohydrate dietary pattern to a rising living standard is on average around 1 (0.96) and 0.8 (0.79) for overweight and obesity, respectively. On the contrary, the average value of EDY in middle HDI countries is always less than one (around 0.5), and it tends to decrease until becoming close to zero (or negative) in the very high-HDI countries.

5. Discussion

The findings this paper highlight the value of providing an economic framework to support epidemiological studies. Regarding the spread of obesity and being overweight in low- and medium-HDI countries, our econometric results support the increasing concerns about the adverse effects of economic development on the ongoing processes of nutrition transition. In these regions, a rising income per capita tends to push populations towards unhealthy Western eating habits. Specifically, a 1% increase in income leads to around a 1% increase in the CDP index and, on average, around a 0.2% and 0.3% increase in the overweight and obesity prevalence, respectively. On the contrary, in high HDI countries, further increases in living standards do not significantly affect the population's dietary pattern and, thus, the spread of the obesity and being overweight problems. Even more promising results come from the very high HDI countries where, on average, the income elasticity of obesity, and that of the dietary pattern, are negative, meaning that there is a positive effect on eating habits of any further improvement in per capita income.

Furthermore, the model that underlies the econometric analysis, albeit extremely simplified, emphasizes the key variables on which public health authorities should operate to tackle the spread of obesity and being overweight. Nutrition information and education programs play a prominent role in promoting healthy eating patterns. However, our model shows that, although essential to improve consumers' awareness about their behavior, information and education may not be enough to change consolidated unhealthy eating habits. On the one hand, there is usually a delay between unhealthy eating habits and the onset of health-related diseases. On the other hand, the consumption of unhealthy high- or ultra-processed foods usually gives the consumer a high immediate (and often addictive) satisfaction. As a result, the value of the product $\rho\eta$ varies with consumer impatience, and it may be very low for those who have strong preference for small immediate rewards over large delayed ones (i.e., consumers with hyperbolic discount functions) [31].

In addition to this, the agro-food industry may operate to increase the value of β, either by effective advertising and marketing strategies or by developing new and powerful additives to improve the foods 'mouth-feel' and 'repeat-appeal' (or addictiveness) [32]. Indeed, as shown in Equation (3), ceteris paribus, a greater awareness of the health effects of the different kinds of foods (in our model, a greater value of η) tends to increase utility and, thus, the consumption, of healthy food (c), and to decrease utility and consumption of the food that promotes overweight and obesity (s). However, as long as the health impact of the unhealthy food—measured by the product $\rho\eta$, i.e., the negative metabolic effect (ρ) times the weight conferred by the consumer to this effect (η)—is smaller than the utility that the consumer gets by eating s (β), even a health-conscious consumer will continue to buy and eat positive amounts of the unhealthy food (and these amounts will be greater the more the value of β is larger than that of the product $\rho\eta$). Finally, eating habits are the results of complex interactions between the cultural, economic and social environment and the consumer's preferences [10]—at both microeconomic (i.e., family and local community) and macroeconomic (i.e., country) levels. Thus, even educated and informed consumers may hardly change their eating habits if they live in an 'obesogenic environment' [33,34].

The findings of our work are, however, subject to at least two main limitations. First, we use a dietary pattern indicator based only on the ratio of simple to complex carbohydrates in the countries' DES. This may lead us to underestimate the real value of *EHD*, which is the negative impact of unhealthy diets on the prevalence of obesity and being overweight. Thus, as highlighted by a recent systematic review on the relationship between food energy density and adult body weight changes [15], further research is needed to develop an indicator able to better capture the complex health effects of high- and ultra-processed foods, which usually combine added sugars with harmful saturated fats and other unhealthy nutritional features (e.g., low fiber, high sodium, and artificial preservatives) in high calorie-dense products.

Second, in our quantitative analysis there is a lack of data on income distribution and all other cultural, economic, and social factors that affect people's eating habits. Poorer and less educated individuals in high HDI countries, for instance, may behave more as the typical consumer of a medium-HDI country, rather than as their wealthier and more educated fellow citizens; or to take another example, gender discrimination due to religious beliefs may distinguish between eating behaviors of populations with otherwise similar levels of economic development. More comprehensive research should, thus, include new variables in both the health production function and the food demand function (including variables on each country's food regulatory framework and food and nutrition public policy and advocacy).

6. Conclusions

In summary, the impact of the global nutrition transition on the overweight and obesity pandemic is a well-established research area that has allowed epidemiologists to link populations' changing eating habits and health outcomes [35]. Although a number of different factors have been identified as key drivers of the more recent transition from healthy to unhealthy dietary patterns, the crucial role of economic development is relatively understood, especially in its quantitative dimension. In this paper we presented an economic framework in which we examine consumer behavior towards healthy and unhealthy foods in the context of increasing disposable income. Our findings corroborate previous research about the causal relationship between the ongoing processes of nutrition transition in the worldwide spread of diet-related diseases, and may help public health scholars in improving effective programs to tackle obesity and being overweight, especially in low and medium HDI countries.

Acknowledgments: We would like to thank three anonymous reviewers for their constructive comments, which helped us to improve the manuscript. All remaining errors are our own.

Author Contributions: Fabrizio Ferretti: conceived the study, developed the theoretical model, collected the data, performed the statistical analysis, analyzed the results, and wrote the paper. Michele Mariani: performed the statistical analysis, analyzed the results, and wrote the paper.

References

1. GBD 2015 Obesity Collaborators. Health effects of overweight and obesity in 195 countries over 25 years. *N. Engl. J. Med.* **2017**, *377*, 13–27. [CrossRef]
2. World Health Organization (WHO). Obesity and overweight—Fact sheet. WHO. Available online: http://www.who.int/mediacentre/factsheets/fs311/en/ (accessed on 6 May 2017).

3. World Health Organization (WHO). *Global Status Report on Non-Communicable Disease*; WHO: Geneva, Switzerland, 2015.
4. Dobb, R. *Overcoming obesity: An initial economic analysis. McKinsey Institute, Discussion Paper—November*; McKinsey Global Institute: Washington, DC, USA, 2014.
5. Keats, S.; Wiggins, S. *Future Diets Implications for Agriculture and Food Prices*, 1st ed.; ODI—Overseas Development Institute: London, UK, 2014.
6. Sun, H.; Ma, Y.; Han, D.; Pan, C.; Xu, Y. Prevalence and trends in obesity among China's children and adolescents, 1985–2010. *PLoS ONE* **2014**, *9*, e105469.
7. Cawley, J. *The Oxford Handbook of the Social Science of Obesity*, 1st ed.; Oxford University Press: Oxford, UK, 2014.
8. Ng, M.; Fleming, T.; Robinson, M.; Thomson, B.; Graetz, N.; Margono, C.; Mullany, E.C.; Biryukov, S.; Abbafati, C.; Abera, S.F.; et al. Global, regional, and national prevalence of overweight and obesity in children and adults during 1980–2013: A systematic analysis for the Global Burden of Disease Study 2013. *Lancet* **2014**, *384*, 766–781. [CrossRef]
9. NCD Risk Factor Collaboration. Trends in adult body-mass index in 200 countries from 1975 to 2014: A pooled analysis of 1698 population-based measurement studies with 19.2 million participants. *Lancet* **2016**, *387*, 1377–1396. [CrossRef]
10. Swinburn, B.; Sacks, G.; Hall, K.; McPherson, K.; Finegood, D.; Moodie, M.; Gortmaker, S. The global obesity pandemic: Shaped by global drivers and local environments. *Lancet* **2011**, *378*, 804–814. [CrossRef]
11. Goryakin, Y.; Suhrcke, M. Economic development, urbanization, technological change and overweight: What do we learn from 244 demographic and health surveys? *Econ. Hum. Biol.* **2014**, *14*, 109–127. [CrossRef] [PubMed]
12. Moore, B.J.; Pi-Sunyer, X. Epidemiology, etiology, and consequences of obesity. In *Textbook of Obesity: Biological, Psychological and Cultural Influences*; Akabas, S.R., Lederman, S.A., Moore, B.J., Eds.; Wiley-Blackwell: New York, NY, USA, 2012.
13. Food and Agricultural Organization (FAO). *Global and Regional Food Consumption Patterns and Trends*; FAO: Rome, Italy, 2003.
14. World Health Organization (WHO). *Diet, Nutrition and the Prevention of Chronic Diseases*; Report of a joint WHO/FAO expert consultation, WHO—Technical Report Series 916; WHO: Geneva, Switzerland, 2003.
15. Stelmach-Mardas, M.; Rodacki, T.; Dobrowolska-Iwanek, J.; Brzozowska, A.; Walkowiak, J.; Wojtanowska-Krosniak, A.; Zagrodzki, P.; Bechthold, A.; Mardas, M.; Boeing, H. Link between food energy density and body weight changes in obese adults. *Nutrients* **2016**, *8*, 229. [CrossRef] [PubMed]
16. World Cancer Research Fund. *Food, Nutrition, Physical Activity and the Prevention of Cancer*; AICR—American Institute for Cancer Research: Washington, DC, USA, 2007.
17. Grossman, M. On the concept of health capital and the demand for health. *J. Polit. Econ.* **1972**, *80*, 223–255. [CrossRef]
18. Wagstaff, A. The demand for health: A simplified Grossman model. *Bull. Econ Res.* **1986**, *38*, 93–95. [CrossRef]
19. Coppola, G. Health, lifestyle and growth. In *Social Exclusion; AIEL Series in Labour Economics*; Parodi, G., Sciulli, D., Eds.; Springer-Verlag: Berlin/Heidelberg, Germany, 2012.
20. Whitney, E.N.; Rolfes, S.R. *Understanding Nutrition*, 14th ed.; Wadsworth Publishing: New York, NY, USA, 2015.
21. Mazidi, M.; Pennathur, S.; Afshinnia, F. Link of dietary patterns with metabolic syndrome: Analysis of the national health and nutrition examination survey. *Nutr. Diabetes* **2017**, *7*, e255. [CrossRef] [PubMed]
22. Stanhope, K.L. Sugar consumption, metabolic disease and obesity: The state of the controversy. *Crit. Rev. Clin. Lab. Sci.* **2015**, *53*, 52–67. [CrossRef] [PubMed]
23. World Health Organization (WHO). Health Topics—Body Mass Index (BMI). WHO-Europe. Available online: http://www.euro.who.int/en/health-topics/disease-prevention/nutrition/a-healthy-lifestyle/body-mass-index-bi (accessed on 12 May 2017).
24. Viscusi, W.K.; William, N.E. Utility functions that depend on health status: Estimates and economic implications. *Am. Econ. Rev.* **1990**, *80*, 353–374.

25. Argyrous, G. Endogenous demand in the theory of transformational growth. In *The Economics of Demand-Led Growth Challenging the Supply-Side Vision of the Long Run*; Setterfield, M., Ed.; Edward Elgar: New York, NY, USA, 2002.
26. Pasinetti, L.L. *Structural Change and Economic Growth*; Cambridge University Press: Cambridge, UK, 1981.
27. Food and Agricultural Organization (FAO). *Food Nutr. Numbers*; FAO: Rome, Italy, 2014.
28. United Nations Development Programme (UNDP). *Human Development Report*; UNDP: New York, NY, USA, 2016.
29. Olsen, J.A. But health can still be a necessity. *J. Health Econ.* **1993**, *12*, 187–191. [CrossRef]
30. Cohen, I.K.; Ferretti, F.; McIntosh, B. A simple framework for analysing the impact of economic growth on non-communicable diseases. *Cogent Econ. Financ.* **2015**, *3*, 1045215. [CrossRef]
31. Story, G.W.; Vlaev, I.; Seymour, B.; Darzi, A.; Dolan, R.J. Does temporal discounting explain unhealthy behaviour? A systematic review and reinforcement learning perspective. *Front. Behav. Neurosci.* **2014**, *8*. [CrossRef] [PubMed]
32. Michael, M. *Salt, Sugar, Fat*; Random House: New York, NY, USA, 2014.
33. Lake, A.; Townshend, T. Obesogenic environments: Exploring the built and food environments. *J. R. Soc. Promot. Health* **2006**, *126*, 262–267. [CrossRef] [PubMed]
34. Popkin, B.M.; Gordon-Larsen, P. The nutrition transition: Worldwide obesity dynamics and their determinants. *Int. J. Obes.* **2004**, *28*, S2–S9. [CrossRef] [PubMed]
35. Popkin, B.M.; Adair, L.S.; Ng, S.W. Global nutrition transition and the pandemic of obesity in developing countries. *Nutr. Rev.* **2012**, *70*, 3–21. [CrossRef] [PubMed]

4

The 1-Week and 8-Month Effects of a Ketogenic Diet or Ketone Salt Supplementation on Multi-Organ Markers of Oxidative Stress and Mitochondrial Function in Rats

Wesley C. Kephart [1], Petey W. Mumford [1], Xuansong Mao [1], Matthew A. Romero [1], Hayden W. Hyatt [1], Yufeng Zhang [2], Christopher B. Mobley [1], John C. Quindry [3], Kaelin C. Young [1,4], Darren T. Beck [1,4], Jeffrey S. Martin [1,4], Danielle J. McCullough [1,4], Dominic P. D'Agostino [5], Ryan P. Lowery [6], Jacob M. Wilson [6], Andreas N. Kavazis [1,4,*] and Michael D. Roberts [1,4,*]

1 School of Kinesiology, Auburn University, Auburn, AL 36849, USA; wck0007@auburn.edu (W.C.K.); pwm0009@auburn.edu (P.W.M.); xzm0012@auburn.edu (X.M.); mzr0049@auburn.edu (M.A.R.); hwh0001@auburn.edu (H.W.H.); moblecb@auburn.edu (C.B.M.); kyoung@auburn.vcom.edu (K.C.Y.); dbeck@auburn.vcom.edu (D.T.B.); jmartin@auburn.vcom.edu (J.S.M.); dmccullough@auburn.vcom.edu (D.J.M.)

2 Department of Biological Sciences, Auburn University, Auburn, AL 36849, USA; yzz0095@auburn.edu

3 Department of Human Health Performance, University of Montana, Missoula, MT 59812, USA; john.quindry@mso.umt.edu

4 Department of Cell Biology and Physiology, Edward via College of Osteopathic Medicine—Auburn Campus, Auburn, AL 36849, USA

5 Department of Molecular Pharmacology and Physiology, University of South Florida, Tampa, FL 33620, USA; dagostino.dominic1@gmail.com

6 Applied Sports Performance Institute, Tampa, FL 33607, USA; rlowery@theaspi.com (R.P.L.); jwilson@theaspi.com (J.M.W.)

* Correspondence: ank0012@auburn.edu (A.N.K.); mdr0024@auburn.edu (M.D.R.)

Abstract: We determined the short- and long-term effects of a ketogenic diet (KD) or ketone salt (KS) supplementation on multi-organ oxidative stress and mitochondrial markers. For short-term feedings, 4 month-old male rats were provided isocaloric amounts of KD (n = 10), standard chow (SC) (n = 10) or SC + KS (~1.2 g/day, n = 10). For long-term feedings, 4 month-old male rats were provided KD (n = 8), SC (n = 7) or SC + KS (n = 7) for 8 months and rotarod tested every 2 months. Blood, brain (whole cortex), liver and gastrocnemius muscle were harvested from all rats for biochemical analyses. Additionally, mitochondria from the brain, muscle and liver tissue of long-term-fed rats were analyzed for mitochondrial quantity (maximal citrate synthase activity), quality (state *3* and *4* respiration) and reactive oxygen species (ROS) assays. Liver antioxidant capacity trended higher in short-term KD- and SC + KS-fed versus SC-fed rats, and short-term KD-fed rats exhibited significantly greater serum ketones compared to SC + KS-fed rats indicating that the diet (not KS supplementation) induced ketonemia. In long term-fed rats: (a) serum ketones were significantly greater in KD- versus SC- and SC + KS-fed rats; (b) liver antioxidant capacity and glutathione peroxidase protein was significantly greater in KD- versus SC-fed rats, respectively, while liver protein carbonyls were lowest in KD-fed rats; and (c) gastrocnemius mitochondrial ROS production was significantly greater in KD-fed rats versus other groups, and this paralleled lower mitochondrial glutathione levels. Additionally, the gastrocnemius pyruvate-malate mitochondrial respiratory control ratio was significantly impaired in long-term KD-fed rats, and gastrocnemius mitochondrial quantity was lowest in these animals. Rotarod performance was greatest in KD-fed rats versus all other groups at 2, 4 and 8 months, although there was a significant age-related decline in performance existed in KD-fed rats which was not evident in the other two groups. In conclusion, short- and long-term KD improves select markers of liver oxidative stress compared to SC feeding, although long-term KD feeding may negatively affect skeletal muscle mitochondrial physiology.

Keywords: ketogenic dieting; ketone salts; skeletal muscle; brain; liver; oxidative stress; mitochondria

1. Introduction

Ketogenic diets (KD) are high fat, moderate protein and low carbohydrate diets that have been associated with a myriad of health benefits including weight loss/management, neurological improvements (e.g., treatment of epilepsy and certain brain cancers) and longevity [1,2]. Rodent models have also indicated that ketogenic dieting increases lifespan [3,4], although the specific mechanisms underpinning these observations have not been well elucidated. Excessive tissue accretion of oxidative stress due to repetitive insults from reactive oxygen species (ROS) are a hallmark signature of the aging process [5,6]. Mitochondria bear the brunt of oxidative damage in the lesions to mitochondrial DNA and are reported to be as much as 10-fold higher than in nuclear DNA [7]. Hence, dietary manipulations that mitigate mitochondrial oxidative stress may serve to mitigate the aging process and optimize cellular function.

Interestingly, oxidative stress defense and improved mitochondrial quantity/quality are potential mechanisms through which KD feeding may confer physiological benefits [8,9]. For instance, hippocampal mitochondrial biogenesis in rodents has been reported after four weeks of KD feeding [10]; this is a phenomenon which could occur via KD-induced AMPK pathway signaling [11,12]. KD feeding has also been shown to decrease ROS and hydrogen peroxide (H_2O_2) production in rodent tissues by increasing uncoupling protein-mediated proton conductance and/or increasing glutathione biosynthesis [10,13–15]. With regard to the later mechanism, Milder and Patel [8] have theorized that KD-induced increases in ROS defense is related to an acute stimulation of 4-hydroxy-2-nonenal (4-HNE) or H_2O_2 which, in turn, stimulates the nuclear factor (erythroid-derived 2)-like 2 (Nrf2) transcription factor to translocate into the nucleus. Nrf2 has specifically been shown to upregulate the mRNA expression glutamate-cysteine ligase (GCL) subunits which is the rate limiting enzyme in glutathione biosynthesis [16,17]. In support of this model, Milder and colleagues [18] reported that KD feeding stimulates H_2O_2 and 4-HNE production in the hippocampus of rodents within a 1–3 days period, and this leads to Nrf2 nuclear translocation within 7 days as well as subsequent increases in the expression of ROS-protective genes that promote oxidative stress resistance during 1–3 weeks of feeding. While it is currently unclear whether these redox adaptations are due to a direct effect of the diet (i.e., dietary ketosis) or an indirect effect of the diet (i.e., weight loss, lower insulin levels, etc.), it is notable that several beneficial physiological effects of KD feeding are independent of weight loss. In this regard, potential antioxidant effects of ketogenic dieting may be stimulated by the consequent metabolites of ketone bodies, beta-hydroxybutyrate (BHB) and acetoacetate (AcAc). For instance, ROS production is decreased and resistance to a H_2O_2-induced stress is conferred when ketones are introduced in cell culture models [19,20]. Thus, it is also possible that exogenous ketone supplementation may also have a direct effect in terms of attenuating ROS production and quenching free radical chain reactions.

Based upon the aforementioned supporting literature, it stands to reason that KD feeding or dietary ketone salt supplementation may mitigate ROS production or attenuate oxidative stress over long-term periods which, in turn, may improve mitochondrial quality. Therefore, the purpose of this investigation was to examine if short-term (i.e., 1 week) and/or long-term (i.e., 8 months) KD feeding or BHB salt supplementation affect skeletal muscle, brain and/or liver measures of oxidative stress and mitochondrial function. Our a priori hypothesis was that KD feeding and ketone salt supplementation would acutely and chronically enhance the expression of endogenous antioxidants and, in long-term rats, this would translate to a reduction in tissue oxidative stress markers and enhanced mitochondrial quantity and quality.

2. Materials and Methods

2.1. Rats in 1 Week Experiment

All experimental procedures were approved by Auburn University's Institutional Animal Care and Use Committee (IACUC, protocol # 2016-2814, approval date 6 January 2016). Male Fisher 344 rats at 4 months of age (~360 g) were purchased (Harlan Laboratories, Indianapolis, IN, USA) and allowed to acclimate in the animal housing facility at Auburn University for 1 week prior to experimentation. During acclimation, rats were provided standard rodent chow (SC; 24% (% kcal) protein, 58% CHO (2.8% fiber *w*/*w*), 18% fat; Teklad Global #2018 Diet, Harlan Laboratories) and water ad libitum in a maintained ambient temperature and constant 12 h light: 12 h dark cycle. For a 1 week period following acclimation, rats were provided isocaloric-isonitrogenous-isofibrous amounts of one of three diets:

(1) 10 rats (SC) were provided with 20 g/day of the aforementioned SC given during the acclimation phase.
(2) 10 rats (KD) were provided with 16 g/day of a commercially designed KD (Harlan Tekland diet #10787; Harlan Laboratories, Indianapolis, IN, USA) that was designed to induce nutritional ketosis and has been used previously by our laboratory [21]. Casein protein (Optimum Nutrition Inc., Downers Grove, IL, USA) and cellulose powder (Allergy Research Group, Alameda, CA, USA) were added to better compensate for between group differences in protein and fiber content (added protein and fiber were 23.5% of the modified diet). The diet specifications (following modifications) were as follows: 4.15 kcal/g, 23% protein, 10% carbohydrate (2.9% fiber *w*/*w*), and 67% fat. Medium chain triglycerides, flaxseed oil and canola oil were prominent fat sources in the parent KD.
(3) 10 rats (SC + KS) were provided with 20 g/day of the aforementioned SC, along with sodium BHB salt (DL-3 sodium hydroxybutyric acid, 5.8 kcal/g; NNB Nutrition, Lewisville, TX, USA) which were added to drinking water for ad libitum consumption with the intent to deliver ~ 2.2 g/day. This dosing schedule was designed with the intent of delivering a human-equivalent dose of 40 g/day dose as a "loading phase" per the body surface area rat-to-human conversions of Reagan-Shaw et al. [22] assuming the average rat weight of 400 g and the average human weight of 80 kg.

Notably, body masses were measured every other day, and food weights were measured daily.

2.2. Rats in 8 Months Experiment

As with the procedures outlined above, 8 months experimental procedures were approved by Auburn University's IACUC (protocol # 2016-2814, approval date 6 January 2016). Male Fisher 344 rats 4 months of age (~360 g) were purchased (Harlan Laboratories, Indianapolis, IN, USA) and allowed to acclimate in the animal housing facility for 1 week prior to experimentation in the same manner as described above. For an 8 months period following acclimation, rats were provided with isocaloric-isonitrogenous-isofibrous amounts of the three diets described above (SC n = 8, KD n = 8, SC + KS n = 8). In the SC + KS group, KS were added to water bottles attempting to deliver ~2.2 g/day for the first week as a "loading phase", then 0.3 g/day as a "maintenance phase" for the remaining duration. This dosing schedule was designed with the intent of delivering a human-equivalent dose of 40 g/day dose during the loading phase and a 10 g/day dose during the maintenance phase per the body surface area rat-to-human conversions of Reagan-Shaw et al. described above. One SC + KS rat inexplicably lost >20% body mass during the first two months of treatment and, thus, was euthanized for humane reasons and not included in the analyses. One SC rat experienced rapid weight loss towards the end of the 8 months intervention. This rat presented large intra-abdominal tumors upon necropsy and was also not included in the analysis. Thus, final n-sizes were SC n = 7, KD n = 8 and SC + KS n = 7. Notably, bodyweights were recorded weekly, food intakes were recorded daily, and water was measured daily in order to ascertain the amount of KS ingested by the SC + KS group.

2.3. Rotarod Performance in 8 Month-Fed Rats

Rotarod performance is used in rodent studies to assess a combination of balance, grip strength, motor coordination and muscular endurance [23]. In 8 month-fed rats, rotarod performance was assessed at 2, 4, 6 and 8 months into the intervention using a single-lane device (Product#: ENV-571R; Med Associates Inc., Saint Albans City, VT, USA). Briefly, all assessments took place during the beginning of the rat light cycle (i.e., 0600–0800) whereby rats were placed on the device and the motorized rotor was initiated at a progressive speed from 4.0 to 40.0 r/min. An automated timer tracked time spent on the rod and, once the rats fatigued and dismounted from the rod, a laser beam break stopped the timer.

2.4. Necropsies and Tissue Preparation in Rats from Both Feeding Experiments

On the morning of necropsies (0500–0600), rats were food-deprived but provided water ad libitum. Rats were then transported from the campus vivarium to the School of Kinesiology and allowed to acclimate for 2–3 h. Thereafter, rats were euthanized under CO_2 gas in a 2 L induction chamber (VetEquip, Pleasanton, CA, USA). Following euthanasia, a final body mass was recorded, and blood was collected from the heart using a 22 gauge syringe. Collected blood was placed in a 6 mL serum separator tube and allowed to clot, centrifuged at 3500 g for 10 min, and resultant serum was aliquoted into 2.7 mL microcentrifuge tubes for storage at −80 °C until analysis. The gastrocnemius, brain, and liver were dissected out. In 1 week-fed rats, approximately 50 mg from each tissue was immediately placed in RNA/DNA Shield (Zymo Research, Irvine, CA, USA) and stored at 4 °C until RNA isolation using Trizol-based methods (described in Section 2.5), whereas the remainder of the tissue was flash frozen in liquid nitrogen and stored at −80 °C until total antioxidant analysis. In 8 month-fed rats, necropsies were carried out exactly as detailed above with the exception being that approximately 800 mg from the right gastrocnemius muscle, 1000 mg of liver and 500 mg of whole-brain (without cerebellum) was immediately used for mitochondria isolation as described below. The remainder of the tissue was flash frozen in liquid nitrogen and stored at −80 °C until Western blotting, GSH/GSSG and total antioxidant capacity analyses described below.

2.5. RNA Isolation, cDNA Synthesis and Real-Time Polymerase Chain Reaction (RT-PCR) for 1 Week-Fed Rat Tissues

Muscle/brain/liver stored in RNA/DNA Shield described above were placed in 10 volumes (500 µL) Ribozol (Ameresco, Solon, OH, USA) in a 2.7 mL microcentrifuge tube and were homogenized with a tight-fitting pestle. Phase separation (for RNA isolation) was achieved according to manufacturer's instructions. Following RNA precipitation and pelleting, pellets were resuspended in 30 µL of RNase-free water, and RNA concentrations were determined in duplicate at an absorbance of 260 nm by using a NanoDrop Lite (Thermo Scientific, Waltham, MA, USA). For cDNA synthesis, 1 µg of muscle/liver/brain RNA was reverse transcribed into cDNA for RT-PCR analyses with a commercial qScript cDNA SuperMix (Quanta Biosciences, Gaithersburg, MD, USA). RT-PCR was performed with gene-specific primers and SYBR green-based methods in a RT-PCR thermal cycler (Bio-Rad, Hercules, CA, USA). Primers were designed with open-sourced software (Primer3Plus, Cambridge, MA, USA), and melt curve analyses demonstrated that one PCR product was amplified per reaction. The forward and reverse primer sequences are as follows: Glutamate-Cysteine Ligase Modifier Subunit (Gclm): forward primer 5′-ACATTGAAGCCCAGGAGTGG-3′, reverse primer 5′-CGATGACCGAGTACCTCAGC-3′; Glutamate-Cysteine Ligase Catalytic Subunit (Gclc): forward primer 5′-GAGATGCCGTCTTACAGGGG-3′, reverse primer 5′-TTGCTACACCCATCC

ACCAC-3′. Catalase (Cat): forward primer 5′-TTAACGCGCAGATCATGCA-3′, reverse primer 5′-CAAGTTTTTGATGCCCTGGT-3′. Glutathione peroxidase (Gpx): forward primer 5′-TCTGCACA CTCCCAGACAAG-3′, reverse primer 5′-AGTCACCCATCACCGTCTTC-3′. Superoxide dismutase 2 (Sod2): forward primer 5′-TTAACGCGCAGATCATGCA-3′, reverse primer 5′-CCTCGGTGAC GTTCAGATTGT-3′. Fold-change values from SC rats were performed using the $2^{-\Delta\Delta CT}$ method where $2^{\Delta CT}$ = (housekeeping gene (HKG) CT − gene of interest CT) and $2^{-\Delta\Delta CT}$ (or fold-change) = ($2^{\Delta CT}$ value for each rat/$2^{\Delta CT}$ group average of SC). Of note, 18S ribosomal rRNA (18S) was used as a HKG given that it remained stable across all treatments (primer sequence: forward primer 5′-AAACGGCTACCACATCCAAG-3′, reverse primer 5′-CCTCCAATGGATCCTCGTTA-3′).

2.6. Tissue Total Antioxidant and Serum BHB Assays for All Rats

Commercial colorimetric assay kits were used to determine muscle/liver/brain total antioxidant capacity (Antioxidant assay kit #709001; Cayman Chemical, Ann Arbor, MI, USA) and serum BHB levels (BHB colorimetric assay kit #700190; Cayman Chemical), respectively, according to manufacturer's instructions. For total antioxidant capacity determination, approximately 100 mg of frozen muscle/brain/liver was homogenized in kit assay buffer and centrifuged according to manufacturer's instructions, and supernatants were assayed. Given that brain tissue in 8 month-fed rats was devoted to mitochondrial assays and Western blotting, brain total antioxidant capacity determination was not performed because of lack of available tissue. Following assay execution, all plates were read in a UV-Vis microplate reader (BioTek Synergy H1 Multi-Mode Reader; BioTek, Winooski, VT, USA) at absorbance readings according to manufacturer's recommendations.

2.7. Western Blot Analysis in 8 Month-Fed Rat Tissues

Muscle/brain/liver was removed from −80 °C storage and crushed on a liquid nitrogen-cooled stage. Approximately 50 mg of tissue from each tissue sample was placed in 500 μL of 1× non-denaturing cell lysis buffer (Cell Signaling, Danvers, MA, USA) with added protease inhibitors (1 μg/mL leupeptin) and phosphatase inhibitors (2.5 mM sodium pyrophosphate, 1 mM β-glycerophoshate, 1 mM sodium orthovanadate) and was homogenized in microcentrifuge tubes using tight-fitting pestles. Samples were centrifuged at 500 *g* for 5 min at 4 °C. Supernatants were then subjected to a protein assay using a commercial bicinchoninic acid assay (Thermo Scientific) and were prepared for Western blotting using 4× Laemmli reducing buffer at 2 μg/μL. Subsequently, 20 μL of prepped samples were loaded onto precast 12% SDS-polyacrylamide gels (Bio-Rad) and were subjected to electrophoresis (200 V at 75 min) using premade 1× SDS-PAGE running buffer (CBS Scientific, San Diego, CA, USA). Proteins were transferred to polyvinylidene difluoride membranes (Bio-Rad), and membranes were stained with Ponceau S following transfers to ensure even loading and transfer between samples. Membranes were then blocked with 5% nonfat milk powder diluted in TBS with 0.1% Tween-20 (TBST) for 1 h at room temperature. Primary antibodies directed against the proteins of interest were incubated with membranes overnight at 4 °C in TBST with 5% BSA added. Primary antibodies were used to detect whole-tissue 4-HNE (Abcam, Cambridge, MA, USA), superoxide dismutase 2 (SOD2; GeneTex, Irvine, CA, USA), Catalase (Cat; GeneTex), glutathione peroxidase (Gpx; GeneTex) and protein carbonyls (Oxyblot kit; EMD Millipore; Bellirica, MA, USA). On the following day, membranes were incubated with anti-rabbit or anti-mouse IgG secondary antibodies diluted in TBST with 5% BSA added (1:2000; Cell Signaling) at room temperature for 1 h prior to membrane development. Membrane development was accomplished by using an enhanced chemiluminescent reagent (EMD Millipore), and band densitometry was achieved with the use of a digitized gel documentation system and associated densitometry software (UVP, Upland, CA, USA). All protein band densities were normalized to Ponceau stain densities. All Western blot analysis data are presented in terms of fold-change from SC rats. Notably, Ponceau staining was used for normalization due to the unknown effects that long-term KD or KS supplementation exerted on putative housekeeping proteins involved in metabolic processes (e.g., GAPDH). Notwithstanding, we have allocated this methodology in past studies examining the effects of KD feeding on skeletal muscle and adipose tissue physiology [9,21,24], and several commentaries exist suggesting that Ponceau normalization for Western blot data is appropriate for models which may affect putative housekeeping protein expression levels [25–27].

2.8. Tissue Mitochondrial Glutathione Assays in 8 Month-Fed Rat Tissues

Muscle/brain/liver mitochondrial oxidized (GSSG) and total glutathione levels were determined using a commercial colorimetric assay (kit #700190; Cayman Chemical) according to the manufacturer's instructions, and reduced glutathione (GSH) levels was extrapolated from these values.

2.9. Mitochondrial Isolation, Respiration Assays, and Mitochondrial ROS Determination in 8 Month-Fed Rat Tissues

The day of necropsies, differential centrifugation was used to isolate gastrocnemius, brain, and liver mitochondria from fresh tissue using techniques described previously [28,29]. Mitochondrial oxygen consumption was measured as described by Messer et al. [30] in a respiration chamber maintained at 37 °C (Hansatech Instruments, Pentney, King's Lynn, UK). Isolated mitochondria were incubated with 1 mL of respiration buffer containing (in mM) 100 KCl, 5 KH_2PO_4, 1 EGTA, 50 MOPS, 10 $MgCl_2$, and 0.2% BSA at 37 °C in a water-jacketed respiratory chamber with continuous stirring. Flux through complex I was measured using 2 mM pyruvate and 2 mM malate, whereas flux through complex II was measured using 5 mM succinate. Rotenone (5 μM) was added to prevent electron backflow to complex I in the succinate-driven experiments. The maximal respiration (state 3), defined as the rate of respiration in the presence of ADP, was initiated by adding 0.25 mM ADP to the respiration chamber containing mitochondria and respiratory substrates. State 4 respiration was recorded following the phosphorylation of ADP. The respiratory control ratio (RCR) was calculated by dividing state 3 by state 4 respiration.

Mitochondrial ROS production was determined using Amplex red (Molecular Probes, Eugene, OR, USA). The assay was performed at 37 °C in 96-well plates with succinate as the substrate. Specifically, this assay was developed on the concept that horseradish peroxidase catalyzes the H_2O_2-dependent oxidation of nonfluorescent Amplex red to fluorescent resorufin red, and it is used to measure H_2O_2 as an indicator of superoxide production. SOD was added at 40 U/mL to convert all superoxide to H_2O_2. Using a multiwell-plate reader fluorometer (BioTek Synergy H1 Multi-Mode Reader; BioTek), we monitored resorufin formation at an excitation wavelength of 545 nm and a production wavelength of 590 nm. The level of resorufin formation was recorded every 5 min for 15 min, and H_2O_2 production was calculated with a standard curve.

2.10. Citrate Synthase Activity Assays in 8 Month-Fed Rat Tissues

Muscle/brain/liver tissue homogenate citrate synthase activities were performed as previously described by our laboratory [9]. Briefly, 40 μg of tissue lysate (obtained from tissue lysis described in Section 2.7) were loaded onto 96-well plates. Subsequently, citrate synthase activity was measured as a function of the increase in absorbance from 5,5′-dithiobis-2-nitrobenzoic acid reduction following the methods described elsewhere [31].

2.11. Statistical Analysis

All statistical analyses were performed using IBM SPSS version 22.0 (IBM, Armonk, North Castle, NY, USA) and all data are presented as means ± standard error. Statistics on most dependent variables in both experiments were performed using one-way analysis of variance (ANOVA) tests with Tukey post hoc tests being performed when ANOVA $p < 0.05$. A two-way repeated measures ANOVA was performed for rotarod performance data in 8 month-fed rats. If group $p < 0.05$ then a Tukey post hoc test was performed to determine main group effects. If a group × time interaction $p < 0.05$ then: (a) one-way ANOVAs were performed with Tukey post hoc tests in order to determine between-group differences at each time point; and (b) repeated measures ANOVAs were performed within each group and Bonferroni post hoc tests were performed if $p < 0.05$ in order to determine within-group changes over time.

3. Results

3.1. Effects of Short-Term Feedings on Body Mass Change, Feed Efficiency and Serum BHB Levels

Days 3, 5 and 7 body masses were significantly different between treatments (all ANOVA $p \leq 0.001$). Specifically, change in body mass at day 3 was significantly lower in KD versus SC and SC + KS rats ($p < 0.001$ and $p < 0.001$, respectively), and this difference persisted at day 5 ($p = 0.010$ and $p = 0.002$, respectively) and day 7 ($p = 0.036$ and $p < 0.001$, respectively) (Figure 1a). Feed efficiency (g body mass gained/kcal consumed) over the 7 days feeding period was significantly different between groups (ANOVA $p = 0.001$). Specifically, KD rats presented significantly lower values compared to SC + KS rats ($p < 0.001$) and differences between KD and SC rats approached significance ($p = 0.070$) (Figure 1b). Serum BHB levels were significantly different between groups (ANOVA $p = 0.035$). Specifically, serum BHB levels were higher in KD versus SC + KS rats ($p = 0.034$), but not different between KD and SC rats ($p = 0.140$) (Figure 1c). Notably, SC + KS rats consumed an average of 0.85 ± 0.03 g/day of sodium beta-hydroxybutyrate over the 1-week intervention through their drinking water.

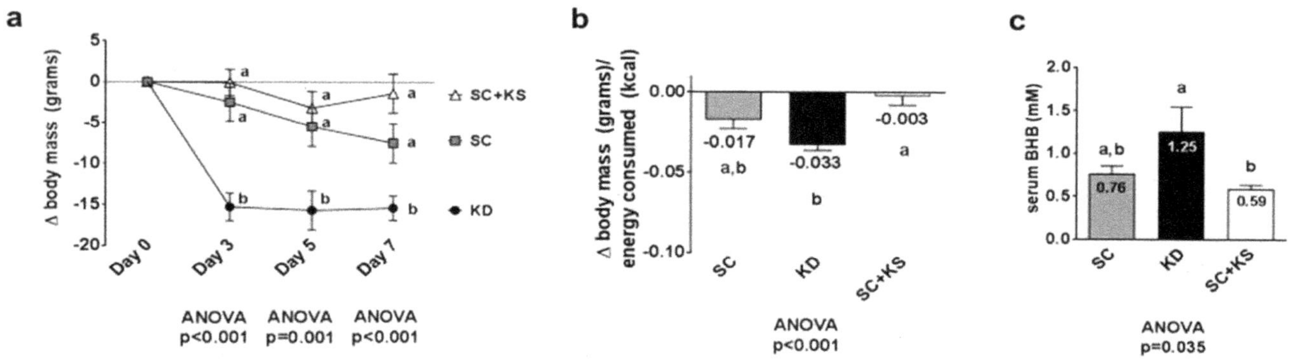

Figure 1. Change in body mass, overall feed efficiency and serum beta-hydroxybutyrate (BHB) levels in 1 week-fed rats. Legend: Change in body mass is presented in panel (**a**). Feed efficiency is presented in panel (**b**). Serum BHB levels are presented in panel (**c**). Data in panel (**a**) are presented as mean ± standard error values (n = 10 per group). In panels (**b**,**c**), all bars are presented as mean ± standard error values and group means are indicated within each bar. For all panels, ANOVA p-values are presented below data, and different lettering ("a" versus "b") indicates significant between-group differences whereas shared lettering ("a" as well as "b" or "a, b") indicates lack of significant between-group differences. Abbreviations: SC, standard chow-fed rats; KD, ketogenic diet-fed rats; SC + KS, standard chow-fed rats with supplemental sodium beta-hydroxybutyrate.

3.2. Effects of Short-Term Feedings on Muscle/Brain/Liver Oxidative Stress-Related mRNAs

Oxidative stress-related genes (i.e., Gclm, Gclc, Gsr, Gpx1, Cat or Sod2) were not differentially expressed in the gastrocnemius, brain or liver (all ANOVA $p > 0.05$; Figure 2a–c). Gastrocnemius antioxidant capacity was significantly different between groups (ANOVA $p = 0.025$; Figure 2d). Specifically, gastrocnemius antioxidant capacity was significantly lower in KD versus SC + KS rats ($p = 0.019$) but was not different between the KD and SC groups ($p = 0.275$) or SC and SC + KS groups ($p = 0.366$). Brain antioxidant capacity was not different between treatments (ANOVA $p = 0.920$; Figure 2d). Liver antioxidant capacity was significantly different between groups (ANOVA $p = 0.040$), although lower values in the SC group approached but were not significant compared to KD ($p = 0.056$) and SC + KS rats ($p = 0.083$) (Figure 2d).

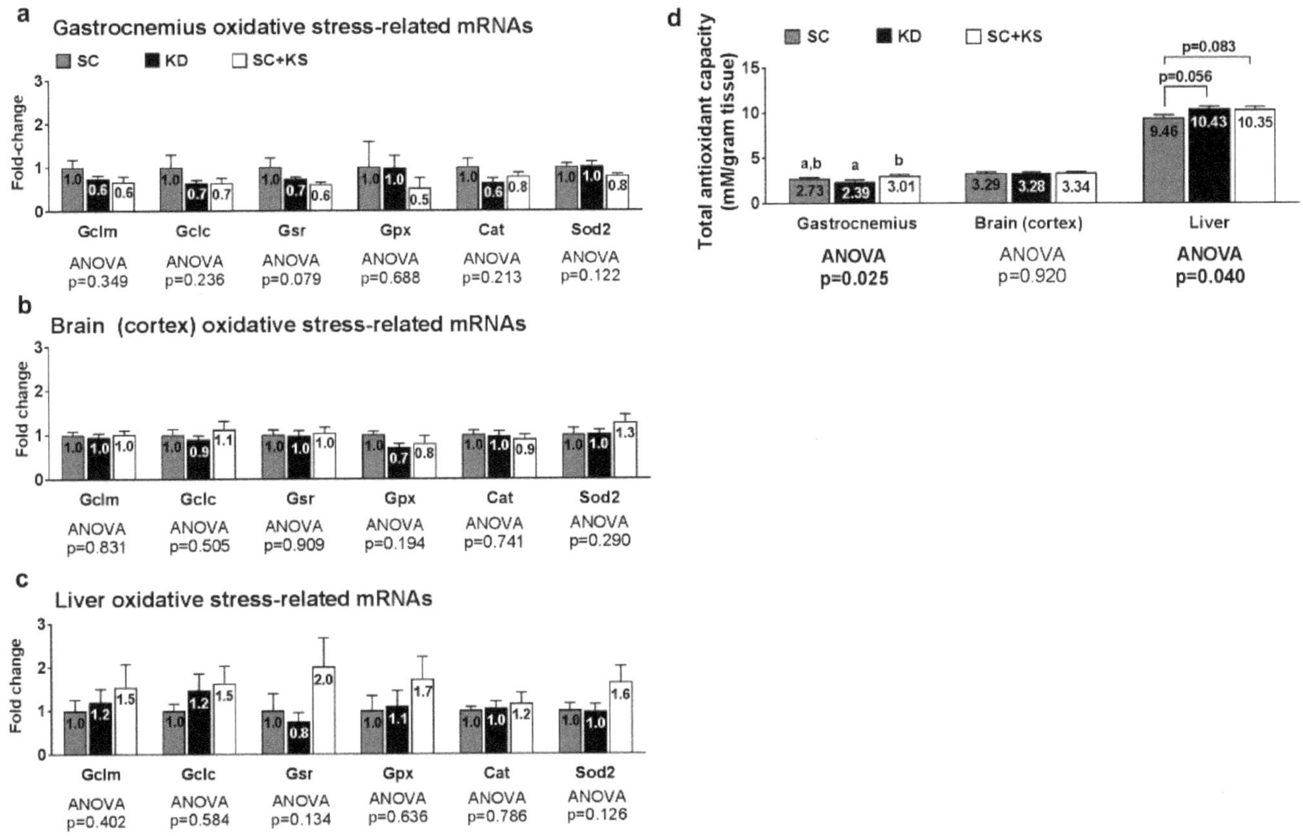

Figure 2. Oxidative stress and endogenous antioxidant-related markers in 1 week-fed rats. Legend: Oxidative stress and endogenous antioxidant related mRNAs are shown for gastrocnemius panel (**a**); brain panel (**b**); and liver panel (**c**). Tissue total antioxidant capacity levels are presented in panel (**d**). Fold-change for each mRNA are expressed relative to the SC group, all bars are presented as mean $\pm$ standard error values (n = 10 per group), group means are indicated within each bar, ANOVA p-values are presented below data, and different lettering in panel D ("a" versus "b") indicates significant between-group differences whereas shared lettering ("a" as well as "b" or "a, b") indicates lack of significant between-group differences. Abbreviations: Gclm, glutamate-cysteine ligase modulatory subunit; Gclc, glutamate-cysteine ligase catalytic subunit; Gsr, glutathione reductase; Gpx1, glutathione peroxidase; Cat, catalase; Sod2, supoeroxide dismutase 2; SC, standard chow-fed rats; KD, ketogenic diet-fed rats; SC + KS, standard chow-fed rats with supplemental sodium beta-hydroxybutyrate.

3.3. Effects of Long-Term Feedings on Body Masses, Feed Efficiency and Serum BHB

Regarding weekly body masses, there were significant differences between groups from weeks 10–30 (all ANOVA $p < 0.05$). Specifically, KD rats weighed less than SC and SC + KS rats from 10 weeks to 30 weeks ($p < 0.05$ at all time points; Figure 3a). Feed efficiency over the 8 months intervention (i.e., g body mass gained/kcal consumed) was significantly different between groups (ANOVA $p < 0.001$). Specifically, KD rats presented significantly feed efficiency values compared to SC + KS rats ($p < 0.001$) and SC rats ($p < 0.001$) (Figure 3b). Serum BHB levels were significantly different between groups (ANOVA $p < 0.001$). Specifically, serum BHB values were higher in KD versus SC rats ($p < 0.001$) and SC + KS rats ($p < 0.001$) (Figure 3c). Notably, SC + KS rats consumed an average of 0.21 $\pm$ 0.02 g/day of sodium beta-hydroxybutyrate salts through their drinking water over the 8 months intervention.

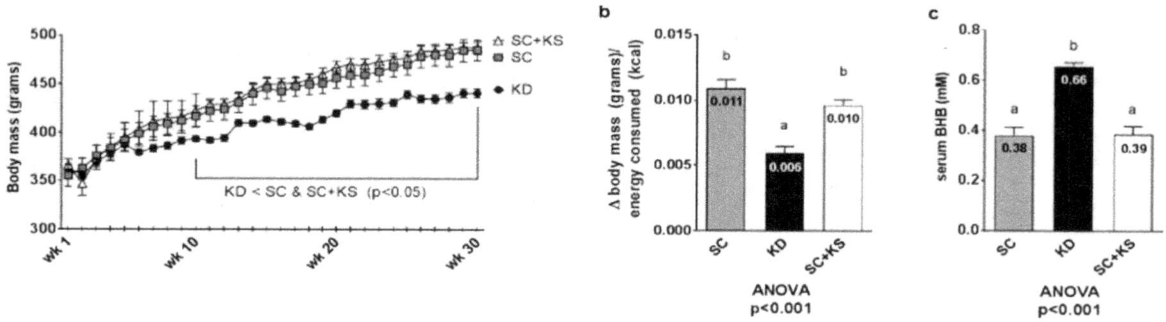

Figure 3. Change in body mass, overall feed efficiency and serum BHB in 8 month-fed rats. Legend: Body mass changes over the intervention are presented in panel (**a**), feed efficiency is presented in panel (**b**) and serum BHB levels are presented in panel (**c**). Data in panel (**a**) are presented as mean ± standard error values (n = 7–8 per group). In panels (**b**,**c**), all bars are presented as mean ± standard error values and group means are indicated within each bar. In panels B and C ANOVA p-values are presented below data, and different lettering ("a" versus "b") indicates significant between-group differences whereas shared lettering ("a" as well as "b" or "a, b") indicates lack of significant between-group differences. Abbreviations: SC, standard chow-fed rats; KD, ketogenic diet-fed rats; SC + KS, standard chow-fed rats with supplemental sodium beta-hydroxybutyrate.

3.4. *Effects of Long-Term Feedings on Rotarod Performance*

There was a significant main group effect ($p < 0.001$) and group × time interaction ($p = 0.005$) for rotarod performance (Figure 4). Regarding the main group effect, rotarod performance was significantly higher in KD rats versus SC ($p = 0.001$) and SC + KS rats ($p = 0.005$). Regarding the group × time interaction: (a) at 2 months, performance was significantly higher in the KD versus the SC ($p < 0.001$) and SC + KS groups ($p = 0.009$); (b) at 4 months, performance was significantly higher in the KD versus the SC ($p = 0.017$) group, and values between the KD versus SC + KS group approached significance ($p = 0.060$); (c) at 8 months, performance was significantly higher in the KD versus the SC ($p = 0.008$) and SC + KS groups ($p = 0.049$); and (d) within the KD group there was a significant time effect ($p = 0.001$) whereby values at 6 months ($p = 0.006$) and 8 months ($p = 0.021$) were significantly lower than 2 months values (notably, there was no time effect within the SC ($p = 0.531$) and SC + KS groups ($p = 0.382$).

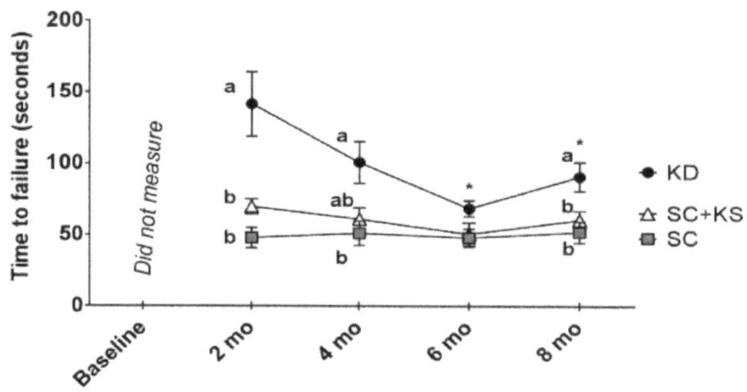

Figure 4. Change in rotarod performance in 8 month-fed rats. Legend: Rotarod performance every 2 months are presented herein. All data are presented as mean ± standard error values (n = 7–8 per group). Given the significant group × tine interaction, post hoc analyses at each time point and within each group were performed. Specifically, different lettering ("a" versus "b") indicates significant between-group differences whereas shared lettering ("a" as well as "b" or "a, b") indicates lack of significant between-group differences, and asterisks indicate significant decreases within the KD rats at 6 and 8 months compared to 2 months values ($p < 0.05$). Abbreviations: SC, standard chow-fed rats; KD, ketogenic diet-fed rats; SC + KS, standard chow-fed rats with supplemental sodium beta-hydroxybutyrate.

3.5. *Effects of Long-Term Feedings on Gastrocnemius Oxidative Stress-Related Proteins and Markers*

Gastrocnemius protein expression levels of Cat (ANOVA p = 0.393), Gpx (ANOVA p = 0.702) and Sod2 (ANOVA p = 0.925) were not differentially expressed between groups (Figure 5a). Likewise, gastrocnemius 4-HNE (ANOVA p = 0.725) and protein carbonyl levels (ANOVA p = 0.504) were not differentially expressed groups (Figure 5b).

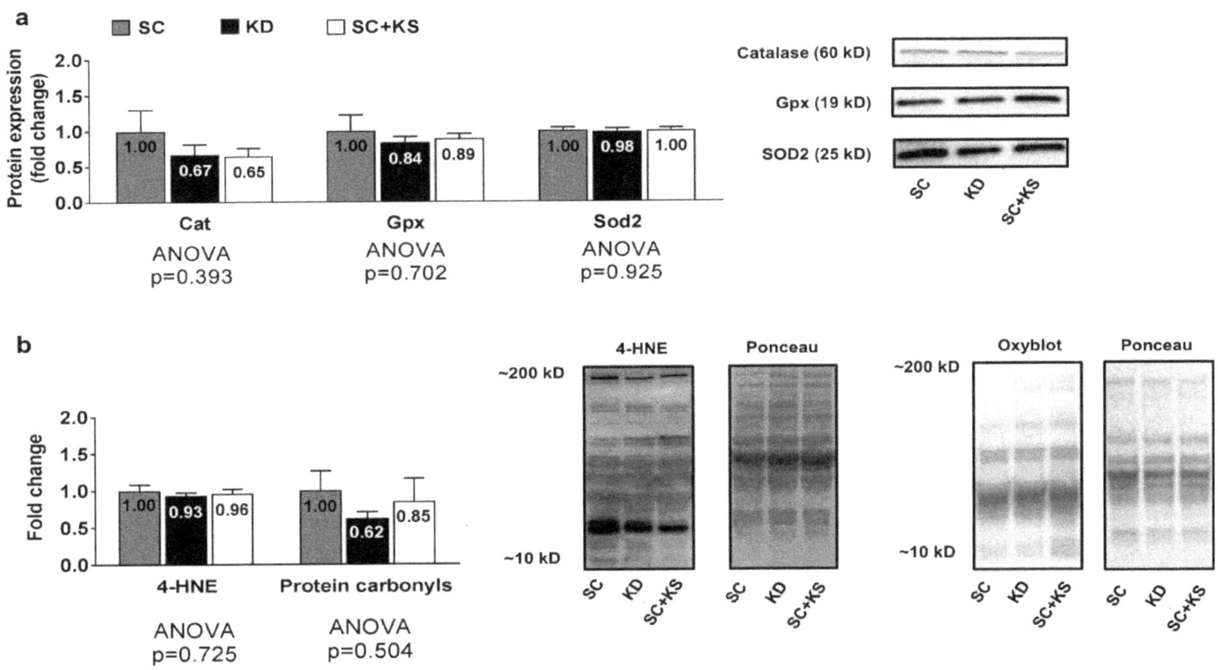

Figure 5. Gastrocnemius oxidative stress-related proteins and markers in 8 month-fed rats. Legend: Gastrocnemius catalase (Cat), glutathione peroxidase (Gpx), and mitochondrial superoxide dismutase (Sod2) protein levels are presented with representative images in panel (**a**). In panel (**b**), tissue 4-hydroxynonenal (4-HNE) and protein carbonyls (Oxyblot) are presented with representative images. Fold-change for each protein are expressed relative to the SC group, all bars are presented as mean ± standard error values (n = 7–8 per group), group means are indicated within each bar and ANOVA p-values are presented below data. Abbreviations: SC, standard chow-fed rats; KD, ketogenic diet-fed rats; SC + KS, standard chow-fed rats with supplemental sodium beta-hydroxybutyrate.

3.6. *Effects of Long-Term Feedings on Brain Oxidative Stress-Related Proteins and Markers*

Brain protein expression levels of Cat (ANOVA p = 0.331), Gpx (ANOVA p = 0.084) and Sod2 (ANOVA p = 0.741) were not differentially expressed between groups (Figure 6a). Likewise, brain 4-HNE (ANOVA p = 0.676) and protein carbonyl levels (ANOVA p = 0.905) were not differentially expressed between groups (Figure 6b).

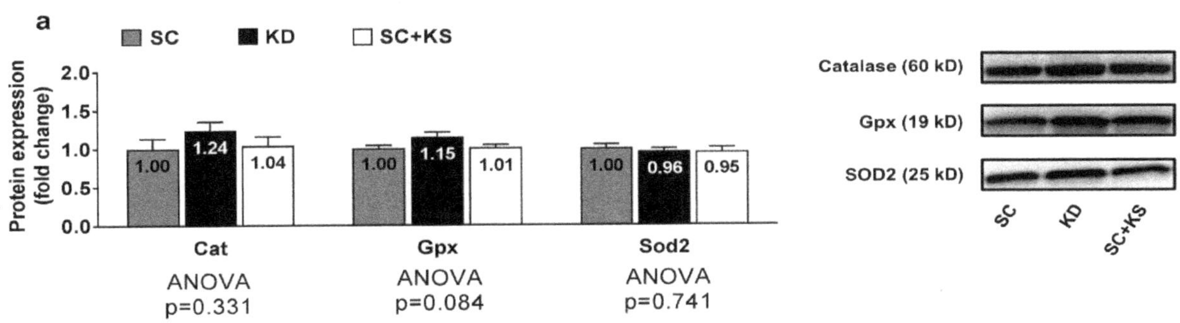

Figure 6. *Cont.*

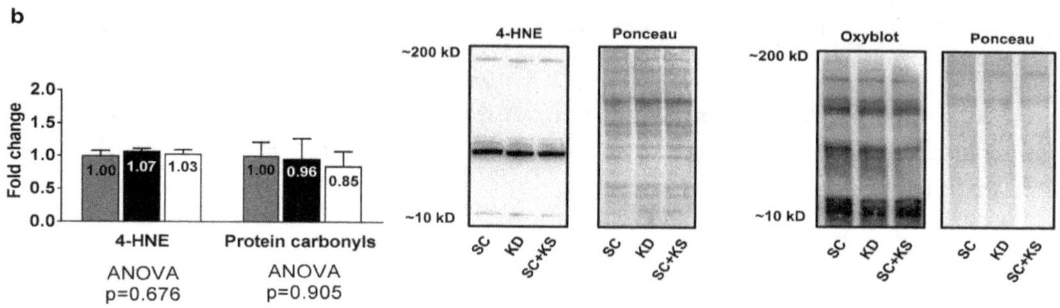

Figure 6. Brain oxidative stress-related proteins and markers in 8 month-fed rats. Legend: Brain catalase (Cat), glutathione peroxidase (Gpx), and mitochondrial superoxide dismutase (Sod2) protein levels are presented with representative images in panel (**a**). In panel (**b**), tissue 4-Hydroxynonenal (4-HNE), and protein carbonyls (Oxyblot) are presented with representative images. Fold-change for each protein are expressed relative to the SC group, all bars are presented as mean ± standard error values (n = 7–8 per group), group means are indicated within each bar and ANOVA p-values are presented below data. Abbreviations: SC, standard chow-fed rats; KD, ketogenic diet-fed rats; SC + KS, standard chow-fed rats with supplemental sodium beta-hydroxybutyrate.

3.7. Effects of Long-Term Feedings on Liver Oxidative Stress-Related Proteins and Markers

Liver protein expression levels of Gpx were greater in the KD versus the SC group (p = 0.004) and high levels approached significance in the KD versus the SC + KS group (p = 0.068) (Figure 7a). Liver protein expression levels of Cat (ANOVA p = 0.932) and Sod2 (ANOVA p = 0.253) were not differentially expressed between groups (Figure 7a). Liver 4-HNE levels were not differentially expressed between groups (ANOVA p = 0.684), although liver protein carbonyls were greater in the SC + KS versus SC (p = 0.034) and KD (p = 0.001) groups (Figure 7b).

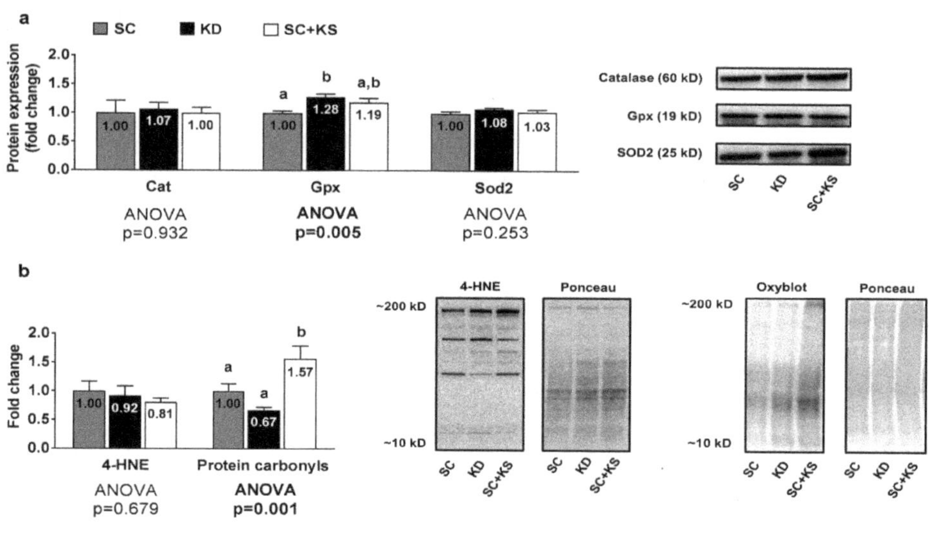

Figure 7. Liver oxidative stress-related proteins and markers in 8 month-fed rats. Legend: Liver catalase (Cat), glutathione peroxidase (Gpx), and mitochondrial superoxide dismutase (Sod2) protein levels are presented with representative images in panel (**a**). In panel (**b**), tissue 4-Hydroxynonenal (4-HNE), and protein carbonyls (Oxyblot) are presented with representative images. Fold-change for each protein are expressed relative to the SC group, all bars are presented as mean ± standard error values (n = 7–8 per group), group means are indicated within each bar, ANOVA p-values are presented below data and different lettering ("a" versus "b") indicates significant between-group differences whereas shared lettering ("a" as well as "b" or "a, b") indicates lack of significant between-group differences. Abbreviations: SC, standard chow-fed rats; KD, ketogenic diet-fed rats; SC + KS, standard chow-fed rats with supplemental sodium beta-hydroxybutyrate.

3.8. Effects of Long-Term Feedings on Tissue Mitochondrial Glutathione, Total Antioxidant Capacity, and ROS Levels

Gastrocnemius mitochondrial oxidized (GSSG) glutathione, reduced (GSH) glutathione and total glutathione were differentially expressed between groups (ANOVA p values = 0.001–0.017; Figure 8a). Specifically, the following was found to occur: (a) GSSG levels were greater in SC-fed versus KD-fed rats (p = 0.018) and trended higher in SC-fed versus SC + KS-fed rats (p = 0.063); (b) GSH levels were greater in the SC versus the KD (p = 0.001) and SC + KS (p = 0.004) groups; and (c) total glutathione levels were greater in the SC versus the KD (p = 0.001) and SC + KS (p = 0.005) groups. Brain mitochondrial GSSG (ANOVA p = 0.294), GSH (ANOVA p = 0.191) and total glutathione (ANOVA p = 0.200) were not differentially expressed between groups (Figure 8b). Liver mitochondrial GSSG (ANOVA p = 0.117), GSH (ANOVA p = 0.699) and total glutathione (ANOVA p = 0.321) were not differentially expressed between groups (Figure 8c). Gastrocnemius total antioxidant capacity levels were not different between groups (ANOVA p = 0.146; Figure 8d). Liver total antioxidant capacity levels were significantly higher in KD versus SC rats (p = 0.028), but not KD versus SC + KS rats (p = 0.216; Figure 8d). Gastrocnemius mitochondrial ROS production was significantly different between groups (ANOVA p = 0.007; Figure 8e). Specifically, ROS values were significantly higher in KD rats versus the SC (p = 0.014) and SC + KS groups (p = 0.015). Mitochondrial ROS production in the brain (ANOVA p = 0.162) and liver (ANOVA p = 0.222) were not different between groups (Figure 8e).

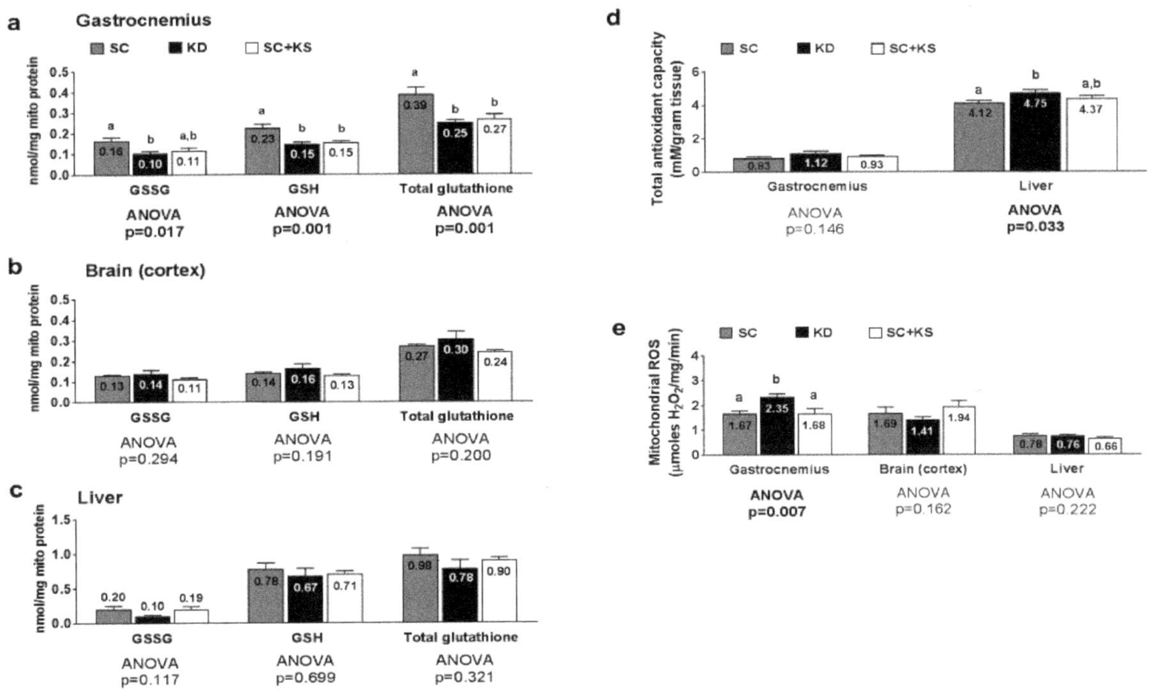

Figure 8. Tissue mitochondrial glutathione, total antioxidant capacity, and ROS levels in 8 month-fed rats. Legend: Gastrocnemius mitochondrial oxidized (GSSG), reduced (GSH) and total glutathione are presented in panel (**a**); Brain mitochondrial oxidized (GSSG), reduced (GSH) and total glutathione are presented in panel (**b**); Liver mitochondrial oxidized (GSSG), reduced (GSH) and total glutathione are presented in panel (**c**); Tissue total antioxidant capacity levels are presented in panel (**d**); Tissue mitochondrial reactive oxygen species production levels are presented in panel (**e**). All bars are presented as mean ± standard error values (n = 7–8 per group), group means are indicated within each bar and ANOVA p-values are presented below data, and different lettering ("a" versus "b") indicates significant between-group differences whereas shared lettering ("a" as well as "b" or "a, b") indicates lack of significant between-group differences. Abbreviations: SC, standard chow-fed rats; KD, ketogenic diet-fed rats; SC + KS, standard chow-fed rats with supplemental sodium beta-hydroxybutyrate.

3.9. Effects of Long-Term Feedings on Gastrocnemius Mitochondrial Function

Between-group differences in gastrocnemius pyruvate-malate state 3 approached significance (ANOVA $p = 0.072$) whereby lower values in KD versus SC rats approached significance ($p = 0.064$) (Figure 9a). Gastrocnemius pyruvate-malate state 4 was not different between groups ($p = 0.119$; Figure 9b). Gastrocnemius pyruvate-malate RCR values were significantly different between groups (ANOVA $p = 0.018$). Specifically, values were significantly lower in KD versus SC rats ($p = 0.030$) and SC + KS versus SC rats ($p = 0.035$) (Figure 9c). Gastrocnemius succinate state 3 (ANOVA $p = 0.706$; Figure 9d), succinate state 4 (ANOVA $p = 0.500$; Figure 9e) and succinate RCR values (ANOVA $p = 0.582$; Figure 9f) were not different between groups.

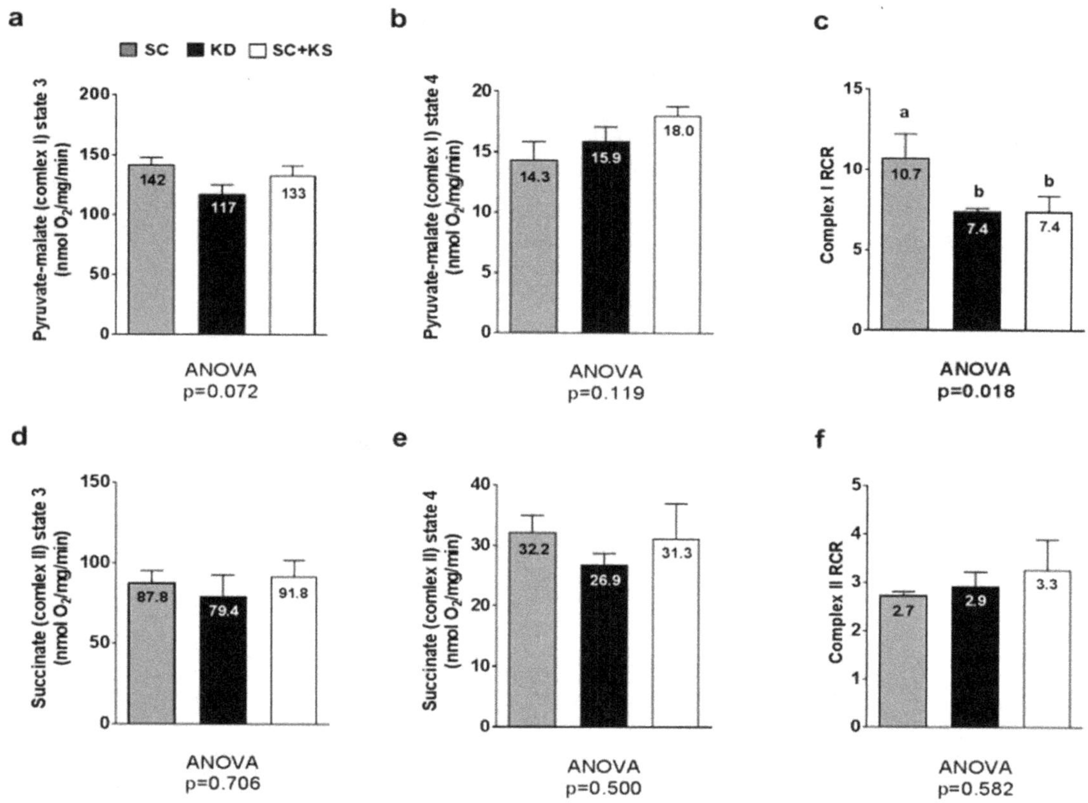

Figure 9. Gastrocnemius mitochondrial function in 8 month-fed rats. Legend: State 3 pyruvate-malate is presented in panel (**a**); State 4 pyruvate-malate is presented in panel (**b**); Pyruvate-malate RCR is presented in panel (**c**); State 3 succinate is presented in panel (**d**); State 4 succinate is presented in panel (**e**); Succinate RCR is presented in panel (**f**). All bars are presented as mean ± standard error values ($n = 7$–8 per group), group means are indicated within each bar and ANOVA p-values are presented below data, and different lettering ("a" versus "b") indicates significant between-group differences whereas shared lettering ("a" as well as "b" or "a, b") indicates lack of significant between-group differences. Abbreviations: SC, standard chow-fed rats; KD, ketogenic diet-fed rats; SC + KS, standard chow-fed rats with supplemental sodium beta-hydroxybutyrate; RCR, respiratory exchange ratio.

3.10. Effects of Long-Term Feedings on Brain and Liver Mitochondrial Function

Brain pyruvate-malate state 3 (ANOVA $p = 0.706$), pyruvate-malate state 4 (ANOVA $p = 0.500$) and pyruvate-malate RCR values (ANOVA $p = 0.582$; Figure 10a) were not different between groups. Notably, brain succinate state 3, state 4 and RCR values are not reported given that a reliable state 4 could not be obtained.

Liver pyruvate-malate state 3 (ANOVA $p = 0.466$), pyruvate-malate state 4 (ANOVA $p = 0.364$) and pyruvate-malate RCR values (ANOVA $p = 0.714$; Figure 10b) were not different between groups.

Liver succinate state 3 (ANOVA $p = 0.246$), succinate state 4 (ANOVA $p = 0.552$) and succinate RCR values (ANOVA $p = 0.112$; Figure 10c) were not different between groups.

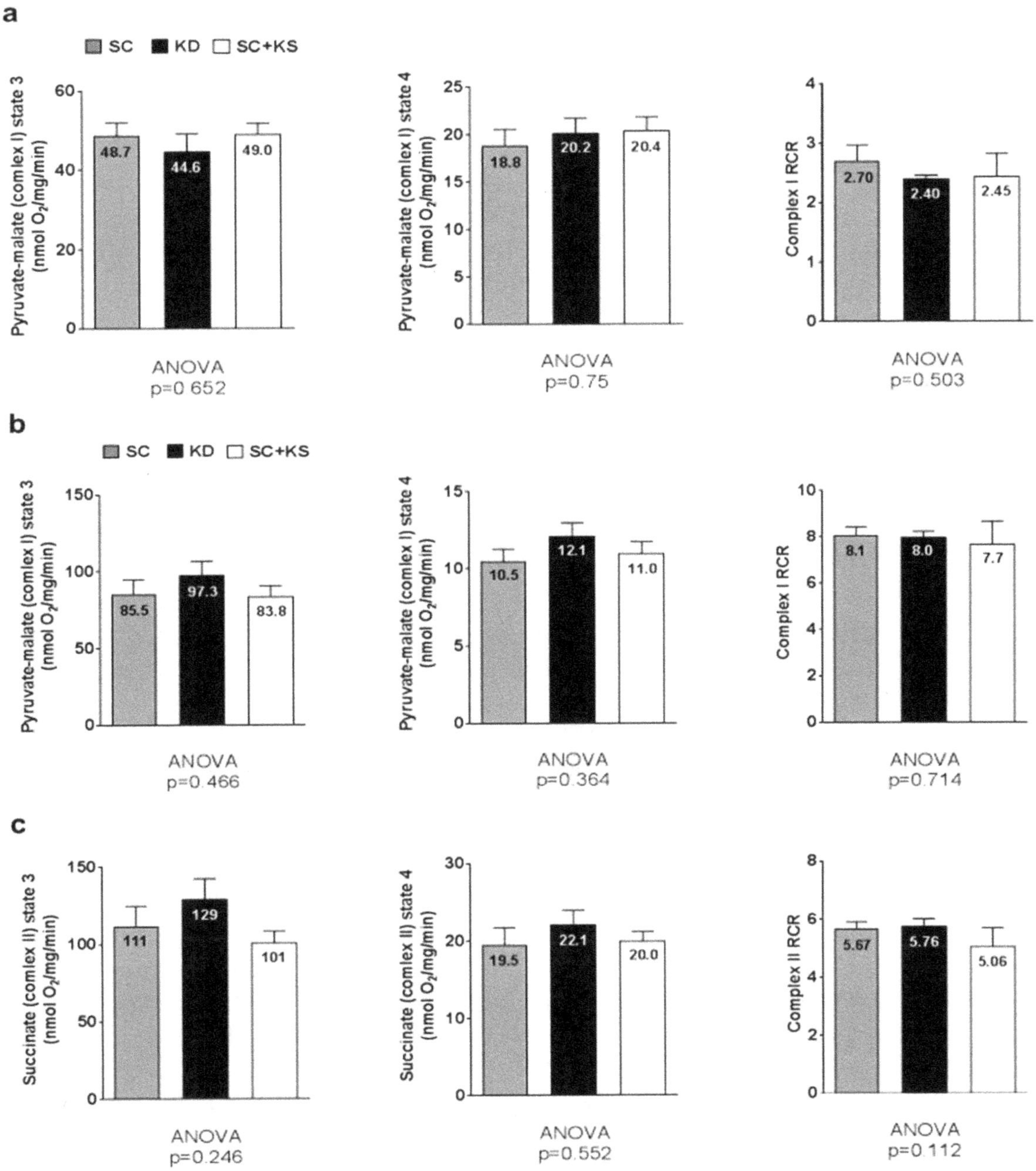

Figure 10. Brain and liver mitochondrial function in 8 month-fed rats. Legend: Brain state 3 and 4 pyruvate-malate and respiratory control ratio (RCR) values are presented in panel (**a**); Liver state 3 and 4 pyruvate-malate and RCR values are presented in panel (**b**); Liver state 3 and 4 succinate and RCR values are presented in panel (**c**). All bars are presented as mean ± standard error values ($n = 7$–8 per group), group means are indicated within each bar and ANOVA p-values are presented below data. Abbreviations: SC, standard chow-fed rats; KD, ketogenic diet-fed rats; SC + KS, standard chow-fed rats with supplemental sodium beta-hydroxybutyrate; RCR, respiratory exchange ratio.

3.11. *Effects of Long-Term Feedings on Tissue Citrate Synthase Activity*

Gastrocnemius citrate synthase activity levels were significantly different between groups (ANOVA $p < 0.001$). Specifically, values were lower in KD versus SC + KS ($p < 0.001$) and SC ($p = 0.009$)

rats (Figure 11). Citrate synthase activity levels in the brain (ANOVA $p = 0.386$) and liver (ANOVA $p = 0.548$) were similar between groups (Figure 11).

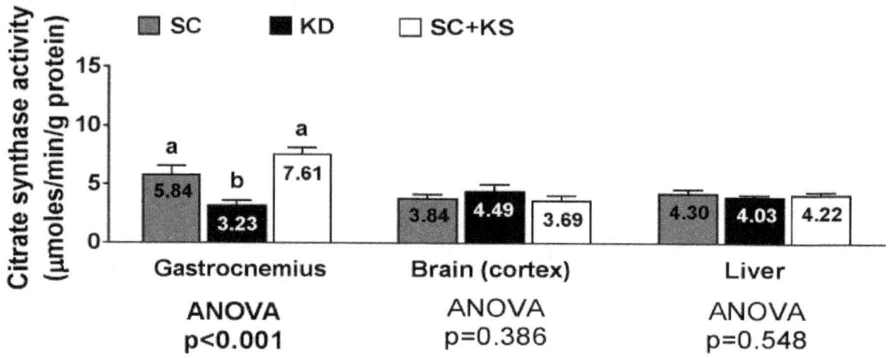

Figure 11. Tissue citrate synthase activity in 8 month-fed rats. Legend: Tissue citrate synthase activity is presented. All bars are presented as mean ± standard error values (n = 7–8 per group), group means are indicated within each bar and ANOVA p-values are presented below data, and different lettering ("a" versus "b") indicates significant between-group differences whereas shared lettering ("a" as well as "b" or "a, b") indicates lack of significant between-group differences. Abbreviations: SC, standard control; KD, ketogenic diet; SC + KS, standard control with supplemental sodium beta-hydroxybutyrate.

4. Discussion

Overall, KD-fed rats exhibited more weight loss (1 week feedings) or an attenuation of weight gain (8 months feedings) compared to the SC and SC + KS groups. In short-term fed rats, serum ketones and liver antioxidant capacity trended higher in KD- versus SC-fed rats, although all muscle, brain and liver oxidative stress-related mRNAs were similar between treatments. In long term-fed rats, serum ketones were greater in KD- versus SC- and SC + KS-fed rats ($p < 0.05$) suggesting that diet, but not the employed KS dosage, induces ketonemia. Moreover, liver total antioxidant capacity and glutathione peroxidase protein levels were 15% and 28% higher, respectively, in long-term KD- versus SC-fed rats ($p < 0.05$), while liver protein carbonyls were lowest in KD-fed rats. Contrary to our hypothesis, gastrocnemius mitochondrial ROS production was ~40% higher in KD-fed rats versus other groups ($p = 0.007$) and this may have been related to significantly lower mitochondrial glutathione levels. Further, pyruvate-malate mitochondrial respiratory control ratio was lower in KD- and SC + KS- versus SC-fed rats ($p < 0.05$), and gastrocnemius mitochondrial quantity was 81% and 136% greater in SC- and SC + KS-fed rats versus KD-fed rats ($p < 0.001$). Rotarod performance was greatest in KD-fed rats versus other groups at 2, 4 and 8 months ($p < 0.05$), although an age-related decline in performance existed in KD-fed rats whereas this was not evident in the other two groups.

4.1. Ketogenic Diet Feeding, But Not Ketone Salt Supplementation, Elevates Serum BHB Levels and Produces Short-Term Weight Loss as Well as a Long-Term Attenuation of Weight Gain

Herein, we report that KD feeding induces short-term weight loss and reduced feed efficiency relative to standard chow feeding. Notably, SC-fed rats also presented weight loss during the 1-week feeding experiment, although KD-induced weight loss was significantly greater. While this finding is difficult to reconcile, we believe that the initial handling of rats (e.g., body mass assessment every other day and food weighing every day) was likely a stressor to all groups of rats in the 1-week study. Hence, we are uncertain as to whether or not this stressor appreciably compromised the molecular markers examined in the 1-week animals. In spite of the aforementioned limitation, our group has previously observed similar outcomes in a separate cohort of rats fed the unmodified KD (i.e., no additional protein or fiber added) over a 6-week period when compared to SC-fed and Western diet-fed rats [24]. Likewise, other studies have reported similar findings using ketogenic diets in rodents [32–34]. While the particular biochemical cascade and subsequent hormonal milieu that occurred during this timeframe was beyond the scope of this study, KD-induced weight loss (or weight gain prevention) may be prompted by chronically low insulin levels and/or due to the bodily loss of biochemical energy via ketone body excretion in the urine [35]. Notably, ketone salt supplementation did not affect body weight or feed efficiency when comparing SC + KS versus SC-fed rats. Ketone ester feedings in mice over a 4-week period has been shown to robustly elevate serum BHB levels, stimulate brown fat activation, elevate resting energy expenditure and promote weight loss in mice [36]. Kesl et al. [37] also reported that 5 and 10 g/kg of KS, which is 8-to-16-fold greater than our employed KS dosage, prevents weight gain in rats although these dosages did not alter serum BHB levels. Providing a mechanistic explanation as to why serum BHB levels are not responsive to exogenous KS versus ketone ester supplementation in rats is difficult to reconcile, but we posit that the lack of significant physiological effects of KS supplementation in both feeding experiments are likely due to the relatively lower KS doses employed in the current study.

4.2. *Short-Term Ketogenic Diet Feeding or Ketone Salt Supplementation Do Not Alter Oxidative Stress-Related Gene Expression in Muscle/Brain/Liver Tissue*

The purpose of the 1 week experiment was to test the theory suggested by Milder and Patel [8] whereby ketogenic diet feeding is posited to increase the mRNA expression of glutathione-related mRNAs (i.e., Gclc and Gclm) after a one week period leading to an enhanced endogenous antioxidant defense system. Additionally, we were interested in examining the effects of KS supplementation given recent findings like that of Shimazu et al. [38] who have reported that BHB acts as an antioxidant in vitro. The data presented herein do not demonstrate altered mRNA expression of either Gclc or Gclm in skeletal muscle, whole brain or liver tissue after 1 week of KD or KS feeding in rats. In addition, we did not observe mRNA alterations in other endogenous antioxidants (i.e., Gsr, Gpx1 and Sod2) or total antioxidant capacity in the assayed tissues. In contrast to our findings, Jarrett and colleagues [14] observed increased GCL activity and elevated protein levels in response to a 3 weeks of KD feeding in rat hippocampal tissue. Discrepancies in our outcomes related to KD feeding could be due to: (a) our investigation of mRNA markers following a one week time course; and/or (b) with regard to our findings in the brain, discordant findings may be related to the region of the brain that was assayed. Notably, we performed all assays in the whole cortical brain while others examining KD-induced alterations in mRNA and protein/enzyme activity have examined the hippocampus. For instance, Ziegler and colleagues [15] also reported that KD feeding over an 8 week period in rats increased Gpx activity increased in the hippocampus, reduced Cat activity in the cerebellum and did not alter these markers in the cortex. Thus, these data collectively suggest that: (a) different brain regions likely express different biochemical responses to KD feeding; and (b) short- or long-term KD feeding does not appreciably alter oxidative stress-related gene expression in skeletal muscle or liver tissue. The lack of appreciable antioxidant effects regarding short-term KS supplementation is likely due to the employed dosage not eliciting increases in serum BHB levels as stated above.

4.3. *Long-Term Ketogenic Diet Feeding Positively Impacts Select Markers of Oxidative Stress in the Liver But Does Not Alter Mitochondrial Quality in Liver or Brain Tissue*

Our findings that the short- and long-term KD feeding increases liver total antioxidant capacity, and long-term KD feeding increases Gpx protein expression levels and decreases liver protein carbonyl levels (numerically versus SC-fed rats and significantly versus SC + KS-fed rats) indicate a potential protective effect of the KD feeding on liver tissue. Several studies have observed that KD feeding increase inflammation and fibroblast growth factor 21-mediated hepatocyte steatosis in rodents [3,39,40]. However, we have previously reported decreased liver inflammatory signaling and triglyceride accumulation with KD feeding in rats whereby the KD was similar to the one utilized in the present study [24]. Milder et al. [18] have also reported an increase in nuclear Nrf2 and a decrease in liver mitochondrial glutathione levels following 3 weeks of KD feeding in rats. While we did not assess nuclear Nrf2 levels in the current study and report that the long-term KD feeding does not alter liver glutathione levels, the contention by Milder et al. that short-term KD feeding leads to long-term increases in oxidative stress defenses may be a potential explanation as to why protein carbonyls were lowest in long-term KD fed animals while Gpx protein and total antioxidant levels were relatively higher in these same animals. It is also plausible that lower liver inflammatory signaling and/or lower triglyceride accumulation, as reported in our past study, could be a contributing mechanism to increased liver oxidative stress protection given the link between ectopic tissue fat accumulation, inflammation and oxidative stress [41].

Interestingly, we also observed that long-term ketone salt supplementation significantly increased liver protein carbonyl levels. While there is currently no literature to date documenting such effects, this suggests that the daily low-dose consumption of ketone salts may induce repetitive bouts of oxidative stress to the liver and this finding warrants further mechanistic investigation. It should also be noted that unaltered brain and liver citrate synthase activity (a well-validated surrogate of mitochondrial density [42]) in KD-fed rats is also discordant with previous literature given that increases in citrate synthase activity have been reported to occur in the hippocampus of KD-fed rodents after a 3-week period [10,43]. Again, however, discrepancies in our findings versus the aforementioned literature may be explained by the long-term nature of our study as well as tissue-specific differences that occur in response to ketogenic diet feedings. Beneficial KD-induced mitochondrial adaptations that occur in the liver or brain, if they do occur, may be transient once the rodents are given an extended period time for dietary adaptation.

4.4. Long-Term Ketogenic Diet Feeding Negatively Impacts Skeletal Muscle Mitochondrial Physiology

While long-term KD feeding did not alter markers of brain and liver mitochondrial quality or quantity, we observed that long-term KD feeding robustly impacts several of these variables in skeletal muscle. Specifically, long-term KD-fed rats expressed lower gastrocnemius glutathione levels, lower gastrocnemius maximal citrate synthase activity, higher gastrocnemius mitochondrial ROS production, and an impairment in gastrocnemius pyruvate-malate respiratory control. Our laboratory has previously investigated skeletal muscle mitochondrial density and mitochondrial quality in 3 months old KD-fed rats following a 6 week dietary intervention [9]. We reported that succinate respiratory control increased in KD-fed rats compared to rats fed a Western diet, suggesting that shorter-term ketogenic dieting may improve lipid oxidation. However, the present study indicates that this mitochondrial adaptation does not persist after 8 months of KD feeding. Regarding the pyruvate-malate respiratory control ratio in skeletal muscle, the depression observed in KD-fed rats may be related to increased concentrations of uncoupling proteins in the gastrocnemius mitochondria. This phenomenon has been observed by others who reported KD-induced uncoupling protein expression increases in brown adipose and neural tissue, respectively [13,44]. Likewise, the KD-induced decrease in gastrocnemius mitochondrial pyruvate-malate respiratory control ratio may also be related to the increased ROS production observed given that ROS-induced mitochondrial damage is implicated in the reduction of mitochondrial function [45–47]. The KD-induced decrease in gastrocnemius citrate synthase activity observed may also be indicative of decrements in skeletal muscle mitochondrial quality or quantity. In this regard, past literature suggests that ketonemia, high fat diet feeding and/or fasting in humans and rodents down-regulates oxidative phosphorylation, lowers skeletal muscle mitochondrial density, or lowers the efficiency mitochondrial respiration [48–50]. The KD-induced increase in gastrocnemius mitochondrial ROS and/or decrease in mitochondrial function and density may have also been due to mitochondrial glutathione levels being low in KD-fed animals. In support of this hypothesis, others have reported that low mitochondrial glutathione levels are associated with increased ROS production and decrements in mitochondrial function [51,52]. Collectively, our results along with other observations in past studies suggest that while short-term ketogenic dieting may enhance mitochondrial biogenesis and/or alter mitochondrial physiology in certain tissues, skeletal muscle may be particularly susceptible to KD-induced alterations in mitochondrial physiology following long-term feeding, and this phenomenon may be due to KD-induced decrements in mitochondrial glutathione levels and/or another unidentified mechanism.

It is notable that, despite the aforementioned observations in the gastrocnemius, KD-fed rats exhibited higher rotarod performance throughout the long-term intervention relative to the other two groups. While rotarod testing does not test maximal aerobic capacity, it does provide a reliable measure of coordination, muscle strength and endurance [23]. Therefore, our rotarod performance data suggest that long-term ketogenic dieting may result in increased skeletal muscle metabolic efficiency (i.e., similar or improved work output with lowered mitochondrial function and/or density in muscle). However, it is notable that rotarod performance robustly decreased with age in KD-fed rats, whereas this did not occur in the SC and SC + KS groups; this being suggestive that long-term KD-induced decrements in mitochondrial function may be a contributor to age-related declines in rotarod performance. In this regard, further research is needed in order to examine: (a) the KD-associated mechanisms that affect mitochondrial function and/or density; and/or (b) if KD feeding affects metabolic efficiency in skeletal muscle.

4.5. Experimental Considerations

Certain limitations are evident in the current study. First, due to resource constraints, short-term tissue analyses herein were only performed at one sacrificial time point which differs from Milder et al. [18] who examined the effects of ketogenic dieting at 1-day, 3-day, 1-week and 3-week sacrificial time points. Second, and as mentioned prior, our brain assays were performed on cortical brain lysates; this is an experimental consideration which likely masked any potential benefit of KD feeding and/or ketone salt supplementation on the hippocampus or other brain regions. Third, it is notable that total antioxidant capacity levels were assayed in different tissues rather than individual antioxidant enzyme activities due to resource constraints. Thus, given that liver antioxidant capacity increases in response to long-term ketogenic dieting, studying the effects of ketogenic dieting on single antioxidant activity levels are warranted. Lastly, it is noteworthy that sedentary rats were studied herein, and this may be a potential reason as to why skeletal muscle mitochondria is negatively impacted with long-term KD feeding. In this regard, we have previously reported that increases in skeletal muscle mitochondrial quality and quantity are not impaired in KD-fed rats that exercised via resistance-loaded voluntary wheel running over a 6-week period [9]. Moreover, elite ultra-endurance athletes that chronically engage in ketogenic-like dieting have been reported to perform equally as well in laboratory-based exercise tests compared to athletes that consume high-carbohydrate diets [53]; this is suggestive that long-term KD athletes do not present functional impairments in skeletal muscle mitochondrial integrity. Hence, again, a future research aim would be to examine if skeletal muscle mitochondrial deficits observed in 8 months KD-fed rats are mitigated with exercise training. One final experimental consideration is the rapid weight loss observed in one long-term SC + KS rat as well as the tumor observed during dissections in one long-term SC-fed rat. While the mechanistic causes of both events were not more thoroughly explored, it is notable that no adverse events were observed in KD-fed rats. Hence, long-term KD feeding in rodents appears to be safe and, with regard to the latter observation, future research is needed in order to determine if KD feeding has anti-tumorigenic effects.

5. Conclusions

In spite of the aforementioned limitations, we posit that these data provide a comprehensive evaluation as to how short-term and long-term KD feeding affect oxidative stress markers, endogenous antioxidant gene and protein expression and mitochondrial function in multiple tissues in rats. Longer-term human studies examining muscle biopsy specimens are needed in order to validate our findings, suggesting that long-term KD feeding appreciably alters mitochondrial physiology.

Acknowledgments: We would like to thank Patricia Rynders, Bettina Schemera and Timothy Knox for their critical assistance with animal husbandry.

Author Contributions: W.C.K. performed most animal husbandry and performed or oversaw most experiments. P.W.M., X.M., M.A.R., H.W.H., Y.Z., C.B.M., J.C.Q., K.C.Y., D.T.B., J.S.M. and D.J.M. critically assisted with experiments, statistical analyses and/or data interpretation. R.P.L., J.M.W., A.N.K. and M.D.R. conceived experimental design and dictated all analytical procedures. W.C.K. and M.D.R. primarily drafted the manuscript and all co-authors edited the manuscript prior to submission.

References

1. Paoli, A.; Rubini, A.; Volek, J.S.; Grimaldi, K.A. Beyond weight loss: A review of the therapeutic uses of very-low-carbohydrate (ketogenic) diets. *Eur. J. Clin. Nutr.* **2013**, *67*, 789–796. [CrossRef] [PubMed]
2. Kulak, D.; Polotsky, A.J. Should the ketogenic diet be considered for enhancing fertility? *Maturitas* **2013**, *74*, 10–13. [CrossRef] [PubMed]
3. Douris, N.; Melman, T.; Pecherer, J.M.; Pissios, P.; Flier, J.S.; Cantley, L.C.; Locasale, J.W.; Maratos-Flier, E. Adaptive changes in amino acid metabolism permit normal longevity in mice consuming a low-carbohydrate ketogenic diet. *Biochim. Biophys. Acta* **2015**, *1852*, 2056–2065. [CrossRef] [PubMed]
4. Simeone, K.A.; Matthews, S.A.; Rho, J.M.; Simeone, T.A. Ketogenic diet treatment increases longevity in kcna1-null mice, a model of sudden unexpected death in epilepsy. *Epilepsia* **2016**, *57*, e178–e182. [CrossRef] [PubMed]
5. Martin, B.; Ji, S.; White, C.M.; Maudsley, S.; Mattson, M.P. Dietary energy intake, hormesis, and health. In *Hormesis*; Springer: Berlin, Germany, 2010; pp. 123–137.
6. Stadtman, E. *The Status of Oxidatively Modified Proteins as a Marker of Aging*; Life Science Research Reports; John Wiley & Sons Ltd.: Hoboken, NJ, USA, 1995; p. 129.
7. Ames, B.N.; Shigenaga, M.K.; Hagen, T.M. Oxidants, antioxidants, and the degenerative diseases of aging. *Proc. Natl. Acad. Sci. USA* **1993**, *90*, 7915–7922. [CrossRef] [PubMed]
8. Milder, J.; Patel, M. Modulation of oxidative stress and mitochondrial function by the ketogenic diet. *Epilepsy Res.* **2012**, *100*, 295–303. [CrossRef] [PubMed]
9. Hyatt, H.W.; Kephart, W.C.; Holland, A.M.; Mumford, P.; Mobley, C.B.; Lowery, R.P.; Roberts, M.D.; Wilson, J.M.; Kavazis, A.N. A ketogenic diet in rodents elicits improved mitochondrial adaptations in response to resistance exercise training compared to an isocaloric western diet. *Front. Physiol.* **2016**, *7*, 533. [CrossRef] [PubMed]
10. Bough, K.J.; Wetherington, J.; Hassel, B.; Pare, J.F.; Gawryluk, J.W.; Greene, J.G.; Shaw, R.; Smith, Y.; Geiger, J.D.; Dingledine, R.J. Mitochondrial biogenesis in the anticonvulsant mechanism of the ketogenic diet. *Ann. Neurol.* **2006**, *60*, 223–235. [CrossRef] [PubMed]
11. McDaniel, S.S.; Rensing, N.R.; Thio, L.L.; Yamada, K.A.; Wong, M. The ketogenic diet inhibits the mammalian target of rapamycin (mtor) pathway. *Epilepsia* **2011**, *52*, e7–e11. [CrossRef] [PubMed]
12. Kennedy, A.R.; Pissios, P.; Otu, H.; Roberson, R.; Xue, B.; Asakura, K.; Furukawa, N.; Marino, F.E.; Liu, F.F.; Kahn, B.B.; et al. A high-fat, ketogenic diet induces a unique metabolic state in mice. *Am. J. Physiol. Endocrinol. Metab.* **2007**, *292*, E1724–E1739. [CrossRef] [PubMed]
13. Sullivan, P.G.; Rippy, N.A.; Dorenbos, K.; Concepcion, R.C.; Agarwal, A.K.; Rho, J.M. The ketogenic diet increases mitochondrial uncoupling protein levels and activity. *Ann. Neurol.* **2004**, *55*, 576–580. [CrossRef] [PubMed]
14. Jarrett, S.G.; Milder, J.B.; Liang, L.P.; Patel, M. The ketogenic diet increases mitochondrial glutathione levels. *J. Neurochem.* **2008**, *106*, 1044–1051. [CrossRef] [PubMed]
15. Ziegler, D.R.; Ribeiro, L.C.; Hagenn, M.; Siqueira, I.R.; Araujo, E.; Torres, I.L.; Gottfried, C.; Netto, C.A.; Goncalves, C.A. Ketogenic diet increases glutathione peroxidase activity in rat hippocampus. *Neurochem. Res.* **2003**, *28*, 1793–1797. [CrossRef] [PubMed]
16. Erickson, A.M.; Nevarea, Z.; Gipp, J.J.; Mulcahy, R.T. Identification of a variant antioxidant response element in the promoter of the human glutamate-cysteine ligase modifier subunit gene. Revision of the are consensus sequence. *J. Biol. Chem.* **2002**, *277*, 30730–30737. [CrossRef] [PubMed]

17. Mulcahy, R.T.; Wartman, M.A.; Bailey, H.H.; Gipp, J.J. Constitutive and beta-naphthoflavone-induced expression of the human gamma-glutamylcysteine synthetase heavy subunit gene is regulated by a distal antioxidant response element/tre sequence. *J. Biol. Chem.* **1997**, *272*, 7445–7454. [CrossRef] [PubMed]
18. Milder, J.B.; Liang, L.P.; Patel, M. Acute oxidative stress and systemic nrf2 activation by the ketogenic diet. *Neurobiol. Dis.* **2010**, *40*, 238–244. [CrossRef] [PubMed]
19. Maalouf, M.; Sullivan, P.G.; Davis, L.; Kim, D.Y.; Rho, J.M. Ketones inhibit mitochondrial production of reactive oxygen species production following glutamate excitotoxicity by increasing nadh oxidation. *Neuroscience* **2007**, *145*, 256–264. [CrossRef] [PubMed]
20. Kim, D.Y.; Davis, L.M.; Sullivan, P.G.; Maalouf, M.; Simeone, T.A.; van Brederode, J.; Rho, J.M. Ketone bodies are protective against oxidative stress in neocortical neurons. *J. Neurochem.* **2007**, *101*, 1316–1326. [CrossRef] [PubMed]
21. Roberts, M.D.; Holland, A.M.; Kephart, W.C.; Mobley, C.B.; Mumford, P.W.; Lowery, R.P.; Fox, C.D.; McCloskey, A.E.; Shake, J.J.; Mesquita, P.; et al. A putative low-carbohydrate ketogenic diet elicits mild nutritional ketosis but does not impair the acute or chronic hypertrophic responses to resistance exercise in rodents. *J. Appl. Physiol.* **2016**, *120*, 1173–1185. [CrossRef] [PubMed]
22. Reagan-Shaw, S.; Nihal, M.; Ahmad, N. Dose translation from animal to human studies revisited. *FASEB J.* **2008**, *22*, 659–661. [CrossRef] [PubMed]
23. Hamm, R.J.; Pike, B.R.; O'Dell, D.M.; Lyeth, B.G.; Jenkins, L.W. The rotarod test: An evaluation of its effectiveness in assessing motor deficits following traumatic brain injury. *J. Neurotrauma* **1994**, *11*, 187–196. [CrossRef] [PubMed]
24. Holland, A.M.; Kephart, W.C.; Mumford, P.W.; Mobley, C.B.; Lowery, R.P.; Shake, J.J.; Patel, R.K.; Healy, J.C.; McCullough, D.J.; Kluess, H.A.; et al. Effects of a ketogenic diet on adipose tissue, liver, and serum biomarkers in sedentary rats and rats that exercised via resisted voluntary wheel running. *Am. J. Physiol. Regul. Integr. Comp. Physiol.* **2016**, *311*, R337–351. [CrossRef] [PubMed]
25. Ghosh, R.; Gilda, J.E.; Gomes, A.V. The necessity of and strategies for improving confidence in the accuracy of western blots. *Expert Rev. Proteomics* **2014**, *11*, 549–560. [CrossRef] [PubMed]
26. Thacker, J.S.; Yeung, D.H.; Staines, W.R.; Mielke, J.G. Total protein or high-abundance protein: Which offers the best loading control for western blotting? *Anal. Biochem.* **2016**, *496*, 76–78. [CrossRef] [PubMed]
27. Gilda, J.E.; Gomes, A.V. Stain-free total protein staining is a superior loading control to beta-actin for western blots. *Anal. Biochem.* **2013**, *440*, 186–188. [CrossRef] [PubMed]
28. Kavazis, A.N.; Smuder, A.J.; Min, K.; Tümer, N.; Powers, S.K. Short-term exercise training protects against doxorubicin-induced cardiac mitochondrial damage independent of HSP72. *Am. J. Physiol. Heart. Circ. Physiol.* **2010**, *299*, H1515–H1524. [CrossRef] [PubMed]
29. Mowry, A.V.; Kavazis, A.N.; Sirman, A.E.; Potts, W.K.; Hood, W.R. Reproduction does not adversely affect liver mitochondrial respiratory function but results in lipid peroxidation and increased antioxidants in house mice. *PLoS ONE* **2016**, *11*, e0160883. [CrossRef] [PubMed]
30. Messer, J.I.; Jackman, M.R.; Willis, W.T. Pyruvate and citric acid cycle carbon requirements in isolated skeletal muscle mitochondria. *Am. J. Physiol. Cell Physiol.* **2004**, *286*, C565–C572. [CrossRef] [PubMed]
31. Kurz, L.C.; Shah, S.; Frieden, C.; Nakra, T.; Stein, R.E.; Drysdale, G.R.; Evans, C.T.; Srere, P.A. Catalytic strategy of citrate synthase: Subunit interactions revealed as a consequence of a single amino acid change in the oxaloacetate binding site. *Biochemistry* **1995**, *34*, 13278–13288. [CrossRef] [PubMed]
32. Bielohuby, M.; Menhofer, D.; Kirchner, H.; Stoehr, B.J.; Muller, T.D.; Stock, P.; Hempel, M.; Stemmer, K.; Pfluger, P.T.; Kienzle, E.; et al. Induction of ketosis in rats fed low-carbohydrate, high-fat diets depends on the relative abundance of dietary fat and protein. *Am. J. Physiol. Endocrinol. Metab.* **2011**, *300*, E65–E76. [CrossRef] [PubMed]
33. Frommelt, L.; Bielohuby, M.; Menhofer, D.; Stoehr, B.J.; Bidlingmaier, M.; Kienzle, E. Effects of low carbohydrate diets on energy and nitrogen balance and body composition in rats depend on dietary protein-to-energy ratio. *Nutrition* **2014**, *30*, 863–868. [CrossRef] [PubMed]
34. Morens, C.; Keijzer, M.; de Vries, K.; Scheurink, A.; van Dijk, G. Effects of high-fat diets with different carbohydrate-to-protein ratios on energy homeostasis in rats with impaired brain melanocortin receptor activity. *Am. J. Physiol. Regul. Integr. Comp. Physiol.* **2005**, *289*, R156–R163. [CrossRef] [PubMed]

35. Hall, K.D.; Chen, K.Y.; Guo, J.; Lam, Y.Y.; Leibel, R.L.; Mayer, L.E.; Reitman, M.L.; Rosenbaum, M.; Smith, S.R.; Walsh, B.T.; et al. Energy expenditure and body composition changes after an isocaloric ketogenic diet in overweight and obese men. *Am. J. Clin. Nutr.* **2016**, *104*, 324–333. [CrossRef] [PubMed]
36. Srivastava, S.; Kashiwaya, Y.; King, M.T.; Baxa, U.; Tam, J.; Niu, G.; Chen, X.; Clarke, K.; Veech, R.L. Mitochondrial biogenesis and increased uncoupling protein 1 in brown adipose tissue of mice fed a ketone ester diet. *FASEB J.* **2012**, *26*, 2351–2362. [CrossRef] [PubMed]
37. Kesl, S.L.; Poff, A.M.; Ward, N.P.; Fiorelli, T.N.; Ari, C.; Van Putten, A.J.; Sherwood, J.W.; Arnold, P.; D'Agostino, D.P. Effects of exogenous ketone supplementation on blood ketone, glucose, triglyceride, and lipoprotein levels in sprague-dawley rats. *Nutr. Metab. (Lond.)* **2016**, *13*, 9. [CrossRef] [PubMed]
38. Shimazu, T.; Hirschey, M.D.; Newman, J.; He, W.; Shirakawa, K.; Le Moan, N.; Grueter, C.A.; Lim, H.; Saunders, L.R.; Stevens, R.D.; et al. Suppression of oxidative stress by beta-hydroxybutyrate, an endogenous histone deacetylase inhibitor. *Science* **2013**, *339*, 211–214. [CrossRef] [PubMed]
39. Dushay, J.; Chui, P.C.; Gopalakrishnan, G.S.; Varela-Rey, M.; Crawley, M.; Fisher, F.M.; Badman, M.K.; Martinez-Chantar, M.L.; Maratos-Flier, E. Increased fibroblast growth factor 21 in obesity and nonalcoholic fatty liver disease. *Gastroenterology* **2010**, *139*, 456–463. [CrossRef] [PubMed]
40. Tendler, D.; Lin, S.; Yancy, W.S., Jr.; Mavropoulos, J.; Sylvestre, P.; Rockey, D.C.; Westman, E.C. The effect of a low-carbohydrate, ketogenic diet on nonalcoholic fatty liver disease: A pilot study. *Dig. Dis. Sci.* **2007**, *52*, 589–593. [CrossRef] [PubMed]
41. Reuter, S.; Gupta, S.C.; Chaturvedi, M.M.; Aggarwal, B.B. Oxidative stress, inflammation, and cancer: How are they linked? *Free Radic. Biol. Med.* **2010**, *49*, 1603–1616. [CrossRef] [PubMed]
42. Larsen, S.; Nielsen, J.; Hansen, C.N.; Nielsen, L.B.; Wibrand, F.; Stride, N.; Schroder, H.D.; Boushel, R.; Helge, J.W.; Dela, F.; et al. Biomarkers of mitochondrial content in skeletal muscle of healthy young human subjects. *J. Physiol.* **2012**, *590*, 3349–3360. [CrossRef] [PubMed]
43. Hughes, S.D.; Kanabus, M.; Anderson, G.; Hargreaves, I.P.; Rutherford, T.; O'Donnell, M.; Cross, J.H.; Rahman, S.; Eaton, S.; Heales, S.J. The ketogenic diet component decanoic acid increases mitochondrial citrate synthase and complex i activity in neuronal cells. *J. Neurochem.* **2014**, *129*, 426–433. [CrossRef] [PubMed]
44. Srivastava, S.; Baxa, U.; Niu, G.; Chen, X.; Veech, R.L. A ketogenic diet increases brown adipose tissue mitochondrial proteins and ucp1 levels in mice. *IUBMB Life* **2013**, *65*, 58–66. [CrossRef] [PubMed]
45. Lee, H.Y.; Choi, C.S.; Birkenfeld, A.L.; Alves, T.C.; Jornayvaz, F.R.; Jurczak, M.J.; Zhang, D.; Woo, D.K.; Shadel, G.S.; Ladiges, W.; et al. Targeted expression of catalase to mitochondria prevents age-associated reductions in mitochondrial function and insulin resistance. *Cell. Metabolism* **2010**, *12*, 668–674. [CrossRef] [PubMed]
46. Anderson, E.J.; Lustig, M.E.; Boyle, K.E.; Woodlief, T.L.; Kane, D.A.; Lin, C.T.; Price, J.W., 3rd; Kang, L.; Rabinovitch, P.S.; Szeto, H.H.; et al. Mitochondrial H_2O_2 emission and cellular redox state link excess fat intake to insulin resistance in both rodents and humans. *J. Clin. Investig.* **2009**, *119*, 573–581. [CrossRef] [PubMed]
47. Sakellariou, G.K.; Pearson, T.; Lightfoot, A.P.; Nye, G.A.; Wells, N.; Giakoumaki, I.I.; Vasilaki, A.; Griffiths, R.D.; Jackson, M.J.; McArdle, A. Mitochondrial ros regulate oxidative damage and mitophagy but not age-related muscle fiber atrophy. *Sci. Rep.* **2016**, *6*, 33944. [CrossRef] [PubMed]
48. Lecker, S.H.; Jagoe, R.T.; Gilbert, A.; Gomes, M.; Baracos, V.; Bailey, J.; Price, S.R.; Mitch, W.E.; Goldberg, A.L. Multiple types of skeletal muscle atrophy involve a common program of changes in gene expression. *Faseb. J.* **2004**, *18*, 39–51. [CrossRef] [PubMed]
49. Sparks, L.M.; Xie, H.; Koza, R.A.; Mynatt, R.; Hulver, M.W.; Bray, G.A.; Smith, S.R. A high-fat diet coordinately downregulates genes required for mitochondrial oxidative phosphorylation in skeletal muscle. *Diabetes* **2005**, *54*, 1926–1933. [CrossRef] [PubMed]
50. Iossa, S.; Lionetti, L.; Mollica, M.P.; Crescenzo, R.; Botta, M.; Barletta, A.; Liverini, G. Effect of high-fat feeding on metabolic efficiency and mitochondrial oxidative capacity in adult rats. *Br. J. Nutr.* **2003**, *90*, 953–960. [CrossRef] [PubMed]
51. Fernandez-Checa, J.C.; Garcia-Ruiz, C.; Ookhtens, M.; Kaplowitz, N. Impaired uptake of glutathione by hepatic mitochondria from chronic ethanol-fed rats. Tracer kinetic studies in vitro and in vivo and susceptibility to oxidant stress. *J. Clin. Investig.* **1991**, *87*, 397–405. [CrossRef] [PubMed]

52. Wilkins, H.M.; Kirchhof, D.; Manning, E.; Joseph, J.W.; Linseman, D.A. Mitochondrial glutathione transport is a key determinant of neuronal susceptibility to oxidative and nitrosative stress. *J. Biol. Chem.* **2013**, *288*, 5091–5101. [CrossRef] [PubMed]

53. Volek, J.S.; Freidenreich, D.J.; Saenz, C.; Kunces, L.J.; Creighton, B.C.; Bartley, J.M.; Davitt, P.M.; Munoz, C.X.; Anderson, J.M.; Maresh, C.M.; et al. Metabolic characteristics of keto-adapted ultra-endurance runners. *Metabolism* **2016**, *65*, 100–110. [CrossRef] [PubMed]

Subjective Satiety Following Meals Incorporating Rice, Pasta and Potato

Zhuoshi Zhang [1], Bernard J. Venn [1], John Monro [2] and Suman Mishra [2,*]

[1] Department of Human Nutrition, University of Otago, P.O. Box 56, Dunedin 9054, New Zealand; zhuoshi.zhang@gmail.com (Z.Z.); bernard.venn@otago.ac.nz (B.J.V.)

[2] New Zealand Institute for Plant & Food Research, Private Bag 11600, Palmerston North 4442, New Zealand; John.Monro@plantandfood.co.nz

* Correspondence: Suman.Mishra@plantandfood.co.nz

Abstract: The satiating capacity of carbohydrate staples eaten alone is dependent upon the energy density of the food but relative satiety when starchy staples are incorporated into mixed meals is uncertain. Our aim was to assess the satiating effects of three carbohydrate staples; jasmine rice, penne pasta, and Agria potato, each consumed within a standard mixed meal. Cooked portions of each staple containing 45 g carbohydrate were combined with 200 g of meat sauce and 200 g of mixed vegetables in three mixed meals. The quantities of staple providing 45 g carbohydrate were: Rice, 142 g; pasta, 138 g and potato 337 g. Participants (n = 14) consumed each of the mixed meals in random order on separate days. Satiety was assessed with using visual analogue scales at baseline and for 3 h post meal. In an area-under-the-curve comparison, participants felt less hungry (mean (SD)) following potato 263 (230) than following rice 374 (237) or pasta 444 (254) mm·min, and felt fuller, more satisfied, and wanted to eat less following the potato compared with the rice and pasta meals (p for all <0.01). The superior satiating effect of potato compared with rice and pasta in a mixed meal was consistent with its lower energy density.

Keywords: carbohydrate; satiety; mixed meal; potato; pasta; rice

---

1. Introduction

The World Health Organization estimates that more than half of the world's adults are overweight or obese and warns of dramatic rises in overweight and obesity in low- and middle-income countries [1]. Overweight and obesity statuses are multifactorial in aetiology with such factors as the food environment, decreased physical activity, inadequate sleep and medication being involved [2,3]. Highly palatable foods that are hard to resist eating are said to be 'hyperpalatable' and are characterized as being inexpensive, highly caloric, fat-laden, potentially addictive and a major contributor to chronic weight gain [4,5]. The involvement of high calorie foods as a contributing factor to overweight and obesity has some credibility as food energy density has been associated with body weight change [6]. A strategy used to reduce dietary energy density has been to add pureed (hidden) vegetables into meals, resulting in a reduction in energy intake [7]. However, the effectiveness of adding fruit and vegetables into diets as a means of reducing overall dietary energy density is questionable as a meta-analysis of the body of literature indicated no long-term effect on weight loss [8]. This may be due to foods such as non-starchy vegetables having a low impact on feelings of satiety when eaten in typical amounts [9]. The authors of the meta-analysis concluded that increasing the fruit and vegetable intake of a diet is unlikely to be a successful weight control strategy because people tend not to decrease their overall dietary energy intake, suggesting that mechanisms underlying participant perceptions of hunger and satiety need to be better understood [8].

At a population level, low energy dense diets of good nutritional quality in Irish children and teenagers have been characterized as having higher intakes of fruits, vegetables, grains, rice, pasta and potato (boiled, baked, mashed); and lower intakes of carbonated beverages and chipped, fried and roasted potatoes [10]. The consumption of low energy dense foods must be accompanied with a concomitant reduction in the intake of high energy dense foods in order for an effect on body weight to be observed [8]. Indeed, the energy density of diets, characterized by a combination of lower fat and higher fruit and vegetable intake, have been associated with long-term weight loss [11]. In an ad libitum dietary intervention in which fat was replaced with either starch- or sugar-rich foods, spontaneous weight loss was achieved with the starchy diet over 2 weeks with the authors suggesting that the starch-based diet was more satiating than the higher fat or sugar diets [12]. Satiety is an important aspect to consider when changing the energy density of meals. When foods were consumed in servings containing 1000 kJ, satiety was inversely related to the energy density of the food, with a strong positive correlation found between the satiety index of food and the serving weight ($r = 0.66$, $p < 0.001$) [13]. The least satiating foods were energy-dense snacks, confectionary and high-fat bakery products; among the starchy foods, white rice and pasta had satiety indices 1.19 and 1.38 times higher than white bread, respectively, with potato having a satiety index over three times (3.23) that of white bread [13].

This evidence is indicative that potato may be of research interest in relation to satiety. In a comparison of instant mashed potato and barley containing 49.5 g and 46.6 g carbohydrate, respectively, there was no difference in satiety between foods although half of the 10 test participants could not finish all of the food [14]. However, people seldom eat single foods so the incorporation of starchy foods into test meals may have more practical relevance. In one such study, 12 participants consumed breakfast meals that included 50–52 g available carbohydrate in the form of baked potato, instant potato, brown rice, white bread and pasta [15]. There was no difference in area-under-the-curve (AUC) hunger or fullness ratings among the meals, with a possible explanation being that a cup of water of variable volume accompanied the food such that the overall water content of the meals plus drink was standardized to 400 mL [15]. This would have evened out differences in energy density among the meals and may have obscured the previously observed effect of energy density on satiety [13]. Therefore, although previous studies are suggestive of a differential effect of starchy foods on satiety, the data are inconsistent, possibly as a consequence of study design. We hypothesized that preserving differences in energy density among meals would maintain differences in feelings of satiety.

Thus, we provided cooked meals for lunch, a usual time for such food to be served, accompanied with a fixed volume of water to drink in order to preserve differences in energy density among meals. Our aims were to assess, in a realistic and normal lunchtime setting, the immediate effect on satiety following meals containing the starchy staple foods; rice, pasta and potato, as part of a mixed meal.

2. Materials and Methods

2.1. Experimental Design

A randomized crossover design was used. On three different days, participants consumed a lunchtime meal comprising minced beef in a Bolognese sauce, mixed vegetables, and a serving of either whole boiled potato, white rice or penne pasta. The order in which participants received the meals was randomized and there was a minimum two-day washout between meals. Participants were asked to keep breakfast consistent on each of the three test days, to avoid consuming any food between breakfast and lunch, and to avoid any food intake for three hours after finishing the test meal, the period during which satiety was measured.

2.2. Recruitment

Volunteers were recruited using a flyer that briefly described the study. In advance of the study each respondent was presented with an information sheet and an informed consent form.

Fourteen healthy volunteers (nine females and five males) were recruited using the following inclusion/exclusion criteria.

2.3. Inclusion Criteria

Age: Aged between 18 and 70.

Sex: Male or female.

Gastrointestinal function: No history of gastrointestinal dysfunction that could have an impact on appetite in the three hours after consuming the meal.

Health: Healthy as gauged by self-assessment and results on the General Health Questionnaire.

Activity: Not involved in prolonged strenuous activity on the day of the trial

Agreement: Subject having given written informed consent to comply with the conditions of the trial.

2.4. Exclusion Criteria

Self-reported intolerance to any of the meal components.

Having a gastrointestinal disorder.

Being involved in a physically demanding work on the day of the trial.

Eligible volunteers who were willing to participate were invited to attend the study at the Plant & Food premises.

Ethical approval was obtained from the New Zealand Health and Disabilities Ethics Committee (HDEC 15/CEN/71). This study was registered on the Australian New Zealand Clinical Trials Registry (www.anzctr.org), registration number ACTRN12615000721505. All participants signed a consent form.

2.5. Test Meal Preparation and Composition

All meals were prepared in advance, frozen as individual meals and reheated before consumption. The carbohydrate foods were cooked and served in equal carbohydrate and calorie portions, and consumed with the standardized meat and vegetable sauce, and 250 mL of water. The meat sauce contained fried beef mince, bacon, onions, chopped celery, thyme, bay leaves and chopped black olives. A commercial pasta sauce (Dairymaid foods, Christchurch, New Zealand) was added and the whole mixture stirred and simmered for 90 min. The mixed vegetables were a commercial frozen mixture consisting of peas, chopped carrots and corn (Heinz Wattie's Ltd., Hastings, New Zealand) and were boiled for 5 min. The pasta (penne; Diamond brand, Wilson Consumer Products, Auckland, New Zealand), rice (Jasmine; SunRice, New South Wales, Australia) and whole potatoes (Agria; Morgan Laurenson Ltd., Palmerston North, New Zealand) were weighed, cooked according to package instructions, and reweighed after cooking. The meals were assembled by placing 200 g vegetables, 200 g Bolognese sauce, and the weight of the rice, penne pasta or whole potato containing 45 g of carbohydrate (Table 1) into aluminum containers which were sealed and frozen until required. Before consumption, the meals were thawed overnight in a refrigerator and heated in a convection oven.

Table 1. Test meal composition.

Meal	Meal Components			Total CHO (g)	Total Energy (kJ)	Energy Density (kJ/g)
	Mince + Sauce (g)	Vegetables (g)	Starchy Staple (g)			
Rice	200	200	142	112	3010	5.55
Pasta	200	200	138	112	3010	5.59
Whole potato	200	200	337	112	3010	4.08

On test days each participant was asked to consume his or her normal breakfast and to refrain from eating between 8 a.m. and 12.00 p.m. (lunch time). Participants were asked to consume a similar breakfast on each of the 3 test days. At lunch time the participants were provided with the test meal and asked to consume it within 20 min.

2.6. Satiety

Satiety was measured using a 100 mm visual analogue scale (VAS) consisting of four questions anchored at either end with the following statements:

- How hungry do you feel? (Not at all hungry–Extremely hungry)
- How full do you feel? (Not at all full–Totally full)
- How strong is your desire to eat? (Not at all strong–Extremely strong)
- How much food do you think you can eat? (Nothing at all–A large amount)

These scales have been recommended in a methodological review of the evaluation of foods for their validity and reliability [16]. The length of the scale was measured from the start to the point that was marked. Participants were asked to rate their hunger/appetite using the VAS immediately before lunch, immediately after lunch and at 1, 2 and 3 h after lunch. The VAS rating for each time was on a separate sheet and participants were instructed not to refer back to ratings of earlier times.

2.7. Sample Size Calculation

In a study on the validity of appetite visual analogue scales, a Table was presented in which sample sizes were given in relation to detectable differences and power [17]. Using this information, 18 subjects would be sufficient to detect a 10% difference in satiety, with 80% power at the 0.05 significance level for a paired design.

2.8. Statistical Analysis

All appetite ratings were recorded in a spreadsheet using the Microsoft Excel for Macintosh (Microsoft® Excel®. Version 15.31. Microsoft Corporation 2017, Redmond, WA, USA). Area under the curve (AUC) was calculated. Results were expressed as means with standard deviation. Random effects regression analysis was used to test for between-treatment differences in AUC satiety responses, with participant id as a random effect and adjusted for randomized order and baseline satiety. Microsoft Stata/MP 14.0 for Macintosh (Stata Corporation, College Station, TX, USA) was used for the regression analysis. p-value of less than 0.05 was set as statistical significance in all analyses.

3. Results

Fourteen adults completed the intervention in a balanced three-arm crossover. The mean (SD) age of the participants was 40.9 (14.6) years with a range of 28–70 years. Eleven participants were of European- and 3 of Asian-descent. The flow of participants through the study is given in Figure 1.

The baseline scores to the satiety questions are given in Table 2. People were randomized to the order in which they received the meals.

At baseline, there was no difference in mean scores of hunger and fullness before eating. There was a lesser desire to eat and people indicated they could eat less on the potato and rice days compared with the pasta day. The main outcomes arising from the visual analogue scale data are given in Table 3. The outcomes are total postprandial AUC over three hours; the difference (mm) between the pre- and post-meal scores (0–15 min); and a rate of return to hunger (15–180 min).

Table 2. Mean (SD) baseline satiety scores of 14 people.

Satiety Measure (mm) *	Pasta	Potato	Rice
Hunger	77.4 (21.9)	77.1 (10.2)	72.9 (19.8)
Fullness	18.9 (16.9)	18.7 (12.1)	19.6 (14.9)
Desire	87.9 (11.1) ^{a}	77.1 (12.5) ^{b}	77.3 (19.1) ^{b}
Quantity	81.9 (11.4) ^{a}	68.9 (11.2) ^{b}	68.6 (19.8) ^{b}

Different superscript letters within a row signify statistically significant. differences. * A high score indicates hunger; fullness, desire to eat; and ability to eat a large quantity.

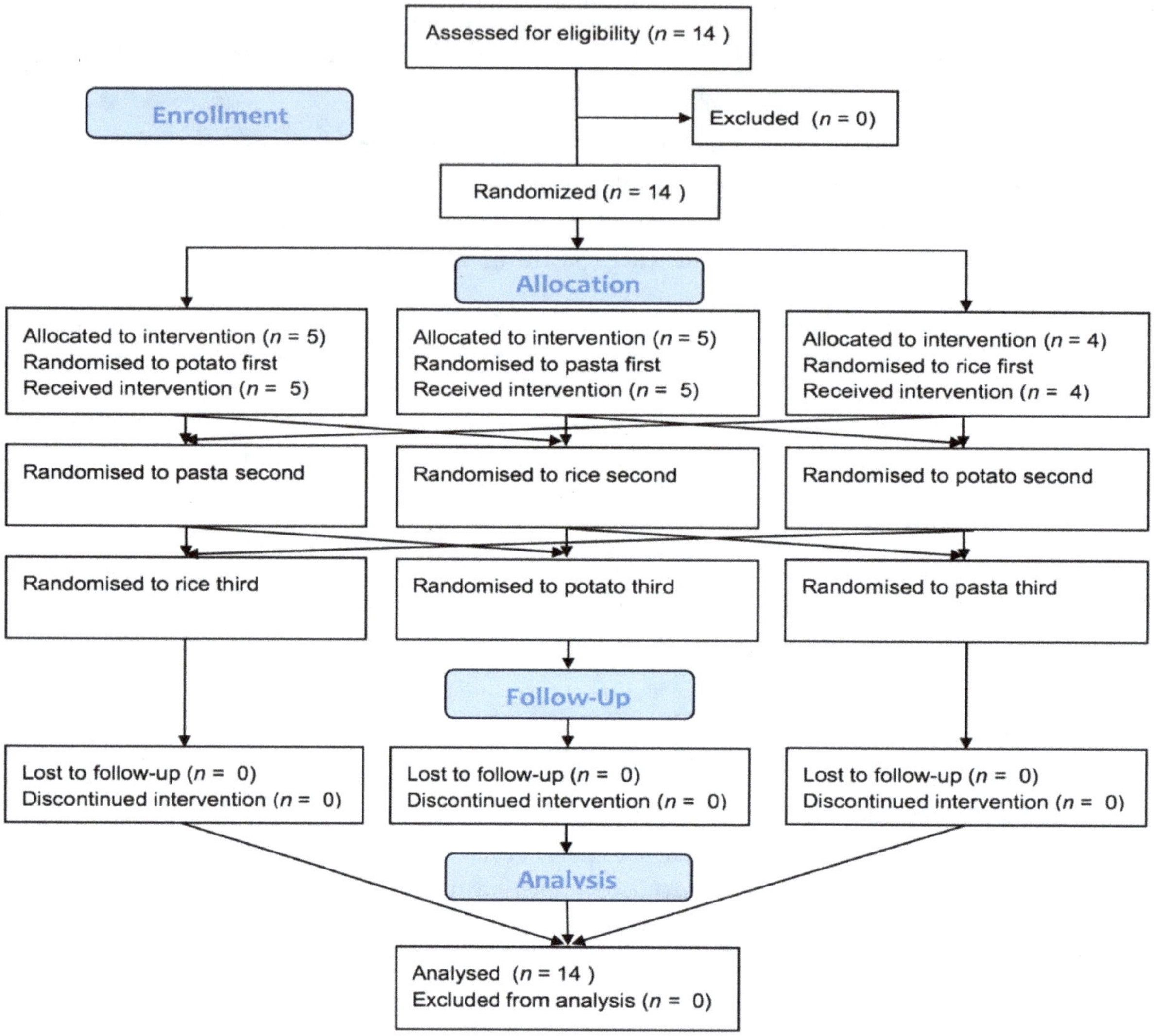

Figure 1. CONSORT diagram showing the flow of participants through the study.

Table 3. Mean visual analogue scale (VAS) outcomes of 14 people in response to four satiety questions.

Satiety Measure 1	Mean (SD)			Mean Difference (95% Confidence Interval) Comparing between Meals Given in the Column Headings above		
	Pasta	Potato	Rice	Pasta vs. Potato	Pasta vs. Rice	Rice vs. Potato
Hunger AUC	448 (254)	264 (230)	376 (236)	184 (105, 263) **$p < 0.001$**	−72 (−151, 8) $p = 0.076$	112 (33, 191) **$p = 0.006$**
Fullness AUC	964 (468)	1120 (345)	954 (423)	−155 (−335, 24) $p = 0.090$	−10 (−189, 170) $p = 0.914$	−165 (−344, 14.3) $p = 0.071$
Desire AUC	427 (220)	210 (190)	361 (218)	217 (147, 287) **$p < 0.001$**	−66 (−136, 4) $p = 0.064$	151 (87, 214) **$p < 0.001$**
Quantity AUC	436 (231)	289 (257)	389 (221)	148 (65, 230) **$p < 0.001$**	−47 (−130, 36) $p = 0.265$	100 (30, 171) **$p = 0.005$**
Change (mm) in VAS scores from commencement of eating to finishing the meal						
Hunger drop 2	76 (18)	72 (15)	71 (16)	3.6 (−2.5, 9.8) $p = 0.249$	−4.6 (−10.9, 1.6) $p = 0.146$	−1.0 (−7.2, 5.2) $p = 0.755$
Fullness rise 2	70.6 (18.3)	75.7 (13.3)	71.4 (19.7)	−5.1 (−8.0, −2.2) **$p = 0.001$**	0.7 (−2.1, 3.7) $p = 0.617$	−4.3 (−7.2, −1.4) **$p = 0.004$**
Desire drop	87.9 (11.1)	77.1 (12.5)	77.3 (19.1)	10.9 (2.3, 19.4) **$p = 0.013$**	−10.6 (−19.2, −2.1) **$p = 0.015$**	0.2 (−8.4, 8.8) $p = 0.961$
Quantity drop	81.9 (11.4)	68.9 (11.2)	68.6 (19.8)	13.0 (5.2, 20.8) **$p = 0.001$**	−13.4 (−21.2, −5.5) **$p = 0.001$**	−0.4 (−8.1, 7.5) $p = 0.929$
Rate of return of VAS scores (mm/h) from eating cessation to 3 h post-baseline						
Hunger return 3	9.8 (6.5)	6.5 (9.0)	10.6 (9.3)	3.2 (−0.1, 6.6) $p = 0.061$	0.9 (−2.5, 4.3) $p = 0.609$	4.1 (0.7, 7.5) **$p = 0.017$**
Fullness return	−10.6 (7.0)	−6.3 (8.5)	−12.2 (9.4)	−4.2 (−8.3, −0.2) **$p = 0.040$**	−1.6 (−5.7, 2.4) $p = 0.425$	−5.9 (−9.9, −1.8) **$p = 0.004$**
Desire return	9.7 (6.1)	5.7 (9.6)	10.2 (8.8)	4.0 (−1.1, 9.1) $p = 0.121$	0.5 (−4.6, 5.6) $p = 0.850$	4.5 (−0.2, 9.2) $p = 0.060$
Quantity return	8.2 (3.9)	3.5 (3.6)	8.6 (6.2)	4.7 (1.5, 7.9) **$p = 0.004$**	0.4 (-2.8, 3.6) $p = 0.803$	5.1 (2.3, 7.9) **$p < 0.001$**

1 AUC Area-Under-the-Curve (cm·min); 2 drop/rise = change in score (mm) from baseline to immediately after finishing the meal; 3 return from a satiated to a less satiated condition over time (mm/h). A positive difference in hunger, desire and quantity represent being hungrier, having greater desire and a feeling of being able to eat more. A negative difference in fullness represents feeling less full. Bolded p-values indicate differences between treatments.

The plots of visual analogue scale data over time are shown in Figure 2.

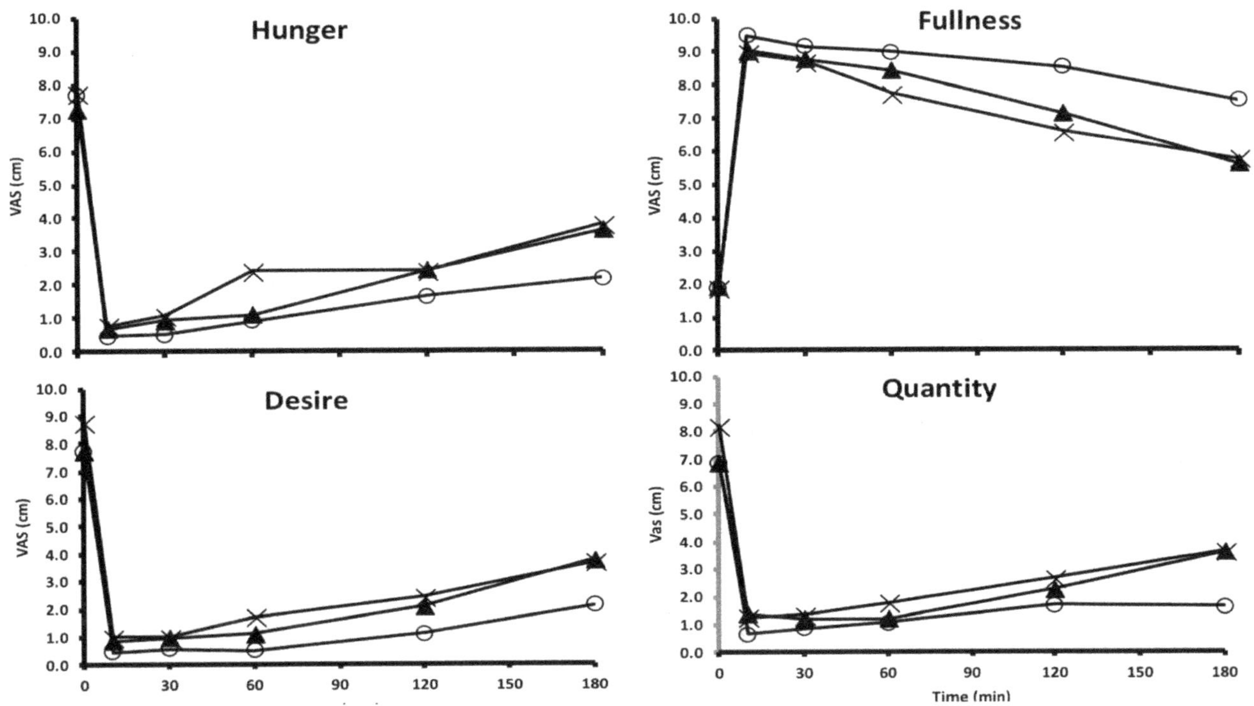

Figure 2. Plots of visual analogue scales (VAS) in response to four questions over time starting at baseline (t = 0) and following the consumption of pasta (×), potato (○) and rice (▲) meals. Data were analyzed by comparing the area-under-the-curve (AUC) among the meals for each of the questions. Interpretation of the data: How hungry do you feel? (Small AUC—Not at all hungry; Large AUC—Extremely hungry). How full do you feel? (Small AUC—Not at all full; Large AUC—Totally full). How strong is your desire to eat? (Small AUC—Not at all strong; Large AUC—Extremely strong). How much do you think you can eat? (Small AUC—Nothing at all; Large AUC—A large amount).

4. Discussion

The study results are indicative that the rice and the pasta meals were equally satiating, whilst participants felt fuller and more satisfied after eating the potato meals compared with the rice and the pasta meals. In this experiment, the comparison among different carbohydrate foods was standardized to an equal carbohydrate content. Similar results have been found when testing foods on an isoenergetic basis in which boiled potatoes eaten alone were more satiating than either rice or pasta eaten alone [13]. The data from the present study in a meal setting, are therefore consistent with differences in satiety found when these foods are eaten alone.

Our findings may be compared with a study in which investigators tested the effects on satiety of consuming meals containing various starchy staples [15]. In that study, desire to eat was lower following baked potato compared with pasta but contrary to our findings, hunger and fullness AUC did not differ among meals containing instant potato, baked potato, brown rice, pasta and white bread [15]. A difference between study designs was that Geleibter et al. standardized the total water content of the meals (food plus water provided as a beverage) whereas we only standardized the volume of water given as an accompanying beverage. Thus, the meals and beverages that Geleibter et al provided presumably tended to be equi-volumetric [15]. This may have obscured a difference in satiety among the meals given that food volume is a determinant of satiety [18]. This is suggestive that if starchy foods are to be exchanged, keeping accompanying drink volume constant may be important when assessing effects on satiety.

With comparable protein, fat, dietary fiber and calorie content, possible explanations for potato being more satiating than rice or pasta are differences in the energy density of the foods. Potatoes have a higher water content and lower energy density than rice or pasta [19]. Therefore, a larger volume of potatoes than rice and pasta needed to be consumed when served in equal carbohydrate portions. A large food volume increases gastric distension and stimulates postprandial satiety [20–22]. When eaten ad libitum, potato, rice and pasta consumed with a pork steak resulted in satiating effects that were not different among the meals despite the total carbohydrate and calorie intake after eating potatoes being significantly less than after eating rice and pasta meals [23]. In a randomized crossover study involving 11 to 13-year-old children, 30–40% less calories ($p < 0.0001$) were consumed after eating ad libitum meals containing boiled and mashed potatoes compared with comparable pasta and rice meals [24]. These observations may have practical and clinical relevance because the amount of carbohydrate consumed directly impacts postprandial glycaemia. If satiety can be maintained whilst consuming a smaller portion of potato compared to other starchy staples, this may offset the potential for a larger glycemic excursion due to potato having a high glycemic index (GI) relative to rice and pasta [25]. A consequence of a smaller portion reduces not only the glycemic load (GI x grams available carbohydrate) but also the energy content of the meal. As suggested, potatoes could be a suitable food option to reduce energy intake whilst maintaining satiety and mitigating postprandial glycaemia as less carbohydrate is consumed [26]. This effect has been observed among an older group consuming an equivalent amount of carbohydrate either as a glucose beverage, instant potato or barley [14]. All 10 participants were able to ingest the beverage but four and five of the participants were unable to eat all of the potato and barley, respectively [14]. Despite the differences in carbohydrate intake of the subset who could not finish their food, as a group mean satiety was greater after potato than after the glucose beverage.

It is interesting to note that the satiating effect of the carbohydrate foods was not clearly related to GI, even though it has been proposed that GI, as an indicator of sustained carbohydrate digestion, is a strong determinant of satiety [27,28]. Potato and jasmine rice are generally considered to be of moderate to high GI, and pasta of low GI, yet the rice and pasta meals did not differ in satiation and the potato meal was more satiating than the pasta meal. The results suggest that the effect of food volume on the proportion of a meal released from the stomach per unit time may have been sufficient to override the effects of differences in digestibility of the carbohydrates. Indeed, the rate of gastric emptying has been found to be affected by food volume and by energy density [29]. There is also a relationship between glycaemia and gastrointestinal motor control indicative that hyperglycemia slows gastric emptying [30]. More research in which blood glucose responses and gastric emptying are measured in conjunction with satiety would be helpful in interpreting the results of the present study.

It has also been found that although the glycemic response to mashed potato was greater compared with rice and pasta when consumed as part of a meal containing vegetables and salmon, the glycemic responses to all three meals were not different [31]. If the same effect has occurred in the present study due to the presence of meat sauce and vegetables, the effects of differences in glycemic response on satiety may have been eliminated leaving food volume as a dominant influence on satiety.

The healthfulness of carbohydrates in the human diet has been examined from a migratory perspective in which carbohydrate-rich staple foods consumed in the country of birth have been replaced by an increased intake of refined carbohydrate, meat and dairy in the adopted country contributing to a higher risk of non-communicable disease [32]. The rice and pasta used in our study were refined and perhaps equivalent whole-grain products would have induced different satiety responses. In previous work there was no difference in satiety found between white and brown rice; brown pasta appeared to be more satiating than white pasta; and boiled potatoes were the most satiating of all of the foods tested [13]. Plant-based starchy and non-starchy foods in general have lower energy density than animal derived foods and foods that are highly possessed with sugar and fat [19]. In practice, a plant-based diet in which starchy foods were recommended to be eaten ad libitum to satiation resulted in a greater reduction in body mass index compared with a usual care control group [33]. Thus, there is evidence to suggest that low energy-dense starchy foods are healthful components of a diet even when eaten ad libitum to satiation.

A potential limitation to our work was the sample size. The study had been powered to detect a difference in satiety among meals and it was sufficient for this purpose. Also, there were no differences at baseline in VAS responses to the questions "How hungry do you feel?" and "How full do you feel?". However, the data were indicative that people had a greater desire to eat; and could eat a larger quantity before the pasta meal compared with the rice and potato meals. We are unsure why this difference occurred as the order in which participants received the meals was randomized and we would not have expected baseline differences to occur. It is unclear whether this is a sample size issue, a chance finding, or whether anticipatory effects could have caused such an outcome. VAS methodology is widely used for assessing satiety [16] but subsequent energy consumption and satiety hormone responses could be informative as objective measurements in future research. A strength of this study was that all test meals were realistic in composition. It provides evidence that reflects real life when meat and vegetables are consumed in combination with starchy staples. A limitation to generalization of this study was that it was not conducted in people who are overweight or obese, a demographic who may have an impaired satiety response [34]. Similar studies undertaken in groups of people who are overweight or obese could provide evidence on which to base dietary recommendations suitable for weight loss.

5. Conclusions

In summary, on an equal carbohydrate basis, potato meals were more satiating than rice or pasta meals. If serving sizes of potato could be reduced such that the satiating properties match that of larger servings of rice or pasta, there would be a caloric intake saving and the potential to bring the glycemic response of high GI potato down to the glycemic responses of the rice and pasta meals, making potatoes an excellent choice of a low energy-dense food with the capacity to satiate.

Author Contributions: Conceptualization, Z.Z. and B.J.V.; Methodology, J.M. and S.M.; Formal Analysis, B.J.V.; Investigation, S.M., J.M., Z.Z. and B.J.V.; Resources, J.M. and S.M.; Data Curation, S.M. and J.M.; Writing-Original Draft Preparation, B.J.V., J.M. and Z.Z.; Writing-Review & Editing, J.M., Z.Z., S.M. and B.J.V.; Supervision, J.M. and B.J.V.; Project Administration, J.M. and S.M.; Funding Acquisition, J.M.

References

1. World Health Organization. Available online: http://www.who.int/topics/obesity/en/ (accessed on 24 August 2018).
2. Wright, S.M.; Aronne, L.J. Causes of obesity. *Abdom. Imaging* **2012**, *37*, 730–732. [CrossRef] [PubMed]
3. Wilding, P.H. Causes of obesity. *Pr. Diabetes Int.* **2001**, *18*, 288–292. [CrossRef]
4. Lerma-Cabrera, J.M.; Carvajal, F.; Lopez-Legarrea, P. Food addiction as a new piece of the obesity framework. *Nutr. J.* **2016**, *15*, 5. [CrossRef] [PubMed]
5. Gearhardt, A.N.; Grilo, C.M.; DiLeone, R.J.; Brownell, K.D.; Potenza, M.N. Can food be addictive? Public health and policy implications. *Addiction* **2011**, *106*, 1208–1212. [CrossRef] [PubMed]
6. Stelmach-Mardas, M.; Rodacki, T.; Dobrowolska-Iwanek, J.; Brzozowska, A.; Walkowiak, J.; Wojtanowska-Krosniak, A.; Zagrodzki, P.; Bechthold, A.; Mardas, M.; Boeing, H. Link between food energy density and body weight changes in obese adults. *Nutrients* **2016**, *8*, 229. [CrossRef] [PubMed]
7. Blatt, A.D.; Roe, L.S.; Rolls, B.J. Hidden vegetables: An effective strategy to reduce energy intake and increase vegetable intake in adults. *Am. J. Clin. Nutr.* **2011**, *93*, 756–763. [CrossRef] [PubMed]
8. Kaiser, K.A.; Brown, A.W.; Bohan Brown, M.M.; Shikany, J.M.; Mattes, R.D.; Allison, D.B. Increased fruit and vegetable intake has no discernible effect on weight loss: A systematic review and meta-analysis. *Am. J. Clin. Nutr.* **2014**, *100*, 567–576. [CrossRef] [PubMed]
9. Gustafsson, K.; Asp, N.G.; Hagander, B.; Nyman, M. Effects of different vegetables in mixed meals on glucose homeostasis and satiety. *Eur. J. Clin. Nutr.* **1993**, *47*, 192–200. [PubMed]
10. O'Connor, L.; Walton, J.; Flynn, A. Dietary energy density and its association with the nutritional quality of the diet of children and teenagers. *J. Nutr. Sci.* **2013**, *2*, e10. [CrossRef] [PubMed]

11. Flood, A.; Mitchell, N.; Jaeb, M.; Finch, E.A.; Laqua, P.S.; Welsh, E.M.; Hotop, A.; Langer, S.L.; Levy, R.L.; Jeffery, R.W. Energy density and weight change in a long-term weight-loss trial. *Int. J. Behav. Nutr. Phys. Act.* **2009**, *6*, 57. [CrossRef] [PubMed]
12. Marckmann, P.; Raben, A.; Astrup, A. Ad libitum intake of low-fat diets rich in either starchy foods or sucrose: effects on blood lipids, factor VII coagulant activity, and fibrinogen. *Metabolism* **2000**, *49*, 731–735. [CrossRef] [PubMed]
13. Holt, S.H.; Miller, J.C.; Petocz, P.; Farmakalidis, E. A satiety index of common foods. *Eur. J. Clin. Nutr.* **1995**, *49*, 675–690. [PubMed]
14. Kaplan, R.J.; Greenwood, C.E. Influence of dietary carbohydrates and glycaemic response on subjective appetite and food intake in healthy elderly persons. *Int. J. Food Sci. Nutr.* **2002**, *53*, 305–316. [CrossRef] [PubMed]
15. Geliebter, A.; Lee, M.I.; Abdillahi, M.; Jones, J. Satiety following intake of potatoes and other carbohydrate test meals. *Ann. Nutr. Metab.* **2013**, *62*, 37–43. [CrossRef] [PubMed]
16. Blundell, J.; de Graaf, C.; Hulshof, T.; Jebb, S.; Livingstone, B.; Lluch, A.; Mela, D.; Salah, S.; Schuring, E.; van der Knaap, H.; et al. Appetite control: methodological aspects of the evaluation of foods. *Obes. Rev.* **2010**, *11*, 251–270. [CrossRef] [PubMed]
17. Flint, A.; Raben, A.; Blundell, J.E.; Astrup, A. Reproducibility, power and validity of visual analogue scales in assessment of appetite sensations in single test meal studies. *Int. J. Obes. Relat. Metab. Disord.* **2000**, *24*, 38–48. [CrossRef] [PubMed]
18. Rolls, B.J.; Castellanos, V.H.; Halford, J.C.; Kilara, A.; Panyam, D.; Pelkman, C.L.; Smith, G.P.; Thorwart, M.L. Volume of food consumed affects satiety in men. *Am. J. Clin. Nutr.* **1998**, *67*, 1170–1177. [CrossRef] [PubMed]
19. The New Zealand Institute for Plant & Food Research Limited and the Ministry of Health (New Zealand). New Zealand FOODfiles 2016. Available online: https://www.foodcomposition.co.nz/downloads/foodfiles-2016-manual.pdf (accessed on 12 November 2018).
20. Deutsch, J.A.; Young, W.G.; Kalogeris, T.J. The stomach signals satiety. *Science* **1978**, *201*, 165–167. [CrossRef] [PubMed]
21. Geliebter, A. Gastric distension and gastric capacity in relation to food intake in humans. *Physiol. Behav.* **1988**, *44*, 665–668. [CrossRef]
22. Poppitt, S.D.; Prentice, A.M. Energy density and its role in the control of food intake: Evidence from metabolic and community studies. *Appetite* **1996**, *26*, 153–174. [CrossRef] [PubMed]
23. Erdmann, J.; Hebeisen, Y.; Lippl, F.; Wagenpfeil, S.; Schusdziarra, V. Food intake and plasma ghrelin response during potato-, rice- and pasta-rich test meals. *Eur. J. Nutr.* **2007**, *46*, 196–203. [CrossRef] [PubMed]
24. Akilen, R.; Deljoomanesh, N.; Hunschede, S.; Smith, C.E.; Arshad, M.U.; Kubant, R.; Anderson, G.H. The effects of potatoes and other carbohydrate side dishes consumed with meat on food intake, glycemia and satiety response in children. *Nutr. Diabetes* **2016**, *6*, e195. [CrossRef] [PubMed]
25. Atkinson, F.S.; Foster-Powell, K.; Brand-Miller, J.C. International tables of glycemic index and glycemic load values: 2008. *Diabetes Care* **2008**, *31*, 2281–2283. [CrossRef] [PubMed]
26. Anderson, G.H.; Soeandy, C.D.; Smith, C.E. White vegetables: Glycemia and satiety. *Adv. Nutr.* **2013**, *4*, 356S–367S. [CrossRef] [PubMed]
27. Brand-Miller, J.; McMillan-Price, J.; Steinbeck, K.; Caterson, I. Dietary glycemic index: Health implications. *J. Am. Coll. Nutr.* **2009**, *28*, 446S–449S. [CrossRef] [PubMed]
28. Brand-Miller, J.C.; Holt, S.H.; Pawlak, D.B.; McMillan, J. Glycemic index and obesity. *Am. J. Clin. Nutr.* **2002**, *76*, 281S–285S. [CrossRef] [PubMed]
29. Hunt, J.N.; Smith, J.L.; Jiang, C.L. Effect of meal volume and energy density on the gastric emptying of carbohydrates. *Gastroenterology* **1985**, *89*, 1326–1330. [CrossRef]
30. Rayner, C.K.; Samsom, M.; Jones, K.L.; Horowitz, M. Relationships of upper gastrointestinal motor and sensory function with glycemic control. *Diabetes Care* **2001**, *24*, 371–381. [CrossRef] [PubMed]
31. Ballance, S.; Knutsen, S.H.; Fosvold, O.W.; Fernandez, A.S.; Monro, J. Predicting mixed-meal measured glycaemic index in healthy subjects. *Eur. J. Nutr.* **2018**. [CrossRef] [PubMed]
32. Holmboe-Ottesen, G.; Wandel, M. Changes in dietary habits after migration and consequences for health: A focus on South Asians in Europe. *Food Nutr. Res.* **2012**, *56*. [CrossRef] [PubMed]
33. Wright, N.; Wilson, L.; Smith, M.; Duncan, B.; McHugh, P. The BROAD study: A randomised controlled trial using a whole food plant-based diet in the community for obesity, ischaemic heart disease or diabetes. *Nutr. Diabetes* **2017**, *7*, e256. [CrossRef] [PubMed]

6

Type-4 Resistant Starch in Substitution for Available Carbohydrate Reduces Postprandial Glycemic Response and Hunger in Acute, Randomized and Double-Blind

Maria L. Stewart [1,*], Meredith L. Wilcox [2], Marjorie Bell [2], Mary A. Buggia [2] and Kevin C. Maki [2]

1 Global Nutrition R & D, Ingredion Incorporated, 10 Finderne Ave, Bridgewater, NJ 08807, USA
2 Midwest Biomedical Research, Center for Metabolic and Cardiovascular Health, 489 Taft Ave Suite 202, Glen Ellyn, IL 60137, USA; mwilcox@mbclinicalresearch.com (M.L.W.); mbell@mbclinicalresearch.com (M.B.); mbuggia@mbclinicalresearch.com (M.A.B.); kmaki@mbclinicalresearch.com (K.C.M.)
* Correspondence: maria.stewart@ingredion.com

Abstract: Resistant starch (RS) is a type of dietary fiber that has been acknowledged for multiple physiological benefits. Resistant starch type 4 (RS4) is a subcategory of RS that has been more intensively studied as new types of RS4 emerge in the food supply. The primary aim of this randomized, double-blind, controlled study was to characterize the postprandial glucose response in healthy adults after consuming a high fiber scone containing a novel RS4 or a low fiber control scone without RS4. Secondary aims included assessment of postprandial insulin response, postprandial satiety, and gastrointestinal tolerance. The fiber scone significantly reduced postprandial glucose and insulin incremental areas under the curves (43–45% reduction, 35–40% reduction, respectively) and postprandial glucose and insulin maximum concentrations (8–10% and 22% reduction, respectively). The fiber scone significantly reduced hunger and desire to eat during the 180 min following consumption and yielded no gastrointestinal side effects compared with the control scone. The results from this study demonstrate that a ready-to-eat baked-good, such as a scone, can be formulated with RS4 replacing refined wheat flour to yield statistically significant and clinically meaningful reductions in blood glucose and insulin excursions. This is the first study to report increased satiety after short-term RS4 intake, which warrants further investigation in long-term feeding studies.

Keywords: resistant starch type 4; dietary fiber; post-prandial; blood glucose; insulin; capillary glucose; venous glucose; glycemic response; satiety; gastrointestinal tolerance

---

1. Introduction

Dietary fiber encompasses a wide range of non-digestible carbohydrates with multiple physiological benefits, and it is noted as a short-fall nutrient in Western diets [1,2]. One such physiological benefit is improved blood glucose control. Postprandial blood glucose management has been well-documented among viscous fibers, such as oat beta-glucan, due to attenuated glucose absorption in the small intestine [3]. Decreased postprandial blood glucose is also observed when fibers, such as resistant starch (RS), replace available carbohydrate in food formulations [4]. Postprandial blood glucose control has long been recognized as a predictor of diabetes development. More recently, poor postprandial blood glucose control correlated with the presence of coronary heart disease [5], thus demonstrating the value of improved postprandial blood glucose control.

As noted previously, RS can reduce postprandial blood glucose, particularly when replacing refined wheat flour in product formulations [4,6]. The majority of clinical research on RS evaluated the effects of resistant starch type-2, which is a granular, native starch, resistant to digestion, and resistant starch type-3, which is a retrograded starch that resists digestion. Fewer clinical studies have been conducted on resistant starch type-4 (RS4, chemically modified starch that resists digestion by intestinal enzymes). The category of RS4 is diverse, with a range of starch bases and chemical modifications existing in the food supply. These attributes can affect functionality in a food product, and digestibility and fermentability after consumption [7]. Due to these differences, it is critical to evaluate food applications and physiological effects of each, specific type of RS4. Within the category of RS4, the most studied type is phosphated distarch phosphate [8–13]. Fewer studies have been conducted on distarch phosphate [14–16], hydroxypropyl distarch phosphate [17,18] and only one study has been conducted on RS4 that is acid hydrolyzed and heat treated, to date [19].

Among the aforementioned studies, the most frequent, primary outcome was postprandial blood glucose. Additional outcomes of the acute studies included satiety, energy expenditure, and substrate utilization. Long-term studies of RS4 examined its effects on blood glucose, blood lipids, and gut microbiota. The primary aim of the present study was to characterize the postprandial blood glucose response in healthy adults to a novel RS4 (acid hydrolyzed and heat treated maize-based RS) in a ready-to-eat baked good. Secondary aims were to evaluate postprandial insulin response, satiety, and gastrointestinal tolerance. We hypothesized that replacement of digestible carbohydrate from refined wheat flour with RS4 would reduce postprandial blood glucose.

2. Materials and Methods

2.1. Study Design and Study Visits

This double-blind, randomized, controlled study was conducted in accordance with the Declaration of Helsinki (2000). The protocol was reviewed and received ethical approval before initiation of the trial (Aspire IRB, Santee, CA, USA; protocol number MB-1702). All subjects provided informed, written consent before any study procedures were conducted. The subjects attended 3 study visits (visit 1, day 7, screening; visit 2 day 0, treatment 1; visit 3, day 7, treatment 2). Female subjects of child bearing ability attended study visits during the follicular phase of their menstrual cycles. On visit 2, subjects were randomly assigned to one of two treatment sequences. Prior to visit 2, subjects completed a 24-h diet record. Subjects arrived to the study center fasted on the morning of visits 2 and 3. Baseline satiety was assessed 30 min prior to study product consumption, and baseline blood samples were taken 15 min prior to study product consumption. Subjects consumed the study scone and 240 mL of water within 10 min. Subjects were offered an additional 178 mL of water after they consumed the study scone. Blood measurements and satiety assessment were conducted during the 180 min following the onset of scone consumption. Prior to visit 3, the subjects were instructed to replicate their diet, based on the 24-h diet record from visit 2. Further details are provided in Section 2.4.

2.2. Study Subjects

Subjects were recruited from the Boca Raton area in Florida, USA. Subjects were enrolled in the study after meeting inclusion (age 18–74 years, body mass index 18.5–29.99 kg/m^2, general good health, women of child bearing potential had to be willing to commit to a medically approved form of contraception for the duration of the study) and exclusion criteria (fasting capillary glucose $\geq$ 5.55 mmol/L, major trauma or surgical event within 3 months of screening, current or recent history of drug or alcohol abuse, $\geq$4.5 kg weight change in past 2 months prior to screening, uncontrolled hypertension, recent use of antibiotics or signs or symptoms of active infection, extreme dietary habits, recent consumption of foods fortified with and/or containing supplements containing probiotics or who had used medications known to influence carbohydrate metabolism, gastrointestinal motility, satiety, appetite, taste, sense of smell, or weight, women only who are currently pregnant or lactating). Subjects agreed to certain study restrictions such as having no plans to change smoking habits or other nicotine use during the study, abstaining from use of tobacco products during study visits, willingness to maintain body weight and habitual diet throughout trial, attempting to replicate the pre-visit 2 diet during the 24 h pre-testing period before visit 3, abstaining from alcohol consumption, and abstaining from vigorous physical activity for 24 h prior and during test visits.

2.3. Study Foods

The fiber scone contained VERSAFIBE™ 2470 resistant starch (Ingredion Incorporated, Bridgewater, NJ, USA), which was the primary source of fiber in the scone. VERSAFIBE™ 2470 resistant starch is a resistant starch type 4 with 70% dietary fiber (AOAC 2009.01). VERSAFIBE™ 2470 resistant starch is produced from food grade high-amylose maize starch. Digestibility of the high-amylose maize starch is decreased through acid hydrolysis and heat treatment, which results in increased RS4 and total dietary fiber (TDF) in the finished product, VERSAFIBE 2470 resistant starch. Because the ingredient is produced from high-amylose maize starch, the nondigestible carbohydrate (fiber) in VERSAFIBE 2470 resistant starch is RS4. There are no nonstarch polysaccharides in the ingredient.

The fiber scone and control scone were matched for weight, fat, protein, sugar and total carbohydrate (Table 1). The portion size was selected based on typical scones in the United States marketplace. Nutrient composition of the scones was analyzed by Medallion Labs (Minneapolis, MN, USA) using standard methods of analysis (fats AOAC 996.06, protein AOAC 992.15, sugar AOAC 977.20, and dietary fiber AOAC 2009.01). Total carbohydrate was determined through calculation by difference. Energy content was calculated using Atwater factors (9 kcal/g fat, 4 kcal/d protein, 4 kcal/g available carbohydrate). Control scone and fiber scone formulations are available in Supplementary Table S1. The fiber and control scones were identical in appearance. The scones were packaged in identical opaque envelopes with a numeric code for identification. Neither the study subjects nor the investigators knew the identity of the scones. The subjects rated the scones on palatability after consumption.

Table 1. Nutrient composition of study scones.

Per Serving, As-Eaten	Control Scone	Fiber Scone
Weight (g)	83.9	84.1
Calories (kcal)	328	270
Fat (g)	16.0	14.4
Saturated fat (g)	5.0	4.7
Protein (g)	7.1	6.1
Total Carbohydrates (g)	42.8	46.4
Available Carbohydrates (g)	38.8	28.9
Dietary Fiber (g) *	4.0	17.5
Sugars (g)	14.8	14.9

* VERSAFIBE™ 2470 resistant starch provided 16.5 g dietary fiber in the Fiber Scone.

2.4. Measurements

2.4.1. Capillary Glucose

The TRUEtrack™ Blood Glucose Monitoring System and the TRUE METRIX® Blood Glucose Meter (Trividia Health Inc., Fort Lauderdale, FL, USA) were used for determination of capillary glucose at screening (visit 1, day 7) and at test visits 2 and 3 (days 0 and 7). At screening, a single fasting glucose test was performed, and at test visits, the capillary glucose was measured at $t = -15 \pm 2$ min, 15, 30, 45, 60, 90, 120 and 180 min $\pm$ 2 min, where $t = 0$ was the start of study product consumption.

The test-retest % CV for tests on different days was similar for the fasting capillary (9.0%) and venous (10.4%) samples.

2.4.2. Venous Glucose and Insulin

Venous samples were drawn from an indwelling catheter that was placed at least 10 min prior to the first sample collected. The catheter was flushed regularly with normal saline to maintain patency. At visits 2 and 3 (days 0 and 7), venous samples for measurement of plasma glucose and insulin concentrations were collected at $t = -15$ min $\pm$ 2 min and at t = 15, 30, 45, 60, 90, 120 and 180 min $\pm$ 2 min, where t = 0 min was the start of study product consumption. The Cleveland Heart Lab (Cleveland, OH, USA) conducted the plasma glucose and insulin analyses. Glucose was measured using a hexokinase/glucose-6-phosphate dehydrogenase enzymatic assay on an automated assay instrument (Roche Cobas Mira Plus Chemistry System, Roche Diagnostic Systems, Indianapolis, IN, USA), and insulin was measured with an electrochemiluminescence immunoassay (Cobas e 411 Immunoassay Analyzer, Roche Diagnostics, Indianapolis, IN, USA) [20].

2.4.3. Satiety Visual Analog Scales (VAS)

At visits 2 and 3 (days 0 and 7), satiety VAS ratings were assessed for fullness, hunger, desire to eat, and prospective consumption at $t = -30$, 30, 60, 90, 120, 150, and 180 min $\pm$ 2 min, where t = 0 min was the start of study product consumption. The questions were "How hungry do you feel?" with anchors at 0 and 100 mm of "Not hungry at all" and "As hungry as I've ever felt"; "How full do you feel?" with anchors of "Not full at all" and "As full as I've ever felt"; "How strong is your desire to eat?" with anchors of "Not at all strong" and "As strong as I've ever felt"; "How much food do you think you can eat?" with anchors of "Nothing at all" and "A large amount."

2.4.4. Gastrointestinal (GI) Tolerability Questionnaire

A GI Tolerability Questionnaire [21] was administered at visits 2 and 3 (days 0 and 7) to assess the presence and severity of selected GI symptoms including nausea, GI rumblings, abdominal pain, bloating, flatulence, and diarrhea during the 0–180 min time period, where t = 0 min was the start of study product consumption. GI symptoms were scored as follows: 0 = none, 1 = no more than usual, 2 = somewhat more than usual, and 3 = much more than usual.

2.4.5. Palatability

At the end of visits 2 and 3 (days 0 and 7), subjects completed a study product palatability questionnaire [22,23] in which they rated the study products on a scale from 1 (dislike extremely) to 10 (like extremely) on appearance, texture, flavor, and overall acceptance of the scones; on a scale from 1 (not at all healthy) to 10 (extremely healthy) on how healthy they thought the scone was; and on a scale from 1 (very little) to 10 (very nutritious) on how nutritious they thought the scone was. Subjects also responded to statements of "I recommend the scone to family and friends" and "I tolerated the muffin well, with no complaints" by marking rating of strongly disagree (−2), disagree (−1), no opinion (0), agree (1), or strongly agree (2).

2.5. Data Analysis

2.5.1. Outcome Variables

The primary outcome variable was the difference between treatment conditions in the incremental area under the curve (iAUC) for venous glucose from 0 to 120 min. The secondary outcome variables were the differences between treatments in the following parameters: venous glucose iAUC from 0 to 180 min; capillary glucose iAUC from 0 to 120 min and from 0 to 180 min; insulin iAUC from 0 to 120 min and from 0 to 180 min; maximal concentrations (Cmax) for glucose (venous and capillary) and insulin (venous); and the hunger, fullness, desire to eat and prospective consumption net incremental area under the curve (niAUC) from 0 to 120 min. For the iAUC calculation of the venous and capillary glucose and venous insulin measures, the pre-consumption measurement at $t = -15$ min was counted as $t = 0$. For the niAUC calculation of the satiety VAS measures, the pre-consumption measurement at $t = -30$ min was counted as $t = 0$. Areas under the curve were calculated using the trapezoidal rule [24].

2.5.2. Sample Size

An evaluable sample of 29 subjects was expected to provide 80% power to detect a difference of 10% in the primary outcome variable of venous glucose $iAUC_{0-120\ min}$ between treatment conditions. This calculation was based on a paired t-test with an expected standard deviation of 18.5% based on previous studies conducted by the investigators. No adjustment to the alpha level was planned for comparisons between treatments for secondary outcome variables. A total of 36 subjects were randomized allowing for anticipated subject attrition.

2.5.3. Statistical Analyses

All tests of significance were assessed at alpha = 0.05, 2-sided. Statistical analyses were conducted using SAS for Windows (version 9.3, Cary, NC, USA). Missing data were not imputed and only observed data were included in the statistical models. Descriptive statistics (number of subjects, mean, standard error of the mean (SEM), standard deviation, median, interquartile limits, minimum and maximum for continuous variables; counts and percentages for categorical variables) were calculated by study product. Baseline comparability of sequence groups was assessed by analysis of variance (ANOVA) with treatment sequence as a fixed effect for continuous variables. For categorical variables, baseline comparability was assessed by chi-square test.

For analyses of the continuous outcome variables and continuous palatability scores, differences in responses between study products were assessed using SAS Proc Mixed repeated measures ANOVA. Initial repeated measures ANOVA models contained terms for treatment, sequence, and period with subject as a random effect. Models were reduced in a stepwise manner until only significant ($p < 0.05$) terms or treatment remained in the model. Assumptions of normality of residuals were investigated for each response measurement. In cases when the normality assumption was rejected at the 1% level with the Shapiro–Wilk test, an analysis using ranks was performed. Differences between study products in the frequency of scores of 2 or greater (somewhat more or much more than usual) on the GI tolerability questionnaire were assessed using McNemar's test.

Sensitivity analyses were performed to assess evidence of any condition by sequence interaction. Because no evidence was present for heterogeneity of response by sequence, the data from the two treatment sequences were pooled for analyses by study product.

3. Results

3.1. Study Subjects

Forty-three persons were screened for the study, but of those, six did not meet the inclusion/exclusion criteria and one met the screening criteria but was later screen failed because of scheduling conflicts with visits 2 and 3. A total of 36 subjects were randomized to a treatment sequence. One subject was terminated from the study before its completion because of inadequate compliance with study instructions. There were 32 subjects included in the glucose and insulin analyses because of missing samples from at least one of the test visits; 35 subjects were included in the satiety VAS, GI tolerability, and palatability analyses. Subject flow through the study is shown in Figure 1.

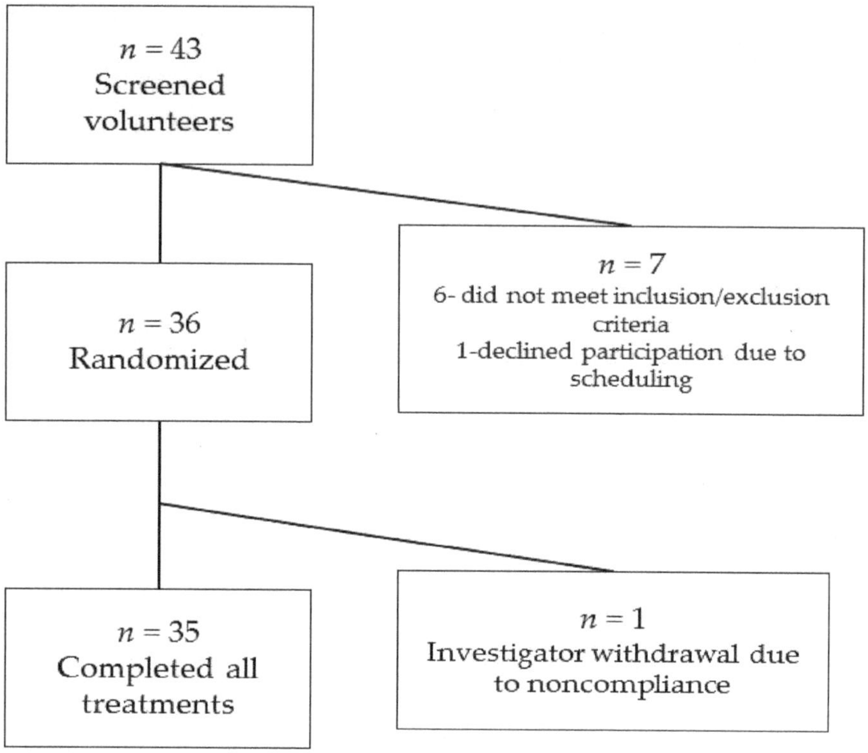

Figure 1. Subject flow through study.

Study subject demographics are reported in Table 2. The subjects were primarily female, with a mean age of 46.2 years and a mean body mass index of 26.1 kg/m^2. Each subject was given a copy of his or her diet record for the 24 h prior to test 1 and asked to replicate intake for the same period prior to test 2. The prior 24-h diet record returned on the day of test 2 was reviewed and any material deviations were noted. None of the subjects had deviations sufficiently large to warrant exclusion from the per protocol analysis in the judgment of the study director.

Table 2. Subject demographics.

Variable	All Participants (n = 35) [1]
Age (y)	46.2 ± 2.2
Sex (male/female)	12/23
Race (white/nonwhite)	22/13
Ethnicity (non-Hispanic/Hispanic)	26/9
Weight (kg)	73.9 ± 2.1
Body mass index (kg/m^2)	26.1 ± 0.5
Fasting capillary glucose (mmol/L)	5.04 ± 0.09

[1] Values for continuous variables are mean ± standard error of the mean; values for categorical values are frequencies.

3.2. Blood Glucose and Insulin

The time-course graph of venous and capillary glucose and venous insulin concentrations is presented in Figure 2, and iAUC and Cmax are shown in Table 3. Venous and capillary glucose iAUC$_{0\text{–}120\text{ min}}$ and iAUC$_{0\text{–}180\text{ min}}$ mean values were all 43–45% lower after consumption of the fiber scone compared to control scone ($p < 0.05$). Venous insulin iAUC$_{0\text{–}120\text{ min}}$ and iAUC$_{0\text{–}180\text{ min}}$ mean values were 35% and 40% lower, respectively, after consumption of the fiber scone compared to control scone ($p < 0.05$). Mean venous and capillary glucose and venous insulin Cmax levels were also significantly lower after consumption of the fiber scone compared to control scone (8%, 10% and 22% lower, respectively; $p < 0.05$).

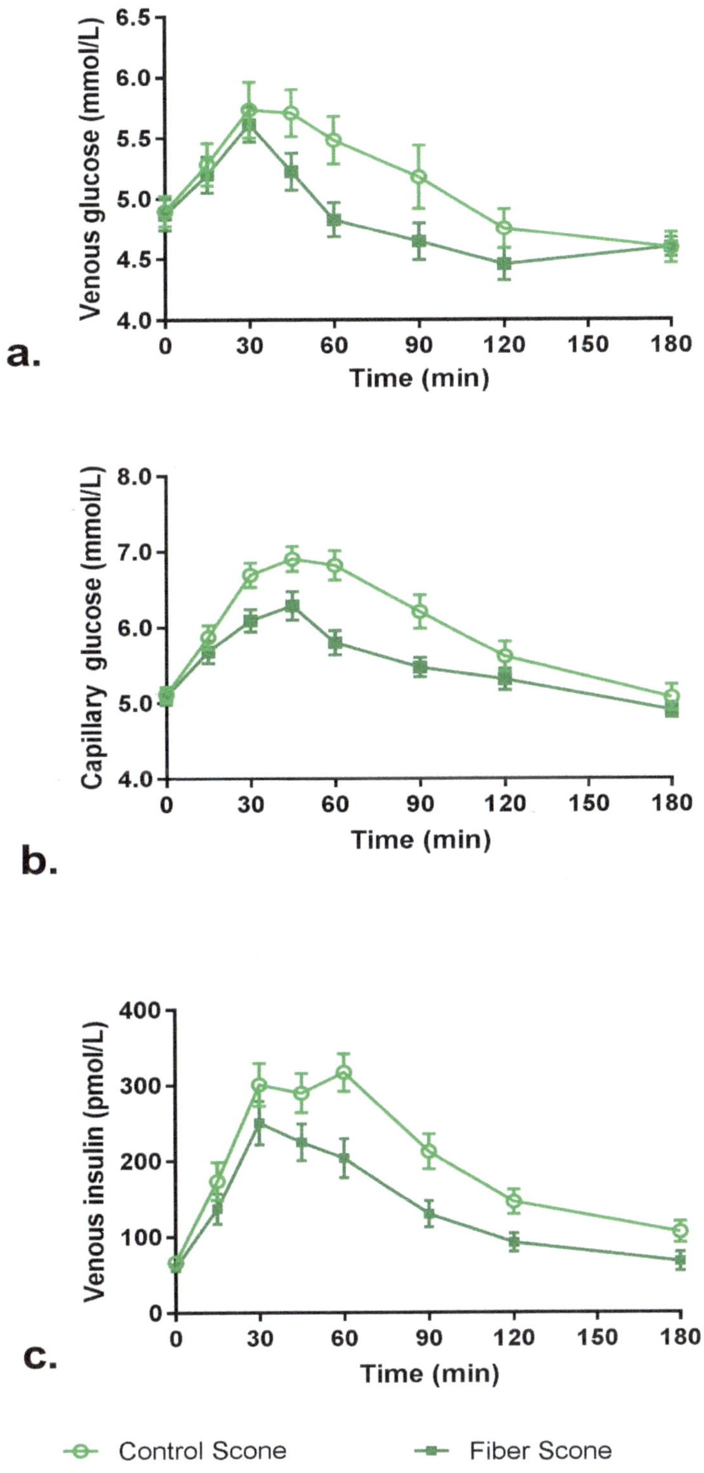

Figure 2. Mean post-prandial glucose and insulin concentrations over 180 min: (**a**) venous glucose; (**b**) capillary glucose (**c**) venous insulin. Error bars represent the standard error of the mean.

Table 3. Post-prandial glucose and insulin iAUC and Cmax (n = 32) [1,2].

Parameter	Control Scone	Fiber Scone	p-Value [3]
Venous blood glucose			
$iAUC_{0–120\ min}$ (min × mmol/L)	69.65 ± 9.05	38.41 ± 5.77	0.0014
$iAUC_{0–180\ min}$ (min × mmol/L) [4]	84.75 ± 11.43	48.29 ± 9.55	0.0039
Cmax (mmol/L) [4]	6.44 ± 0.18	5.88 ± 0.12	0.0039
Capillary blood glucose			
$iAUC_{0–120\ min}$ (min × mmol/L) [4]	139.14 ± 14.60	79.75 ± 8.10	0.0004
$iAUC_{0–180\ min}$ (min × mmol/L) [4]	171.88 ± 19.65	94.63 ± 10.66	0.0003
Cmax (mmol/L) [4]	7.49 ± 0.19	6.72 ± 0.16	0.0002
Venous insulin			
$iAUC_{0–120\ min}$ (min × pmol/L)	19,229 ± 1865	12,592 ± 1686	0.0005
$iAUC_{0–180\ min}$ (min × pmol/L)	23,850 ± 2138	14,192 ± 1901	<0.0001
Cmax (pmol/L) [4]	392 ± 28	305 ± 26	0.0008

[1] iAUC = incremental area under the curve, Cmax = maximum concentration. [2] Values are mean ± standard error of the mean. [3] p-values derived from repeated measure analysis of variance (ANOVA) with subject included as a random effect. [4] Values were ranked prior to ANOVA.

3.3. Satiety VAS Scores

Results for niAUC satiety VAS scores are shown in Table 4. Hunger and desire to eat $niAUC_{0–180\ min}$ mean values were significantly lower after consumption of the fiber scone compared to control scone ($p < 0.05$). Fullness and prospective consumption $niAUC_{0–180\ min}$ mean values did not differ significantly between study products.

Table 4. Satiety visual analog scores (n = 35) [1,2].

Parameter	Control Scone	Fiber Scone	p-Value [3]
Hunger $niAUC_{0–180\ min}$ (mm × min)	−1173 ± 896	−2840 ± 780	0.0316
Fullness $niAUC_{0–180\ min}$ (mm × min)	3926 ± 753	4028 ± 898	0.8858
Desire to eat $niAUC_{0–180\ min}$ (mm × min)	−1184 ± 918	−3046 ± 773	0.0135
Prospective consumption $niAUC_{0–180\ min}$ (mm × min)	−2098 ± 799	−2847 ± 672	0.1619

[1] mm = millimeters, min = minutes, niAUC = net incremental area under the curve; [2] Values are mean ± standard error of the mean; [3] p-values derived from repeated measures analysis of variance with subject included as a random effect.

3.4. GI Tolerability Questionnaire

Results for the analyses of the frequency of scores of 2 or greater (somewhat more than usual and much more than usual) on the components of the GI tolerability questionnaire are shown in Table 5. There were no significant differences between study products in the number of subjects with ratings of somewhat more than usual or much more than usual for nausea, bloating, GI rumblings, flatulence, abdominal pain, or diarrhea.

Table 5. Gastrointestinal Tolerability: Frequency of scores ≥ 2 (n = 35) [1,2,3].

Parameter	Control Scone	Fiber Scone	p-Value [4]
Nausea	0 (0) [3]	0 (0)	1.000
Bloating	1 (2.9)	0 (0)	1.000
GI Rumblings [4]	4 (11.4)	1 (2.9)	0.2482
Flatulence	1 (2.9)	0 (0.0)	1.000
Abdominal Pain	0 (0.0)	0 (0.0)	1.000
Diarrhea	0 (0.0)	0 (0.0)	1.000

[1] GI = gastrointestinal; [2] Scoring system: 0 = none, 1 = no more than usual, 2 = somewhat more than usual, 3 = much more than usual; [3] Values are n (%); [4] p-value generated from McNemar's test for frequencies of values ≥ 2.

3.5. Study Product Palatability

Results for the analyses of study product palatability are shown in Table 6. There was no significant difference between study products for any of the characteristics evaluated on the palatability questionnaire including appearance, texture, flavor, acceptance, healthiness or nutritiousness of the fiber scone and control scones. There were also no significant differences between study products for subjects' agreement with the statements "I recommend the scone to family and friends" and "I tolerated the scone well, with no complaints".

Table 6. Palatability Evaluation (n = 35) [5].

Parameter	Control Scone	Fiber Scone	p-Value [6]
Appearance [1]	7.74 ± 0.32	7.63 ± 0.32	0.4875
Texture [1]	6.97 ± 0.34	6.40 ± 0.36	0.0743
Flavor [1]	7.11 ± 0.04	6.69 ± 0.43	0.1185 [7]
Acceptance [1]	7.17 ± 0.36	6.77 ± 0.43	0.2271 [7]
Healthy [2]	5.91 ± 0.46	5.71 ± 0.44	0.4205
Nutritious [3]	5.57 ± 0.44	5.23 ± 0.44	0.2092 [7]
Recommend [4]	0.17 ± 0.20	0.09 ± 0.21	0.5712
Tolerated [4]	0.89 ± 0.20	0.97 ± 0.16	0.8601 [7]

[1] Scoring system: 1 (dislike extremely) to 10 (like extremely) on the appearance, texture, flavor, and overall acceptance of the scones; [2] Scoring system: 1 (not at all healthy) to 10 (extremely healthy); [3] Scoring system: 1 (very little) to 10 (very nutritious). [4] "I recommend the scone to family and friends" and "I tolerated the scone well, with no complaints" by marking rating of −2 (strongly disagree), −1 (disagree), 0 (no opinion), +1 (agree), or +2 (strongly agree); [5] Values are mean ± standard error of the mean; [6] p-value derived from repeated measures analysis of variance (ANOVA) that included subject as a random effect; [7] Individual values were ranked prior to ANOVA.

4. Discussion

The present study demonstrates that replacing a portion of refined wheat flour in a food with RS4 can reduce postprandial glucose and insulin concentrations and increase selected measures of satiety. The blood glucose and insulin findings align with results from a previous study administering the same RS4 in a muffin top to healthy adults [19]. In the present study, the percent reductions in $iAUC_{0–120\ min}$ glucose (venous and capillary) and $iAUC_{0–120\ min}$ insulin were greater than in the previously published study, which may be attributed to the higher dietary fiber content of the RS4-containing scone in the present study. Both study foods replaced a portion of refined wheat flour with VERSAFIBE 2470 resistant starch. This replacement resulted in an increase in TDF content and a decrease in available carbohydrate content which contributed to the reduced glucose and insulin responses. The absolute blood glucose values typically differ when measured intravenously or through capillary sampling, with capillary sampling typically displaying lower variation [25]. It is expected that the venous values will be a bit lower than the capillary values because capillary blood will have a value intermediate between that of venous and arterial blood. The present data from individual time points align with this previous observation.

The intended application of the novel RS4 in the present study is to replace digestible starch (e.g., wheat flour) in food products. Accordingly, the study was designed to provide data on the glycemic and insulinemic responses to food products prepared with non-resistant starch (control) or RS4 resistant starch. Therefore, the trial was designed in a manner that matched total carbohydrate content and portion size rather than available carbohydrate content. This deliberate choice in study design provides information relevant to the intended application of the ingredient studied (RS4). Glycemic response, which was evaluated in the present study, is often confused with glycemic index, which requires that the control food and test food be matched for 50 g available carbohydrate. These two concepts have been discussed in detail elsewhere [26].

Other types of RS4 have also been effective in lowering blood glucose compared to a control treatment. Four acute studies of RS4 containing distarch phosphate or phosphated distarch phosphate demonstrated reduction in postprandial blood glucose when administered in a beverage [8,14], a bar [9], and a cookie [16]. An acute study of maize hydroxypropyl distarch phosphate RS4 (38 g) in pancakes administered to healthy adults reported a significant reduction in postprandial glucose and insulin compared to control (0–180 min) [17]. A similarly designed study using the same RS4 (40 g) in pancakes reported no difference in blood glucose or insulin values over 180 min [18]. It should be noted that the RS4-containing pancake in both studies provided 0 g fiber. The inconsistency in blood glucose response to different RS4s emphasizes the need for evaluating health effects from consuming specific types of RS4, especially as new RS4s are developed.

Three studies examined the effect of a different type of RS4 on acute satiety response [11,14,18], and each study examined a different type of RS4. Satiety ratings in response to wheat phosphated distarch phosphate in a bar (10 g) [11] and potato distarch phosphate in a beverage (30 g) [14], and maize hydroxypropyl distarch phosphate in pancakes (40 g) [18], did not differ from those in control treatments. In contrast, the present study demonstrated that acid-hydrolyzed and heat-treated RS4 reduced hunger and desire to eat during the 180 min following consumption. The mechanism of action for this short-term effect is unclear and warrants further research. Additionally, long-term studies of RS4 on energy intake and weight management are needed to understand the full range of responses to consumption of this fiber.

Effects of long-term intake of wheat-based RS4 (phosphated distarch phosphate) were examined in two studies and published in three articles [10,12,13]. Martinez et al. (2010) compared the effects of high amylose maize resistant starch (RS2) and wheat phosphated distarch phosphate (RS4) on the gut microbiota [10]. While both types of RS impacted the gut microbiota, their effects were distinct, which reinforces the hypothesis that different types of RS may yield different health effects. A study in the Hutterite community, which has a high prevalence of metabolic syndrome, demonstrated that inclusion of RS4 did not affect measures of glycemic health, but improved blood lipids, waist circumference, and body composition [12]. The amount of RS4 or fiber consumed was not reported, which limits the ability to draw conclusions on long-term intake. An analysis of a subsample from the aforementioned study reported changes in gut microbiota composition and increased fecal short-chain fatty acid concentrations, suggesting that the gut microbiota may be a mediator for the changes in metabolic biomarkers [13]. This paper reported mean nutrient intake at baseline and after the two intervention periods. However, this was a subsample of the previous study and it is unclear whether the dietary data applies to the larger group in the previously published paper.

The glycemic response findings in the present study are supported by results from many previous studies of RS4. This study demonstrates that a reduction in post-prandial blood glucose and insulin can be achieved using an RS4 that is created through a novel chemical modification (acid hydrolyzed and heat-treated, instead of phosphate cross-linked). This is the first study to report significantly increased satiety (hunger, desire to eat) after consuming RS4. There are a few limitations of this study: (1) the study was conducted in healthy individuals, so we cannot draw conclusions related to chronic disease risk or management of existing conditions such as diabetes mellitus; and (2) the study foods (low fiber scone and high fiber scone) may not be culturally relevant to all countries and, thus, additional research is needed to evaluate glycemic and satiety response to culturally appropriate foods. Future research should examine the long-term effects of different RS4s to better understand the range of health effects from these ingredients.

5. Conclusions

In conclusion, this study demonstrated that a baked good, fortified with RS4 (acid hydrolyzed and heat treated maize starch) that replaced available carbohydrate from wheat flour, reduced postprandial plasma glucose response (venous and insulin) and correspondingly reduced plasma insulin. The study foods were administered in a practical portion size, emulating what consumers might find in the marketplace. This is the first study to report changes in two measures of satiety, hunger and desire to eat, after consuming RS4. The high fiber scone was well-tolerated and did not change gastrointestinal symptoms. Resistant starch type 4 has the potential for helping to fill the fiber gap in the Western diets while improving glycemic health.

Acknowledgments: This study was funded by Ingredion Incorporated.

Author Contributions: M.L.S. conceived and designed the study and contributed to writing the paper; K.C.M. was the study director and contributed to study design. M.B. completed the statistical analysis. M.A.B. was the principal investigator and supervising physician, she contributed to study design, data collection and data interpretation. M.L.W. contributed to writing the paper. All authors have reviewed and approved the paper.

References

1. Dahl, W.J.; Stewart, M.L. Position of the academy of nutrition and dietetics: Health implications of dietary fiber. *J. Acad. Nutr. Diet.* **2015**, *115*, 1861–1870. [CrossRef] [PubMed]
2. Stephen, A.M.; Champ, M.M.; Cloran, S.J.; Fleith, M.; van Lieshout, L.; Mejborn, H.; Burley, V.J. Dietary fibre in Europe: Current state of knowledge on definitions, sources, recommendations, intakes and relationships to health. *Nutr. Res. Rev.* **2017**, *30*, 1–42. [CrossRef] [PubMed]
3. Tosh, S.M. Review of human studies investigating the post-prandial blood-glucose lowering ability of oat and barley food products. *Eur. J. Clin. Nutr.* **2013**, *67*, 310–317. [CrossRef] [PubMed]
4. Robertson, M.D. Dietary-resistant starch and glucose metabolism. *Curr. Opin. Clin. Nutr. Metab. Care* **2012**, *15*, 362–367. [CrossRef] [PubMed]
5. Jiang, J.; Zhao, L.; Lin, L.; Gui, M.; Aleteng, Q.; Wu, B.; Wang, S.; Pan, B.; Ling, Y.; Gao, X. Postprandial blood glucose outweighs fasting blood glucose and hba1c in screening coronary heart disease. *Sci. Rep.* **2017**, *7*, 14212. [CrossRef] [PubMed]
6. Lockyer, S.; Nugent, A.P. Health effects of resistant starch. *Nutr. Bull.* **2017**, *42*, 10–42. [CrossRef]
7. Maningat, C.C.; Seib, P.A. RS4-type resistant starch: Chemistry, functionality and health benefits. In *Resistant Starch: Sources, Applications and Health Benefits*; Shi, Y.C., Maningat, C.C., Eds.; John Wiley & Sons: Chichester, UK, 2013; pp. 43–77.
8. Haub, M.D.; Hubach, K.L.; Al-Tamimi, E.K.; Ornelas, S.; Seib, P.A. Different types of resistant starch elicit different glucose reponses in humans. *J. Nutr. Metab.* **2010**, *2010*, 230501. [CrossRef] [PubMed]
9. Al-Tamimi, E.K.; Seib, P.A.; Snyder, B.S.; Haub, M.D. Consumption of cross-linked resistant starch ($RS4_{XL}$) on glucose and insulin responses in humans. *J. Nutr. Metab.* **2010**, *2010*, 651063. [CrossRef] [PubMed]
10. Martínez, I.; Kim, J.H.; Duffy, P.R.; Schlegel, V.L.; Walter, J. Resistant starches types 2 and 4 have differential effects on the composition of the fecal microbiota in human subjects. *PLoS ONE* **2010**, *5*, e15046. [CrossRef] [PubMed]
11. Karalus, M.; Clark, M.; Greaves, K.A.; Thomas, W.; Vickers, Z.; Kuyama, M.; Slavin, J. Fermentable fibers do not affect satiety or food intake by women who do not practice restrained eating. *J. Acad. Nutr. Diet.* **2012**, *112*, 1356–1362. [CrossRef] [PubMed]
12. Nichenametla, S.N.; Weidauer, L.A.; Wey, H.E.; Beare, T.M.; Specker, B.L.; Dey, M. Resistant starch type 4-enriched diet lowered blood cholesterols and improved body composition in a double blind controlled cross-over intervention. *Mol. Nutr. Food Res.* **2014**, *58*, 1365–1369. [CrossRef] [PubMed]
13. Upadhyaya, B.; McCormack, L.; Fardin-Kia, A.R.; Juenemann, R.; Nichenametla, S.; Clapper, J.; Specker, B.; Dey, M. Impact of dietary resistant starch type 4 on human gut microbiota and immunometabolic functions. *Sci. Rep.* **2016**, *6*, 28797. [CrossRef] [PubMed]
14. Haub, M.D.; Louk, J.A.; Lopez, T.C. Novel resistant potato starches on glycemia and satiety in humans. *J. Nutr. Metab.* **2012**, *2012*, 478043. [CrossRef] [PubMed]
15. Dahl, W.J.; Ford, A.L.; Ukhanova, M.; Radford, A.; Christman, M.C.; Waugh, S.; Mai, V. Resistant potato starches (type 4 RS) exhibit varying effects on laxation with and without phylum level changes in microbiota: A randomised trial in young adults. *J. Funct. Foods* **2016**, *23*, 1–11. [CrossRef]
16. Stewart, M.L.; Zimmer, J.P. A high fiber cookie made with resistant starch type 4 reduces post-prandial glucose and insulin responses in healthy adults. *Nutrients* **2017**, *9*, 237. [CrossRef] [PubMed]

17. Shimotoyodome, A.; Suzuki, J.; Kameo, Y.; Hase, T. Dietary supplementation with hydroxypropyl-distarch phosphate from waxy maize starch increases resting energy expenditure by lowering the postprandial glucose-dependent insulinotropic polypeptide response in human subjects. *Br. J. Nutr.* **2011**, *106*, 96–104. [CrossRef] [PubMed]
18. Gentile, C.L.; Ward, E.; Holst, J.J.; Astrup, A.; Ormsbee, M.J.; Connelly, S.; Arciero, P.J. Resistant starch and protein intake enhances fat oxidation and feelings of fullness in lean and overweight/obese women. *Nutr. J.* **2015**, *14*, 113. [CrossRef] [PubMed]
19. Stewart, M.L.; Zimmer, J.P. Post-prandial glucose and insulin response to high-fiber muffin top containing resistant starch type 4 in healthy adults: A double-blind, randomized, controlled trial. *Nutrition* **2018**, in press.
20. Cassidy, J.P.; Luzio, S.D.; Marino, M.T.; Baughman, R.A. Quantification of human serum insulin concentrations in clinical pharmacokinetic or bioequivalence studies: What defines the "best method"? *Clin. Chem. Lab. Med.* **2012**, *50*, 663–666. [CrossRef] [PubMed]
21. Maki, K.C.; Rains, T.M.; Kelley, K.M.; Cook, C.M.; Schild, A.L.; Gietl, E. Fibermalt is well tolerated in healthy men and women at intakes up to 60 g/d: A randomized, double-blind, crossover trial. *Int. J. Food Sci. Nutr.* **2013**, *64*, 274–281. [CrossRef] [PubMed]
22. Mialon, V.S.; Clark, M.R.; Leppard, P.I.; Cox, D.N. The effect of dietary fibre information on consumer responses to breads and "English" muffins: A cross-cultural study. *Food Qual. Preference* **2002**, *13*, 1–12. [CrossRef]
23. Baixauli, R.; Salvador, A.; Martínez-Cervera, S.; Fiszman, S.M. Distinctive sensory features introduced by resistant starch in baked products. *LWT Food Sci. Technol.* **2008**, *41*, 1927–1933. [CrossRef]
24. Brouns, F.; Bjorck, I.; Frayn, K.N.; Gibbs, A.L.; Lang, V.; Slama, G.; Wolever, T.M. Glycaemic index methodology. *Nutr. Res. Rev.* **2005**, *18*, 145–171. [CrossRef] [PubMed]
25. Wolever, T.M.; Vorster, H.H.; Bjorck, I.; Brand-Miller, J.; Brighenti, F.; Mann, J.I.; Ramdath, D.D.; Granfeldt, Y.; Holt, S.; Perry, T.L.; et al. Determination of the glycaemic index of foods: Interlaboratory study. *Eur. J. Clin. Nutr.* **2003**, *57*, 475–482. [CrossRef] [PubMed]
26. Augustin, L.S.; Kendall, C.W.; Jenkins, D.J.; Willett, W.C.; Astrup, A.; Barclay, A.W.; Bjorck, I.; Brand-Miller, J.C.; Brighenti, F.; Buyken, A.E.; et al. Glycemic index, glycemic load and glycemic response: An International Scientific Consensus Summit from the International Carbohydrate Quality Consortium (ICQC). *Nutr. Metab. Cardiovasc. Dis.* **2015**, *25*, 795–815. [CrossRef] [PubMed]

7

Metabolic Effects of High Glycaemic Index Diets: A Systematic Review and Meta-Analysis of Feeding Studies in Mice and Rats

Grace J. Campbell [1,*], Alistair M. Senior [2] and Kim S. Bell-Anderson [1]

[1] Charles Perkins Centre, School of Life and Environmental Sciences, University of Sydney, Sydney, NSW 2006, Australia; kim.bell-anderson@sydney.edu.au

[2] Charles Perkins Centre, School of Mathematics and Statistics, University of Sydney, Sydney, NSW 2006, Australia; alistair.senior@sydney.edu.au

* Correspondence: grace.campbell@sydney.edu.au

Abstract: Low glycaemic index (LGI) diets are often reported to benefit metabolic health, but the mechanism(s) responsible are not clear. This review aimed to systematically identify studies investigating metabolic effects of high glycaemic index (HGI) versus LGI diets in mice and rats. A meta-analysis was conducted to calculate an overall effect size, Hedge's standardised mean differences (hereafter *d*), for each trait, with moderator variables considered in subsequent meta-regressions. Across 30 articles, a HGI diet increased five of the seven traits examined: body weight ($d = 0.55$; 95% confidence interval: 0.31, 0.79), fat mass ($d = 1.08$; 0.67, 1.49), fasting circulating insulin levels ($d = 0.40$; 0.09, 0.71), and glucose ($d = 0.80$; 0.35, 1.25) and insulin ($d = 1.14$; 0.50, 1.77) area under the curve during a glucose tolerance test. However, there was substantial heterogeneity among the effects for all traits and the small number of studies enabled only limited investigation of possible confounding factors. HGI diets favour body weight gain, increased adiposity and detrimentally affect parameters of glucose homeostasis in mice and rats, but these effects may not be a direct result of GI per se; rather they may be due to variation in other dietary constituents, such as dietary fibre, a factor which is known to reduce the GI of food and promote health via GI-independent mechanisms.

Keywords: glycaemic index; glycaemic index; mice; rats; metabolism; glucose homeostasis

---

1. Introduction

Obesity is a chronic lifestyle disease that is brought about by many factors, the easiest of which to identify are diet and behaviour. Increased consumption of "Western" diets combined with increased sedentary behaviours are thought to be major contributors to the rapid rise in the prevalence of obesity worldwide [1]. Obesity is defined as an excess accumulation of fat mass and is associated with insulin resistance, increasing risk for type 2 diabetes mellitus, cardiovascular disease and some cancers. Diet is key to addressing this urgent public health issue, and the delineation of mechanisms linking dietary patterns and metabolic health is needed to establish optimal nutrition for individuals and populations.

Dietary guidelines recommend that carbohydrate, including sugars, starch and fibre, contribute roughly half the calories of our daily energy intake [2,3]. The nutritional importance of the subtypes of carbohydrate and their distinct physiological effects on health are not fully known. However, it is generally recommended that intake of added sugars be limited and wholegrain and fibre content increased [4,5]. Changes in food-processing technology since the Industrial Revolution have resulted in an increased supply and consumption of refined starchy foods, which feature heavily in a "Western" diet and are also associated with increased energy density, reduced fibre density and micronutrient dilution.

Starch can be further categorised as rapidly digestible starch (RDS), slowly digestible starch (SDS), or resistant starch (RS) based on the rate of digestion in the body. The two types of digestible starch (DS) are often distinguished based on their effect on postprandial blood glucose levels, with RDS quickly increasing and then decreasing blood glucose levels, and SDS inducing a slight rise that is maintained over a longer duration [6]. RS is the portion of carbohydrate that escapes digestion in the small intestine, and passes to the large intestine where it undergoes microbial fermentation, resulting in production of short chain fatty acids. RS may also be considered a source of fibre, as opposed to a form of carbohydrate, according to relatively new definitions of fibre [7].

The glycaemic index (GI) is used to compare different carbohydrate containing foods based on their effects on postprandial blood glucose levels in humans [8,9]. High glycaemic index (HGI) carbohydrates have a dramatic effect on blood glucose, with a quick release of glucose into the blood stream and a similarly quick dispersal. Low glycaemic index (LGI) carbohydrates result in a more gradual release of glucose that is digested and absorbed over a greater period of time. Hence, HGI carbohydrates consist mainly of RDS and LGI less so. The association between LGI and health is commonly criticized because a number of other factors lower GI, such as increased fat, protein and fibre content. While increased fibre, such as RS, within a diet can lower the GI of food [10], the well-documented beneficial effect of fibre on glucose homeostasis may be independent of its effects on postprandial glycaemia, and may act via other mechanisms such as those due to interactions among diet, microbiome and host.

Perhaps due to the more gradual perturbation in blood glucose levels, LGI foods lead to better control of blood glucose levels compared to HGI foods, particularly in type 2 diabetic patients [11,12]. To better understand this mechanism, the effect of both HGI and LGI diets on blood glucose homeostasis have been studied in humans and animals. Animal studies are essential for deeper investigation of molecular mechanisms attributed to the GI, and help isolate these effects of the environment, or diet, from genetic variability. While there have been several studies investigating the effect of dietary GI on rodent metabolism, these studies report somewhat contradictory results and it is unclear if these heterogeneous results are due to differences in experimental design and methodology, such as diet, or simply sampling variance. In this review, studies in mice and rats were identified and, after subjecting them to pre-set inclusion and exclusion criteria, data relating to macronutrient composition, carbohydrate source and their effect on metabolic characteristics were extracted and effect sizes derived providing the first meta-analysis of the effect of high glycaemic index diets in mice and rats.

2. Methods

2.1. Eligibility Criteria and Literature Search

The method for this review was adapted from Ainge et al. 2011 [13] and, as such, complied with the Cochrane Guidelines, Version 5.0.1 Part 2-General Methods for Cochrane Reviews [14]. In order to minimise bias during the search, a set of specific inclusion and exclusion criteria was specified a priori (Table 1). These criteria were obtained based on the set question this review aimed to answer: "What is the effect of a high versus low glycaemic index diet on metabolic characteristics in mice and rats?" As the aim was to observe the effect of GI, carbohydrate was required to contribute the majority of the energy composition. Additionally, sufficient protein content was necessary in order for the mice and rats to remain healthy and produce their own protein [15–17].

Table 1. Inclusion and exclusion criteria. This criterion was used to assess all articles and determine their eligibility for inclusion in this review. HGI, high glycaemic index; LGI, low glycaemic index.

Inclusion Criteria	Exclusion Criteria
Mice or rat studies	Transgenic animal models
Experiments performed in live whole animals	Cell cultures
HGI diet	No control diet (controls include chow or LGI)
Carbohydrates >50% of energy content	Diet of unknown macronutrient composition
Proteins >19% of energy content	Use of HGI supplement such as sugars to non-HGI diet
In English	Review, conference abstract or supplementary stub article

Four databases, PubMed, Web of Science, Medline and Scopus, were searched for papers containing a HGI diet fed to either mice or rats (Table 2). Boolean operators, alternate phrases and spellings, truncated search terms and quotation marks were used to ensure the search completed was as comprehensive and specific as possible. This search was conducted on 3 January 2017.

Table 2. Search criteria and initial results. These specific terms were used to search four databases, with the number of results yielded stated. HGI, high glycaemic index; GI, glycaemic index.

Search Term	("high glycemic*" OR "high glycaemic*" OR "high-glycemic*" OR "high-glycaemic*" OR "HGI" OR "H-GI" OR "H GI" OR "high GI" OR "high-GI" OR "simple carbohydrate*" OR "simple-carbohydrate*" OR "high carbohydrate*" OR "high-carbohydrate*" OR "high glucose*" OR "high-glucose*" OR "higher GI*" OR "higher-GI*" OR "higher glycemic*" OR "higher-glycemic*" OR "higher glycaemic*" OR "higher-glycaemic*") AND (mice OR rat) AND ("GI" OR "glycemic*" OR "glycaemic*")				
Database	PubMed	Web of Science	Scopus	Medline	Total
Results	175	422	228	254	1079

Once duplicate articles had been removed, each article's abstract was subjected to the inclusion and exclusion criteria as described above. The remaining articles were then similarly screened based on their methodology. The reference lists of all articles that fit the inclusion and exclusion criteria were obtained and these articles similarly screened. Where information was missing, it was assumed that the article did not meet the specified standards on that point. For example, if the article did not state the macronutrient composition, it was assumed that it would not meet the requirements and was excluded.

2.2. Data Extraction

The full texts of the final articles were examined and requisite information was extracted, including the specific animals and diets used, and any measurement that could be used to determine the effects of the experiment on body weight, body adiposity, energy intake or glucose homeostasis. Glucose homeostasis measures included were fasting blood glucose levels, fasting plasma or serum insulin levels and the area under the curves (AUCs) for glucose and insulin during glucose tolerance tests (GTTs), leading to a total of seven traits. Data were collated primarily from text and/or tables, but where unavailable was extracted from graphs using GetData Graph Digitizer software v2.26.0.20 (GetData, Kogarah, Australia). To maximize the differences between HGI and LGI fed animals, the latest time point for each trait for each study, or subgroup of animals for studies with multiple cohorts, was used. Any data lacking sample size or a measure of sample distribution, such as standard deviation or standard error of the mean, were not included.

For each of the examined traits for each group of animals on a HGI or LGI diet, the mean trait value, a measure of error such as standard error of the mean, standard deviation or 95% confidence interval (CI) and the sample size were extracted. All measures of variation were back calculated to standard deviation for calculation of the effect size. Where a range for the sample size was given, the minimum value was used to ensure that the results were not given undeserved weighting.

Data for seven moderator variables were also extracted for each group of animals: species, sex, length of diet, dietary fat content, starting age, length of fasting time, and use of anaesthesia.

Three were categorical factors (species, sex and use of anaesthesia) and four were continuous variables (length of diet, dietary fat content, starting age and length of fasting time). All categorical factors were recorded as binary variables; mouse or rat, male or female, yes or no respectively. Continuous variables were recorded as an integer, with length of diet and starting age recorded in days, dietary fat content as a percentage of the dietary energy content, and length of fasting time in hours. Where a range was provided for any of the continuous factors, the midpoint was used. An age of "adult" was assumed to be 18 weeks or 126 days, and a fasting time of "overnight" was assumed to be 15 h unless other clarifying information was given. Two papers did not provide starting age and as such were not included in that particular meta-regression. The raw data are available in Table S1. All continuous variables were scaled to standard deviations and centred via z-transformation.

2.3. Effect Size Calculation and Meta-Analysis

For each experimental comparison within a study, we calculated Hedge's d (hereafter d) and its sampling variance following equations 1–4 in Nakagawa et al. 2015 [18]. We calculated d such that positive values suggest that the trait of interest was greater in the HGI group than the LGI group of animals. All effect size calculations and meta-analyses were implemented using the statistical programming language *R* v3.3.1 (The R Foundation, Vienna, Austria) [19]. The seven traits were analysed separately, but in an identical way. To estimate the overall effect size for each trait we first implemented a random-effects meta-analysis (REMA), using the "rma.mv" function in the *R* package *metafor* (Maastricht University, Maastricht, Netherlands) [20]. Each REMA fitted d as the response along with its sampling variance, as well as a matrix denoting the estimated covariance among effect sizes that were based on contrasts with the same control group of animals, following the method of Besson et al. 2016 [21]. This type of covariance is sometimes called non-independence due to shared control or "stochastic dependency" [22,23]. Statistical significance of the overall effect of the diet was identified when the 95% CI did not span 0. d values of 0.3, 0.5 and 0.8 were considered small, moderate and large differences, respectively [18]. Excluding p-values, all statistical results are reported to two decimal places. We report statistical heterogeneity, that is, variation among studies in the reported effect of diet on each trait, as τ and assess its statistical significance using Cochran's Q test [24]. τ is interpretable as the standard deviation of the effect sizes, that is, differences in study outcomes that is not attributable to sampling.

In a second step, we explored possible drivers of heterogeneity by fitting random-effects meta-regression (REMR) to explore factors that affected the magnitude of the reported effects. REMR were fitted in the same way as the REMA described above, but with moderator variables included. The effect of each moderator variable on each trait was evaluated in a separate model. The restriction of limited sample sizes precluded the consideration of multiple predictors simultaneously, thus each moderator was evaluated individually. The moderators chosen were those considered most crucial to the methodology, and as such were also those most likely reported. Due to limited sample sizes, only those moderators that were disclosed in most papers could be analysed.

We evaluated the impact of publication bias, which is a systematic under-representation of effect sizes owing to the process of peer-review and publishing, using a trim and fill analysis with the "trimfill" function in *metafor*. Trim and fill analyses were applied to the residuals of the REMA for each trait following the method of Nakagawa et al. 2012 [25]. All *R* code is presented in Text S1.

2.4. Methodological Quality Assessment (MQA)

To assess the quality and validity of the articles, we performed a MQA twice by independent researchers (G.J.C. and K.S.B.-A.). The criteria were obtained from Ainge et al. 2011 [13] and as such were a modified Downs and Black "Quality Index" (QI) (Table 3) [26]. There were two categories, each with three sections. These criteria were further modified for this review with an additional 4 criteria added to the Design and Outcomes section within the Reporting category, and one removed from the

Confounding section in the Internal Validity category. There were further slight modifications to the specific questions in order to tailor it to this review.

Table 3. Methodological Quality Assessment questions. MQA questions modified from Ainge et al. 2011 [13] and Downs and Black 1998 [26]. GTT, glucose tolerance test; GI, glycaemic index.

Modified Downs and Black Quality Index
Reporting
General
1. Were the hypotheses, aims or objectives of the study clearly described in the introduction? [a] 2. Were the main outcomes to be measured clearly described in the introduction or methods section?
Animal Characteristics
3. Was animal species/strain and sex specified? [a] 4. Was the animal age at commencement of the study specified? [a] 5. Have the animal weights at commencement of the study been specified or given graphically? [a] 6. Have the animal starting numbers been specified? [a] 7. Have the housing details been specified, including temperature, light cycle and group housing? Design and Outcomes 8. Were the interventions of interest clearly described? 9. Were the main findings of the study clearly described? 10. Were estimates of the random variability in the data for the main outcomes clearly described, such as through standard deviation or standard error of the mean? [a] 11. Have all important adverse events that may be a consequence of the intervention been reported? 12. Have the actual probability values been reported for the main outcomes, except where probability value is less than 0.05? [a] 13. Were all blood tests, GTTs performed without anaesthetic? [b] 14. Were all GTTs performed after a maximum 5 h fast? [b] 15. Were the diet matched both in terms of macronutrient composition and fibre content? [b] 16. Was a difference in GI of the two diets shown, either quantitatively or qualitatively? [b]
Internal Validity
Bias
17. Was an attempt made to blind those measuring the main outcomes of the intervention? 18. Were the statistical tests used to assess the main outcomes appropriate? 19. Were the main outcomes measures used accurate (valid and reliable)?
Confounding
20. Was it stated in the text that the animals were randomised to intervention groups? [a] 21. Was there adequate adjustment for confounding in the analyses from which the main findings were drawn?
Power
22. Was the paper of sufficient power to detect a clinical important effect where the probability value for a difference being due to chance is less than 5%?

[a] Modified questions; [b] Additional questions.

For the quality assessment, if a specific point was not addressed in the article, such as blinding or the sample size for the power calculation, the article achieved a 0 for that question. The qualification of the final MQA question, concerning power, was determined using the software program G*Power v3.1.9.2 (Heinrich-Heine-Universität, Düsseldorf, Germany) [27]. A one tailed unpaired t-test post-hoc analysis was performed with the effective size of a difference of 1.0 mM for plasma glucose, α, the probability of incorrectly rejecting the null hypothesis, set to 0.05, and the accepted power threshold of above 0.8. That is, an accepted threshold of β, the probability of incorrectly retaining the null hypothesis, of below 0.2.

3. Results

3.1. Article Selection

Twenty-two articles were identified from the initial search, with an additional eight from the manual search of reference lists. The systematic search procedure with the number of articles included and excluded at each point is depicted in Figure 1. The end result was 30 articles, with 15 [28–42] involving mice, 13 [43–55] involving rats and two [56,57] with experiments performed on both species. Of the articles that contained pertinent results, all contained information regarding the change or comparison of body weight or fat, and most examined some measure of glucose homeostasis. Each study also included a LGI diet as a comparison for the HGI diet; only two also included a chow diet as a control [28,46] and neither reported the in vivo postprandial glycaemic response to chow, which would have led to severely underpowered analyses; thus, only LGI control diets were analysed. No study used the standard rodent diets from the American Institute of Nutrition (AIN), AIN-93, as control diets. The average study quality was moderate with a range of 8–18 and a median of 14, and a range of 10–16 with a median of 12 for mice and rats, respectively.

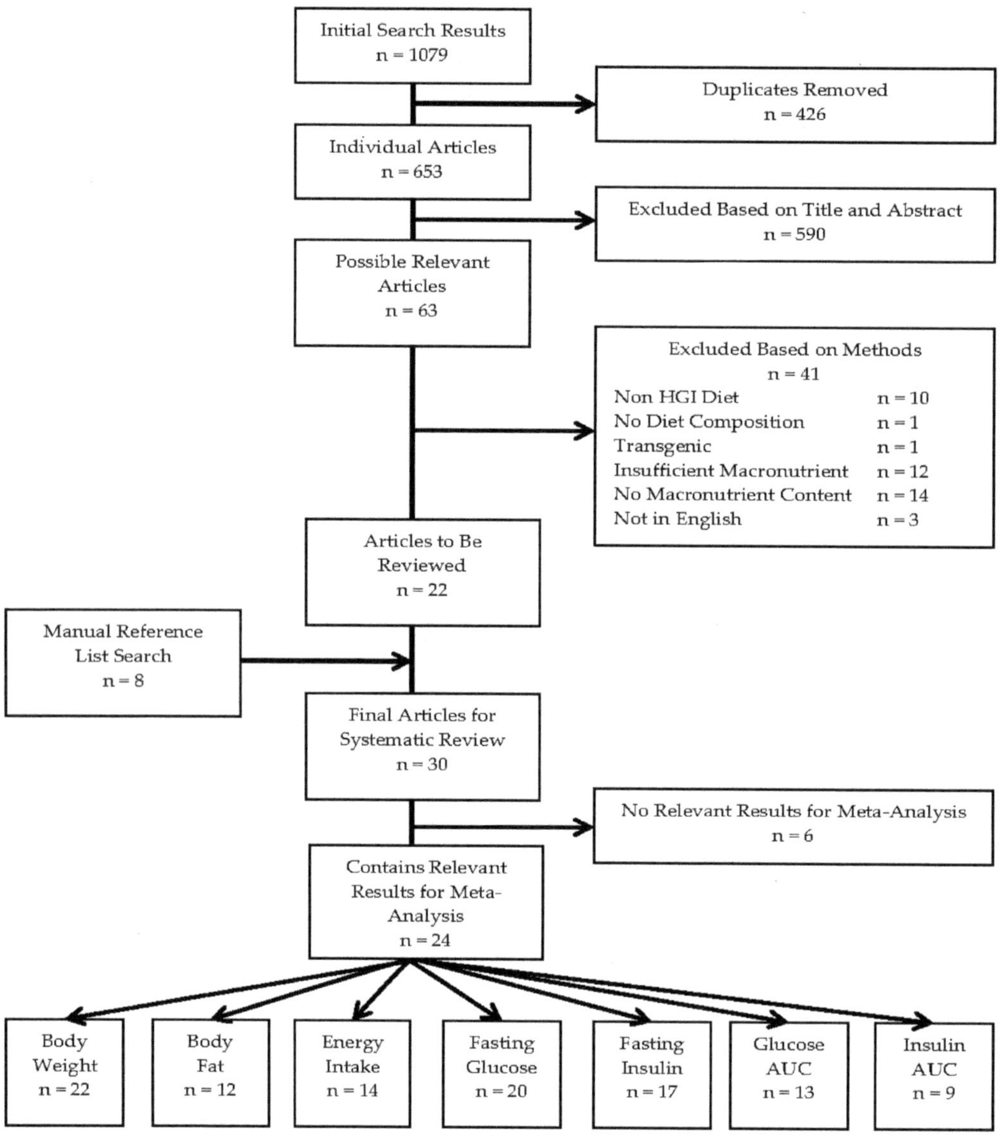

Figure 1. Flow of the study selection process for this systematic review. A flow diagram of article numbers included and excluded at each step of the systematic review process. Adapted from Ainge et al. 2011 [13]. *n*, number of articles; HGI, high glycaemic index; AUC, area under the curve.

3.2. Meta-Analysis

The meta-analyses of the extracted results, in terms of body weight, body adiposity and energy intake, and the results in relation to key measures of glucose homeostasis, are depicted in Figures 2 and 3, respectively. These results are shown dissected in terms of species, sex, length of diet, dietary fat content, starting age, fasting time and use of anaesthesia to illustrate some of the factors influencing results. Five of the seven traits showed an increased effect in male animals fed a HGI diet. Fasting blood glucose was only significantly increased by HGI feeding in male mice, and no significant effects were detected in energy intake. A funnel plot of the effect sizes for each trait is shown in Figure S1.

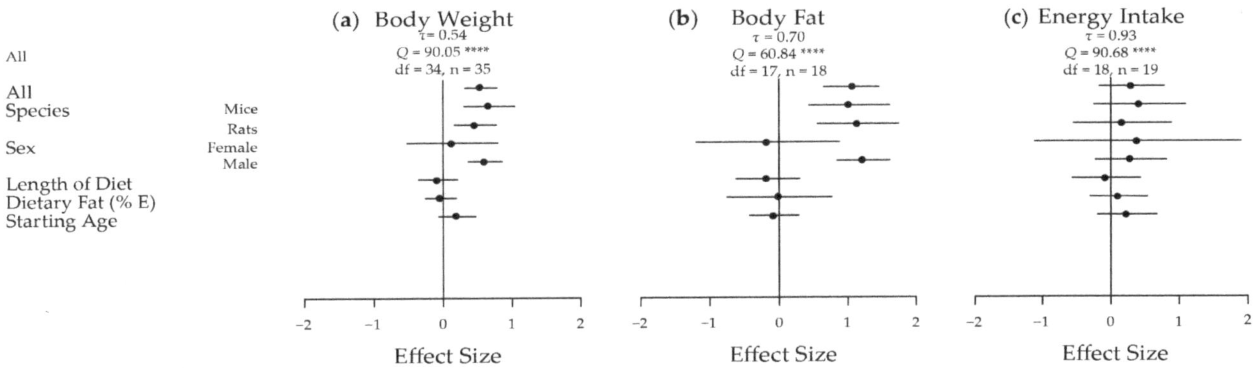

Figure 2. Meta-analysis of the extracted results for body weight, body fat and energy intake in high versus low glycaemic index fed animals. A plot of the calculated effect size and sampling variance for each of the three traits either as a whole or broken down by confounding factor: (**a**) Body Weight; All, Length of Diet and Dietary Fat $n = 35$, Mice $n = 14$, Rats $n = 21$, Female $n = 4$, Male $n = 31$, Starting Age $n = 32$; (**b**) Body Fat; All, Length of Diet and Dietary Fat $n = 18$, Mice $n = 9$, Rats $n = 9$, Female $n = 2$, Male $n = 16$, Starting Age $n = 17$; and (**c**) Energy Intake; All, Length of Diet and Dietary Fat $n = 19$, Mice $n = 10$, Rats $n = 9$, Female $n = 2$, Male $n = 17$, Starting Age $n = 18$. n, number of effect sizes; *df*, degrees of freedom; E, energy. **** $p < 0.0001$

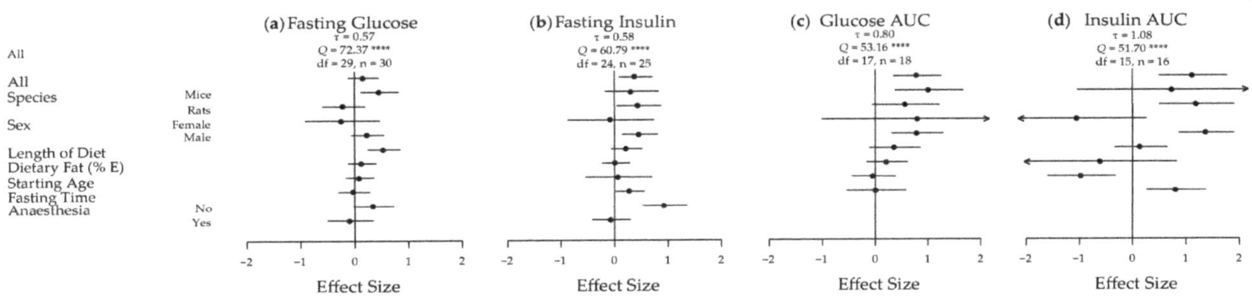

Figure 3. Meta-analysis of the extracted results for measures of glucose homeostasis in high versus low glycaemic index fed animals. A plot of the calculated effect size and sampling variance for each of the four traits either as a whole or broken down by confounding factor: (**a**) Fasting Glucose; All, Length of Diet, Dietary Fat and Fasting Time $n = 30$, Mice $n = 16$, Rats $n = 14$, Female $n = 4$, Male $n = 26$, Starting Age $n = 27$, No Anaesthesia $n = 17$, Anaesthesia $n = 13$; (**b**) Fasting Insulin; All, Length of Diet, Dietary Fat and Fasting Time $n = 25$, Mice $n = 9$, Rats $n = 16$, Female $n = 3$, Male $n = 22$, Starting Age, $n = 23$, No Anaesthesia $n = 12$, Anaesthesia $n = 13$; (**c**) Glucose AUC; All, Length of Diet, Dietary Fat and Fasting Time $n = 18$, Mice $n = 9$, Rats $n = 9$, Female $n = 1$, Male $n = 17$, Starting Age $n = 17$; and (**d**) Insulin AUC; All, Length of Diet, Dietary Fat and Fasting Time $n = 16$, Mice $n = 2$, Rats $n = 14$, Female $n = 2$, Male $n = 14$, Starting Age $n = 14$. AUC, area under the curve; n, number of effect sizes; *df*, degrees of freedom; E, energy. **** $p < 0.0001$

3.2.1. Body Weight

Overall, there was a moderate and statistically significant increase in body weight in HGI fed animals relative to LGI fed animals ($d = 0.55$; 95% CI: 0.31, 0.79) (Figure 2a). Significant heterogeneity was present across the studies ($\tau = 0.54$, $Q = 90.05$, degrees of freedom (df) = 34, $p < 0.0001$) necessitating further analysis. When subset, this effect was significant and large in males ($d = 0.61$; 0.36, 0.86) but not in females ($d = 0.13$; −0.52, 0.47). The overall effect was also slightly greater in mice ($d = 0.67$; 0.30, 1.04) than in rats ($d = 0.47$; 0.16, 0.78). Starting age, length of diet and percentage of dietary fat as energy were not estimated to have any effect on the magnitude of the effect of diet on body weight. The effect on body weight was most prominent in ad libitum studies, and as most of the studies were indeed ad libitum, the results reflected this. For example, rats fed ad libitum HGI diets exhibited a much greater body weight than those fed a LGI diet in many of the studies [43,45,47,50,51,57], but, in contrast, rats fed energy-restricted HGI diets lost a greater proportion of body weight than those fed an energy-restricted LGI diet [50].

3.2.2. Body Fat Mass

Body fat mass also had a large and significant increase in HGI compared to LGI fed animals overall ($d = 1.08$; 0.67, 1.49) (Figure 2b), again there was significant heterogeneity amongst effects ($\tau = 0.70$, $Q = 60.84$, $df = 17$, $p < 0.0001$). This effect was also large and significant in mice ($d = 1.02$; 0.43, 1.62), rats ($d = 1.15$; 0.56, 1.75) and males ($d = 1.23$, 0.84, 1.62). Again, there were no significant differences in females and no moderation of the effect was observed with continuous variables. In specific studies, a HGI diet induced significantly greater body fat mass [28–33,35–37,42] by as much as 93% [56] compared with mice on a LGI diet. Specifically, visceral and subcutaneous fat depots were heavier [30,31], and epididymal adipocytes were larger [56], in HGI fed mice.

3.2.3. Energy Intake

Energy intake was not significantly different in any subset (overall $d = 0.31$; −0.17, 0.78) (Figure 2c), and again no moderation was seen with the continuous variables. Significant heterogeneity existed amongst the effects ($\tau = 0.93$, $Q = 90.68$, $df = 18$, $p < 0.0001$). Interestingly, a LGI diet increased energy output in faeces as measured by bomb calorimetry [29,32,42], compared to a HGI diet in the three papers that measured energy excretion to help inform energy balance.

3.2.4. Fasting Blood Glucose Levels

While fasting blood glucose levels were not significantly different overall ($d = 0.17$; −0.11, 0.45) (Figure 3a), significant heterogeneity was present ($\tau = 0.57$, $Q = 72.37$, $df = 29$, $p < 0.0001$). Mice had a moderate significant high fasting blood glucose ($d = 0.47$; 0.12, 0.82) in response to HGI feeding, and a statistically significant moderately positive effect of length of time on the diet was also seen ($d = 0.55$; 0.25, 0.85). This suggests that the longer the animals were on the diet, the greater the difference in mean fasting blood glucose levels between the HGI and LGI fed animals.

3.2.5. Fasting Circulating Insulin Levels

Fasting insulin was moderately and significantly affected overall ($d = 0.40$; 0.09, 0.71) (Figure 3b), with significant heterogeneity ($\tau = 0.58$, $Q = 60.79$, $df = 24$, $p < 0.0001$). Similar magnitude effects were seen in rats ($d = 0.46$; 0.04, 0.87) and males ($d = 0.48$; 0.14, 0.81). A large effect was seen in the subset of animals that were not anesthetized ($d = 0.94$; 0.54, 1.35). The difference in fasting insulin levels between diets also became greater with fasting time ($d = 0.30$; 0.03, 0.56).

3.2.6. Glucose and Insulin AUC

Glucose AUC in response to a GTT was significantly increased in HGI fed animals with a large difference seen overall ($d = 0.80$; 0.35, 1.25) (Figure 3c). Again, significant heterogeneity was present ($\tau = 0.80$, $Q = 53.17$, $df = 17$, $p < 0.0001$). Large effects were observed in mice ($d = 1.02$; 0.38, 1.67) and in males ($d = 0.80$; 0.31, 1.29). Insulin AUC in response to a GTT was significantly and largely increased by a HGI diet overall ($d = 1.14$; 0.50, 1.77) (Figure 3d), in rats ($d = 1.20$; 0.50, 1.90) and in males ($d = 1.39$; 0.87, 1.90). Similar to fasting insulin, a large statistically significant effect was observed for fasting time on insulin AUC ($d = 0.82$; 0.27, 1.37), with significant heterogeneity ($\tau = 1.08$, $Q = 51.70$, $df = 15$, $p < 0.0001$). A large negative significant effect was also seen for starting age on insulin AUC ($d = -0.96$; -1.60, -0.32). This implies that the older the animals are when they are placed on the experimental GI diets, the smaller the difference is between insulin AUC during a GTT between HGI and LGI diets, suggesting early exposure has a significantly more dramatic effect on insulin AUC.

3.2.7. Publication Bias

Trim and fill analysis detected no missing studies for four of the examined traits: body weight, energy intake, fasting glucose and glucose AUC. For both body fat and fasting insulin, it was calculated that there were four studies missing to the left side of the funnel (Figure S1b,e). After adjustment for these missing studies, the overall effects for body fat and fasting insulin where decreased by 0.25 to 0.84, and by 0.27 to 0.13, respectively. In the case of fasting insulin, this adjusted mean effect constitutes a small effect, as opposed to a moderate effect. Insulin AUC was estimated to have one missing study from the left of the funnel (Figure S1g), which reduced the effect size by 0.07 and led to an adjusted overall effect of 1.06, not altering the qualitative interpretation of the magnitude of the effect, similar to body fat.

3.3. MQA

The animal and diet characteristics for each of the studies are shown in Tables 4 and 5 for mice and rats, respectively, listed by year. The results for the MQA are shown in Tables 6 and 7 for mice and rats, respectively. The average score, out of 22, for each species was 13.3 and 12.2, respectively, to one decimal place. There was a small amount of variation in the quality of the articles, with the vast majority having a score between 11 and 16, inclusive [28–30,32,34–37,41–45,47,49–52,54–57], and a lowest score of 8 [38] and highest of 18 [31].

4. Discussion

This systematic review and meta-analysis provides evidence that male mice and rats fed HGI diets increase body weight, body adiposity, and parameters of glucose homeostasis compared to animals fed LGI diets. These findings highlight the importance of determining the effect of different carbohydrate subtypes on metabolic health, as while slowing carbohydrate bioavailability might be key, the LGI diets were also typically high in fibre such as RS which may exert mechanisms on metabolism independent of effects on postprandial glycaemia. Unfortunately, we were not able to analyse the effect of dietary fibre on metabolic outcomes across the studies in our meta-analysis as fibre content was typically not quantified in the original reporting articles, with only two paper specifying fibre content [34,57]. This lack of information was taken into consideration when determining the quality of the papers through question 15 of the MQA. This study, as a systematic review and meta-analysis, has examined the current state of rodent GI studies in an unbiased way, and has shown that, overall, better controlled studies are required in the future to properly elucidate the effect of GI alone on metabolism.

The current literature has been shown to be insufficient in regards to examining the specific effect of GI on metabolism. Only seven traits could be examined, and only seven moderators included in analyses due to the limit reported data. To examine any other effects or correlations, significant improvement in current reporting standards is required, as any other analyses conducted on the current literature would be severely underpowered. This reviews' calculated correlations are important new findings that can be used to plan future studies.

Table 4. Mouse animal and diet characteristics for intervention studies that compared LGI and HGI diets. The key information from each article using mice is shown. - denotes missing data. Approximate (~) starting weights are taken from graphs [a]. Carb, carbohydrates; HGI, high glycaemic index; LGI, low glycaemic index; E, energy; *n*, sample size; AP, amylopectin; AL, amylose; M, male; DS, digestible starch; RS, resistant starch; F, female.

Article	Carb in HGI Diet	Carb in LGI Diet	*n*	Starting Age	Sex	Strain	Starting Weight (g)	Length of Diet	Carb (% E)	Protein (% E)
Walker, 2002 [28]	Mazaca wax 100% AP	Hi-Maize 60% AL 40% AP	12	6 weeks	M	CBA/T6	24.6 ± 0.2	10 weeks	67	22
Pawlak, 2004 [56]	100% AP	60% AL 40% AP Hi-Maize	12	11 weeks	M	C57BL/6J	26.98 ± 0.37	9 weeks	69	20
Scribner, 2007 [29]	100% AP	60% AL 40% AP	9	5 weeks	M	129S2/SvPas	~17.5	25 weeks	68	19
So, 2007 [30]	DS Amioca 0% RS	RS Hi-Maize 60% RS	24 HGI or 16 LGI	3 weeks	M	C57BL/6	~17	8 weeks	69	20
Scribner, 2008 [31]	100% AP	60% AL 40% AP	16	5 weeks	M	129SvPas	~20	10 or 38 weeks	68	19
Zhou, 2008 [57]	Amioca 100% corn AP	Hi-Maize 260	-	Adult	M	C57BL/6J	-	19 days	64 [a]	19.3 [a]
Isken, 2009 [32]	100% AP	30% AP	10 or 8	16 or 44 weeks	M	C57BL/6	~23	20 or 26 weeks	65	23
Van Schothorst, 2009 [33]	100% AP	~60% AL 40% AP	50	9 weeks	M	C57BL/6JOlaHsol	25.68 ± 0.23 HGI or 25.63 ± 0.2 LGI	13–14 weeks	50	20
Anderson, 2010 [34]	Pregelatinized starch	Native starch	7	6–8 weeks	F	C57BL/6J	18.5 ± 0.2	22 weeks	68 HGI or 65 LGI	18 HGI or 22 LGI
Colbert Coate, 2010 [36]	Waxy maize 100% AP	high-AL-res 40% AP	6–8	6–8 weeks	M	C57BL/6	~22	16 weeks	65	20
Isken, 2010 [35]	100% AP	30% AP	10	16 weeks	M	C57BL/6J	~25	6 or 20 weeks	65	23
Van Schothorst, 2011 [37]	100% AP	~60% AL and ~40% AP	50	9 weeks	M	C57BL/6	25.7 ± 0.2 HGI or 25.6 ± 0.2 LGI	13–14 weeks	50	20
Uchiki, 2012 [38]	100% AP	30% AP 70% AL	-	16 months	-	C57BL/6	-	7.5 months	65	21
Weikel, 2012 [39]	100% AP (Amioca)	70% AL 30% AP (Hylon VII)	10	5 or 16 months	M	C57BL/6	-	26 or 46 weeks	65	21
Birarda, 2013 [40]	100% AP (Amioca)	70% AL 30% AP (Hylon VII)	-	5 months	M	C57BL/6	-	12 months	65	21
Rowan, 2014 [41]	100% AP (Amioca)	70% AL 30% AP (Hylon VII)	9–12	11 weeks	M	C57BL/6	~26	33 weeks	65	21
Kleckner, 2015 [42]	Amioca waxy 100% AP	H-Maize 260 60% AL	-	6–8 weeks	M	C57BL/6	~26	16 weeks	66.5	20.1

[a] Based on Ain-93G [58].

Table 5. Rat animal and diet characteristics for intervention studies that compared LGI and HGI diets. The key information from each article using rats is shown. - denotes missing data. Approximate (~) starting weights are taken from graphs. Articles using two different strains or sexes are across two rows, with the defining characteristics in bold. Only new information is entered in the second row. Carb, carbohydrates; HGI, high glycaemic index; LGI, low glycaemic index; E, energy; *n*, sample size; SHR, spontaneously hypertensive rats; AL, amylose; M, male; SD, Sprague-Dawley; AP, amylopectin; F, female.

Article	Carb in HGI Diet	Carb in LGI Diet	*n*	Starting Age	Sex	Strain	Starting Weight (g)	Length of Diet	Carb (% E)	Protein (% E)
Byrnes, 1995 [43]	Waxy cornstarch (0% AL)	Hi-Maize 60% AL	-	8 weeks	M	SD	250–300	8 weeks	60	22
				3–4 weeks	-	Wistar	50–90	4, 8 or 12 weeks		
Higgins, 1996 [44]	100% glucose or 100% AP (waxy corn)	Hi-Maize 60% AL	18	6 weeks	M	Wistar	200	8, 16 or 52 weeks	67	22
Lerer-Metzger, 1996 [45]	French toast (wheat starch)	Mung bean starch	14	6 weeks	M	SD	155	5 weeks	59	22 HGI or 24 LGI
Suga, 2000 [46]	60% glucose	60% fructose	-	-	F	SD	240–280	2 weeks	60	29
Widdup, 2000 [47]	Glucose	Hi-Maize 60% AL	-	6 weeks	M	Wistar	180 ± 2	6 weeks	65	22
Pawlak, 2001 [48]	Waxy corn 100% AP	Hi-Maize 60% AL	-	6–7 weeks	-	Wistar	215 ± 6	7 weeks	69	20
Pawlak, 2004 [56]	100% AP	60% AL Hi-Maize	12	6 weeks	M	SD	50–55	18 weeks	69	20
			7	7 weeks			-	3 weeks per diet		
Kopilas, 2007 [49]	50% Sucrose	50% LGI Starch	-	6 weeks	M	SHR	-	6 weeks	67.7^{b}	20.8^{b}
Zhou, 2008 [57]	Amioca 100% corn AP	Hi-Maize 260	50	-	M	SD	-	10 days	64^{a}	19.3^{a}
			10		F			32 days		
Aziz, 2009 [50]	100% AP	70% AL cornstarch or Cornstarch	10–12	Adult	M	SD	250	4 weeks	64^{a}	19.3^{a}
Belobrajdic, 2012 [51]	Low AL maize	High AL maize starch	8	9 weeks	M	SD	329 ± 5	4 weeks	64^{a}	19.3^{a}
Ble-Castillo, 2012 [52]	67% digestible cornstarch	67% native banana starch	30 total	7 weeks	M	Wistar	180–200	8 weeks	75.6	21.8
Stavrovskaya, 2013 [53]	High (65%) sucrose	Low (0%) sucrose	8	8 weeks	M	FBNF1	188 ± 2	8 weeks	68	21
Gugusheff, 2015 [54]	Dextrinised starch	Gel crisp starch	14	-	F	Wistar	200	70weeks	63	21
Thompson, 2016 [55]	Amioca corn (high AP)	Resistant starch (high AL)	50	19 days	F	SD	~40	8 weeks	50	20

[a] Based on Ain-93G [58]; [b] Based on Ain-76A [58].

Table 6. Mouse Methodological Quality Assessment. Each article using mice was given a score of 0 or 1 for each question. MQA, methodological quality assessment.

Article	Reporting Questions																Internal Validity Questions					Total
Author, Year	**1**	**2**	**3**	**4**	**5**	**6**	**7**	**8**	**9**	**10**	**11**	**12**	**13**	**14**	**15**	**16**	**17**	**18**	**19**	**20**	**21**	**22**	
Walker, 2002 [28]	1	1	1	1	1	1	0	0	1	1	0	1	1	0	0	0	0	1	1	0	0	0	**12**
Pawlak, 2004 [56]	1	1	1	1	1	1	0	1	0	1	1	1	1	0	0	1	0	1	1	1	1	0	**16**
Scribner, 2007 [29]	0	1	1	1	1	1	0	1	1	1	0	1	1	1	0	0	0	1	1	1	1	0	**15**
So, 2007 [30]	1	1	1	1	1	1	1	1	1	1	0	1	1	0	0	0	1	1	1	0	0	1	**16**
Scribner, 2008 [31]	1	1	1	1	1	1	0	1	1	1	0	1	1	1	0	1	0	1	1	1	1	1	**18**
Zhou, 2008 [57]	0	1	1	0	0	0	1	1	1	1	0	1	1	1	0	0	0	1	1	0	0	0	**11**
Isken, 2009 [32]	1	1	1	1	1	1	1	1	0	1	0	1	1	0	0	1	0	1	1	0	0	0	**14**
Van Schothorst, 2009 [33]	1	1	1	1	1	1	1	1	1	1	0	1	1	1	0	1	0	1	1	0	0	1	**17**
Anderson, 2010 [34]	1	1	1	1	1	1	0	1	1	1	0	0	0	0	0	1	0	1	0	1	0	0	**12**
Colbert Coate, 2010 [36]	1	1	1	1	1	1	0	1	1	1	0	1	1	0	0	0	0	1	1	0	0	0	**13**
Isken, 2010 [35]	0	1	1	1	1	1	1	1	1	1	0	1	1	0	0	1	0	1	1	0	0	0	**14**
Van Schothorst, 2011 [37]	0	1	1	1	1	1	1	1	1	1	0	1	1	1	0	1	0	1	1	0	0	1	**16**
Uchiki, 2012 [38]	0	1	0	1	0	0	0	1	1	1	0	1	1	0	0	0	0	0	0	1	0	0	**8**
Weikel, 2012 [39]	0	1	1	1	0	1	0	1	1	1	0	0	1	0	0	0	0	1	0	0	0	0	**9**
Birarda, 2013 [40]	1	1	1	1	0	0	0	1	1	1	0	1	0	0	0	0	0	1	0	0	0	0	**9**
Rowan, 2014 [41]	1	1	1	1	1	1	0	0	0	1	0	1	1	0	0	0	0	1	1	0	0	0	**11**
Kleckner, 2015 [42]	1	1	1	1	1	0	1	1	1	1	0	1	1	0	0	1	0	1	1	0	1	0	**15**
							Total																**Mean**
17	**11**	**17**	**16**	**16**	**13**	**13**	**7**	**15**	**14**	**17**	**1**	**15**	**15**	**5**	**0**	**8**	**1**	**16**	**13**	**5**	**4**	**4**	**13.3**

Table 7. Rat Methodological Quality Assessment; each article using rats was given a score of 0 or 1 for each question. MQA, methodological quality assessment.

Article	**Reporting Questions**																**Internal Validity Questions**						**Total**
Author, Year	**1**	**2**	**3**	**4**	**5**	**6**	**7**	**8**	**9**	**10**	**11**	**12**	**13**	**14**	**15**	**16**	**17**	**18**	**19**	**20**	**21**	**22**	
Byrnes, 1995 [43]	1	1	1	1	1	0	0	1	1	1	0	1	1	0	0	1	0	1	0	0	0	0	**12**
Higgins, 1996 [44]	1	1	1	1	1	1	1	1	1	1	0	1	1	0	0	0	0	1	1	1	0	1	**16**
Lerer-Metzger, 1996 [45]	1	1	1	1	1	1	0	0	1	1	0	1	0	0	0	1	0	1	0	1	0	1	**13**
Suga, 2000 [46]	1	1	1	0	1	0	0	0	0	1	0	0	0	1	1	0	0	1	1	0	1	0	**10**
Widdup, 2000 [47]	1	1	1	1	1	0	1	1	1	1	0	1	1	0	0	0	0	1	1	0	0	0	**13**
Pawlak, 2001 [48]	1	1	0	1	1	0	0	1	0	1	0	1	1	0	0	0	0	1	0	1	0	0	**10**
Pawlak, 2004 [56]	1	1	1	1	0	0	0	1	1	0	1	1	1	0	0	0	0	0	1	1	1	0	**12**
Kopilas, 2007 [49]	1	1	1	1	0	0	1	1	1	1	0	1	0	0	0	0	0	1	0	0	1	0	**11**
Zhou, 2008 [57]	0	1	1	0	0	1	1	1	0	1	0	1	1	1	0	0	0	1	1	0	0	0	**11**
Aziz, 2009 [50]	1	1	1	0	1	1	1	1	1	1	0	1	1	0	0	1	0	1	0	0	0	0	**13**
Belobrajdic, 2012 [51]	1	1	1	1	1	1	1	1	1	1	0	1	0	0	0	0	0	1	1	1	0	0	**14**
Ble-Castillo, 2012 [52]	1	1	1	1	1	0	1	1	0	1	0	1	1	0	0	0	0	1	0	0	0	0	**11**
Stavrovskaya, 2013 [53]	0	0	1	1	1	1	0	1	1	1	0	1	0	0	0	0	0	0	1	1	0	0	**10**
Gugusheff, 2015 [54]	1	1	1	0	1	1	1	1	1	1	0	1	1	0	0	1	0	1	1	0	0	1	**15**
Thompson, 2016 [55]	1	1	1	1	1	1	1	0	0	1	0	1	0	0	0	1	0	0	0	1	0	1	**12**
	Total																						**Mean**
15	13	14	14	11	12	8	9	12	10	14	1	14	9	2	1	5	0	12	8	7	3	4	12.2

Animal studies are key to dissecting the mechanisms underlying the health benefits of a LGI diet, but it seems isolating the effect of postprandial glycaemia while controlling for other physiological properties of LGI foods is not widespread. The glycaemic potential of most foods is indicated by starch digestibility and glucose absorption from the gut. A number of things could affect the GI including: type of starch, fibre viscosity, the food matrix, cooking, processing and macronutrient composition. The majority of articles in this review based their GI diets on the percentages of amylose or amylopectin in the starch. It has been reported that the commonly used low GI Hi-Maize amylose starch contains up to 60% RS [59]. RS reduces the available energy density of the diet and may have important effects on gut hormone secretion as it modifies the motility of the gastrointestinal tract and interacts with the gut microbiome. RS represents energy that is consumed but not available to the host, and would explain reports of increased energy content in faecal output in LGI fed animals [29,32,42]. Several articles also used RS and a control of a HGI starch. However, during the search for articles, we did not include a search term specific to RS as this review aimed to isolate articles that tested diets with differing GI, rather than RS content. This was regardless of the fact that many articles seemed to view these two concepts as synonymous. However, based on the premise for a systematic review, any articles that met the criteria were included in this review regardless of the RS content of their diets. It is important to note that most of the LGI diets contained RS at levels that could not be achieved in human diets, which may be a differentiator of human and animal studies.

There is no standard for GI testing in animals. As shown in the MQA, only eight mouse and five rat papers showed some difference in the GI of the diets, with most others merely assuming a difference in GI based on differing levels of RS as discussed above, or the GI of the carbohydrate sources as measured in humans. Some studies contained no basis for the high versus low GI diets, other than claiming them to be so. Of the studies that did discuss a proven difference in GI, most conducted a meal tolerance test that has similarities to the standard GI practice in humans, however they were key differences in methodology that showed no study accurately measured GI in vivo. In humans, ten subjects are tested in a cross-over design where they consume the tested meal over 12 min, have their blood glucose tested over the following 2 h, and the AUC compared to an identical test with glucose matched for the amount of carbohydrate in the meal by weight [60]. Three studies examined GI in vitro [34,45,54], which has been shown to be similar to GI measured in vivo in humans [6]. Of these three, one [34] used a reference food of white bread to calculate an approximate GI, another [45] also conducted a meal tolerance test, and the last [54] performed an additional in vivo GI test in rats, but did not state the methodology. Of the eleven papers that performed meal tolerance tests, two [31,50] performed the tests in a cross-over design as would be done in human. Three papers [33,37,50], with two of these from the same study, used a reference food, although one study used glucose in the diet frame as opposed to straight glucose and while the other did test straight glucose, it was compared to the carbohydrate source as opposed to the diet itself. Three provided the diets in terms of carbohydrate content [43,50,55], as is done in humans, as opposed to food weight. Only three papers used at least 10 animals for the test [33,37,45], and the time to eat ranged considerably with two as gavages [55], three eating for 15 min [33,37,45], and the remaining tests having the animals eat for 5 min [32,35,42,43]. Most studies did test the blood glucose over two hours [32,33,35,37,43,50,54,55]. While the meal tolerance tests were able to show a qualitative difference in glycaemic response, without following the standard methodology, particularly in terms of using a glucose reference, the GI could not be quantified for any diet. Regrettably no study examined the GI of standard diets, however, recently in our laboratory we successfully implemented GI testing in mice and found that both chow and high corn starch diets, similar to AIN-93, are actually relatively HGI [61].

Unfortunately, many articles lacked specific details relating to diet composition. We included six articles where the macronutrient content was stated, but not explicated to whether this percentage was of weight or energy [29–31,35,38,40]. Criteria for this review required carbohydrate contribution to energy greater than 50%, and, as protein, fat and carbohydrates have different energy densities, if the given content was of weight, some articles may not have actually met these criteria; accordingly, these articles were excluded. A further article [43] did not state the protein content at all, and it was only through being cited in another paper [44] that this information could be found and the original article [43] included. Future studies should report animal diet ingredients for confirmation that the diets meet all nutritional needs of the animals and enable reproducibility of experimental results.

Only one [46] of the HGI diets was paired with a control that was matched for both digestible macronutrient composition and fibre, including resistant starch, content, but this study had several limitations. Of all studies included in the meta-analysis, it was one of two studies that did not state the starting age of animals, one of only five using females, and was the shortest study overall, with rats exposed to the diet for only two weeks [46]. Of note, the rats from this paper were subjected to electrode induced lesions on the ventromedial nucleus of their hypothalamus, which would severely impact their metabolism [46]. Additionally, as this is a highly invasive surgery, even the sham rats would be significantly and adversely affected.

In the meta-regression, there were considerable differences between the sexes. Of the 30 articles included, five papers detailed experiments on female animals, one of which used mice [34] and four used rats [46,54,55,57]. This makes it difficult to be sure that there is really a sex difference in response to HGI feeding as the data suggest. Traditionally, female animals, as opposed to male, have been thought to present additional variation due to the continually changing hormonal environment through the oestrous cycle. One of the papers that used female rats also used male rats in a parallel experiment, however the sample size for female rats was five times smaller leading to insufficient power [57]. Ideally, equivalent studies should be performed, and results compared, in both sexes of mice and rats as it is becoming increasingly apparent that there are distinct metabolic differences between the sexes [62,63] necessitating the investigation of both sexes in order to gain full understanding of any metabolic factors. The dearth of female studies is most likely a crucial contributor to the lack of significant results for this subgroup for any of the traits.

Several articles did not use conventional animal strains. A "conventional" animal strain refers to those used in the majority of papers, such as C57BL/6 mice, and Albino Wistar or Sprague-Dawley rats, being the most well studied and hence understood. C57BL/6 mice are commonly used in metabolic studies, as they are susceptible to diet-induced obesity and hyperglycaemia. The animals studied within this systematic review that were not deemed "typical" include CBA/T6 [28] and 129S2/SvPas [33] mice, and spontaneously hypertensive [49], and partial pancreatomised [56] rats. The issue with the last is obvious, as any hormones the pancreas produces, not limited to insulin, would be decreased and therefore would alter the entire systemic environment. The experiments from that article [56] involving non-pancreatomised rats were still included in this meta-analysis, as were the experiments involving streptozotocin [45,57], gold thioglucose [28] or leptin [47] injections or surgery to induce lesions on the ventromedial nucleus of the hypothalamus [46] as a sensitivity test showed removing these data did not affect the analytical outcomes. A few studies [43,44,47,48] also involved inserting cannulas into the animals' jugular vein and/or carotid artery but as this is a relatively short surgery and the animals were given sufficient recovery time, the impact on metabolic results should be minimal. All of these animal strains and treatments have the potential to confound any and all results; regardless, results reported in these animals were generally consistent with those reported across most studies in this review. For this reason, as well as the limited number of total studies, it was decided not to investigate the effects broken down by the many different species during the meta-analysis.

The animal age at commencement of study and the length of study varied considerably. Most of the mice studies [32–42,56,57] utilized adult animals, ranging in age from 8 weeks to 16 months at the start of the study, while several rat studies used animals that were 6 weeks old or younger [43–45,47–49,55,56]. Two rat studies did not provide the starting age of animals, thus their developmental state is unknown [46,54]. One of these studies [54] is a study of the maternal effect of diet, so it could be assumed that the rats were mature, but the other [46] gave no age indication, and only lasted for two weeks, thus these rats may not be fully developed even at the completion of the study. Most of the mice studies were relatively long studies, consisting of interventions lasting at least 16 weeks [29,31,32,34–36,38–42] compared to the majority of rat studies lasting only 4–8 weeks, with only four lasting longer than eight weeks [43,44,54,56]. Due to the young age and short length of study, it is possible that the animals in some of these experiments [30,43,45–49,52,53,55,56] are still in an adolescence period and hence the results may not reflect the generalized effects of HGI or LGI diets. Indeed, the results of the meta-analysis show that early and longer exposure significantly increase the effect of HGI diets on insulin AUC and fasting glucose, respectively. This should be taken into account when planning a GI animal experiment.

The MQA question on power relied on sample size, hence the eight studies that did not provide sample size [38,40,42,43,46–49,57] received a potentially lower MQA score for this lack of information. Of all 30 articles, only eight had sufficient power [30,31,33,37,44,45,54,55] with a sample size of 14 or greater per group. Most of the studies had a sample size of 8–12, with the smallest sample size of six [36] and highest of 50 [33,37,55,57]. The insufficient replication in the papers with smaller sample sizes is indicative of less reliable results which require further investigation before a valid conclusion can be made and accepted. However, as the calculation for the effect size, and the associated estimate of sampling variance which was included in the analyses, was dependant on the sample size, our analyses accounted for differences among studies arising due to precision. Thus, all studies were included in the meta-analysis to avoid this bias.

Two questions we added to the MQA were regarding use of anaesthetic and fasting time. Most studies refrained from using anaesthesia, with only three studies using anaesthetic during non-terminal blood sampling [34,45,51]. No study used anaesthesia for GTTs. Anaesthesia affects brain metabolism and can affect serum concentrations of circulating proteins and metabolites [64], thus use of anaesthesia for metabolic studies is not desirable as it may impair the accurate measurement of postprandial changes in glucose and metabolic hormones such as insulin. The time frame used for acceptable fasting was 5 h. Excessive fasting, such as overnight for mice or greater than 18 h for rats, can artificially induce larger differences in the data [64]. Increased fasting time was shown to increase the effect of HGI on fasting insulin or insulin AUC to a small or large extent respectively. Fasting insulin was also affected by anaesthesia, with an absence of anaesthesia correlating with a large difference between HGI and LGI fed animals, and those subjected to anaesthesia showing no significant difference between the diets. Thus, use of anaesthesia may mask effects and fasting time may exaggerate effects on glucose metabolism and are important considerations in metabolic studies.

Most of the articles included measured some parameter of glucose homeostasis. The majority measured only blood glucose and insulin levels, with a few performing GTTs of some form. Only one paper conducted a euglycaemic clamp [48]; however, the findings are questionable given that the insulin levels reported were too high for animal survival, with a peak at 4200 pmol/L [48] compared with a typical peak being an average of 1200 pmol/L [65–67]. Additionally, the glucose metabolism calculations in this paper were not physiological [48]. All results in this paper therefore, must be seen as questionable.

The two articles by Van Schothorst et al. [33,37] contained one study, split over two papers. While the results were not duplicated as such, the continuation of a single study across the two articles is worth noting since it leads to a replication of similar findings included in this review from the two papers. The only relevant trait discussed in the latter paper [37], body weight, was already reported for the larger group of mice in the first article [33] and so was not included in the meta-analysis to avoid duplication.

5. Conclusions

This is the first systematic review and meta-analysis of the effects of GI on rodent metabolism. A HGI diet fed to male mice and rats increases body weight, adiposity, fasting insulin levels, and the AUCs for glucose and insulin levels during a GTT, to a greater extent than a LGI diet. There are too few studies in female animals to be confident of effects; future experiments should at least include females, if not specifically investigate the effects of GI diets in females given that the maternal nutritional environment is critical for the development of chronic diseases later in life. From these articles, it is difficult to conclude whether the beneficial health effects of a LGI diet are due to alterations in postprandial glycaemia per se, as dietary composition was considerably variable, particularly with respect to digestible macronutrient composition, fibre and resistant starch.

Acknowledgments: The method and approach for this review were based on those of Ainge et al. 2011 [13] with assistance from the author Kieron Rooney. We thank Kieron Rooney, Jennie Brand-Miller and Damien Belobrajdic for providing critical reviews of this manuscript. This research received no specific grant from any funding agency, commercial or not-for-profit sectors.

Author Contributions: G.J.C. and K.S.B.-A. conceived, designed and performed the experiments; G.J.C. and A.M.S. analysed the data; and G.J.C. and K.S.B.-A. wrote the paper. All authors have read and approved the final manuscript.

Abbreviations

AIN	American Institute of Nutrition
AUC	area under curve
CI	confidence interval
df	degrees of freedom
DS	digestible starch
GI	glycaemic index
GTT	glucose tolerance test
HGI	high glycaemic index
LGI	low glycaemic index
MQA	methodological quality assessment
QI	quality index
RDS	rapidly digestible starch
REMA	random-effects meta-analysis
REMR	random-effects meta-regression
RQ	respiratory quotient
RS	resistant starch
SDS	slowly digestible starch

References

1. World Health Organization. *Overweight and Obesity*; WHO Press Global Health Observatory: Geneva, Switzerland, 2013.
2. Mann, J.; Cummings, J.H.; Englyst, H.N.; Key, T.; Liu, S.; Riccardi, G.; Summerbell, C.; Uauy, R.; van Dam, R.M.; Venn, B.; et al. FAO/WHO scientific update on carbohydrates in human nutrition: Conclusions. *Eur. J. Clin. Nutr.* **2007**, *61* (Suppl. S1), S132–S137. [CrossRef] [PubMed]
3. Trumbo, P.; Schlicker, S.; Yates, A.A.; Poos, M. Dietary reference intakes for energy, carbohydrate, fiber, fat, fatty acids, cholesterol, protein and amino acids. *J. Am. Diet. Assoc.* **2002**, *102*, 1621–1630. [CrossRef]
4. World Health Organization. *Guideline: Sugars Intake for Adults and Children*; WHO Press: Geneva, Switzerland, 2015.
5. Seal, C.J.; Nugent, A.P.; Tee, E.S.; Thielecke, F. Whole-grain dietary recommendations: The need for a unified global approach. *Br. J. Nutr.* **2016**, *115*, 2031–2038. [CrossRef] [PubMed]
6. Englyst, K.N.; Englyst, H.N.; Hudson, G.J.; Cole, T.J.; Cummings, J.H. Rapidly available glucose in foods: An in vitro measurement that reflects the glycemic response. *Am. J. Clin. Nutr.* **1999**, *69*, 448–454. [PubMed]
7. McCleary, B.V. Dietary fibre analysis. *Proc. Nutr. Soc.* **2003**, *62*, 3–9. [CrossRef] [PubMed]

8. Jenkins, D.J.A.; Kendall, C.W.C.; Augustin, L.S.A.; Franceschi, S.; Hamidi, M.; Marchie, A.; Jenkins, A.L.; Axelsen, M. Glycemic index: Overview of implications in health and disease. *Am. J. Clin. Nutr.* **2002**, *76*, 266S–273S. [PubMed]
9. Jenkins, D.J.A.; Wolever, T.M.S.; Taylor, R.H. Glycemic index of foods: A physiological basis for carbohydrate exchange. *Am. J. Clin. Nutr.* **1981**, *34*, 362–366. [PubMed]
10. Mackowiak, K.; Torlinska-Walkowiak, N.; Torlinska, B. Dietary fibre as an important constituent of the diet. *Postepy Higieny i Medycyny Doswiadczalnej* **2016**, *70*, 104–109. [CrossRef]
11. Brand-Miller, J.; Hayne, S.; Petocz, P.; Colagiuri, S. Low-glycemic index diets in the management of diabetes: A meta-analysis of randomized controlled trials. *Diabetes Care* **2003**, *26*, 2261–2267. [CrossRef] [PubMed]
12. Wolever, T.M.S.; Jenkins, D.J.A.; Vuksan, V.; Jenkins, A.L.; Buckley, G.C.; Wong, G.S.; Josse, R.G. Beneficial effect of a low glycaemic index diet in type 2 diabetes. *Diabet. Med.* **1992**, *9*, 451–458. [CrossRef] [PubMed]
13. Ainge, H.; Thompson, C.; Ozanne, S.E.; Rooney, K.B. A systematic review on animal models of maternal high fat feeding and offspring glycaemic control. *Int. J. Obes.* **2011**, *35*, 325–335. [CrossRef] [PubMed]
14. Higgins, J.; Green, S. *Cochrane Handbook for Systematic Reviews of Interventions*; Version 5.0.2; The Cochrane Collaboration: London, UK, 2009.
15. Goettsch, M. Comparative protein requirement of the rat and mouse for growth, reporduction and lactation using casein diets. *J. Nutr.* **1960**, *70*, 307–312.
16. Sheehan, P.M.; Clevidence, B.A.; Reynolds, L.K.; Thye, F.W.; Ritchey, S.J. Carcass nitrogen as a predictor of protein requirement for mature female rats. *J. Nutr.* **1981**, *111*, 1224–1230. [PubMed]
17. White, B.D.; Porter, M.H.; Martin, R.J. Effects of age on the feeding response to moderately low dietary protein in rats. *Physiol. Behav.* **2000**, *68*, 673–681. [CrossRef]
18. Nakagawa, S.; Poulin, R.; Mengersen, K.; Reinhold, K.; Engqvist, L.; Lagisz, M.; Senior, A.M.; O'Hara, R.B. Meta-analysis of variation: Ecological and evolutionary applications and beyond. *Methods Ecol. Evol.* **2015**, *6*, 143–152. [CrossRef]
19. R Core Team. *R: A Language and Environment for Statistical Computing*; R Foundation for Statistical Computing: Vienna, Austria, 2016.
20. Viechtbauer, W. Conducting meta-analyses in R with the metafor package. *J. Stat. Softw.* **2010**, *36*, 1–48. [CrossRef]
21. Besson, A.A.; Lagisz, M.; Senior, A.M.; Hector, K.L.; Nakagawa, S. Effect of maternal diet on offspring coping styles in rodents: A systematic review and meta-analysis. *Biol. Rev. Camb. Philos. Soc.* **2016**, *91*, 1065–1080. [CrossRef]
22. Nakagawa, S.; Noble, D.W.; Senior, A.M.; Lagisz, M. Meta-evaluation of meta-analysis: Ten appraisal questions for biologists. *BMC Biol.* **2017**, *15*, 18. [CrossRef] [PubMed]
23. Noble, D.W.; Lagisz, M.; O'Dea R, E.; Nakagawa, S. Nonindependence and sensitivity analyses in ecological and evolutionary meta-analyses. *Mol. Ecol.* **2017**, *26*, 2410–2425. [CrossRef] [PubMed]
24. Seehra, J.; Pandis, N.; Koletsi, D.; Fleming, P.S. Use of quality assessment tools in systematic reviews was varied and inconsistent. *J. Clin. Epidemiol.* **2015**, *69*, 179–184.e5. [CrossRef] [PubMed]
25. Nakagawa, S.; Santos, E.S.A. Methodological issues and advances in biological meta-analysis. *Evol. Ecol.* **2012**, *26*, 1253–1274. [CrossRef]
26. Downs, S.; Black, N. The feasibility of creating a checklist for the assessment of the methodological quality both of randomised and non-randomised studies of health care interventions. *J. Epidemiol. Community Health* **1998**, *52*, 377–384. [CrossRef] [PubMed]
27. Faul, F.; Erdfelder, E.; Buchner, A.; Lang, A.G. Statistical power analyses using G*power 3.1: Tests for correlation and regression analyses. *Behav. Res. Methods* **2009**, *41*, 1149–1160. [CrossRef] [PubMed]
28. Walker, C.G.; Bryson, J.M.; Phuyal, J.L.; Caterson, I.D. Dietary modulation of circulating leptin levels: Site-specific changes in fat deposition and ob mRNA expression. *Horm. Metab. Res.* **2002**, *34*, 176–181. [CrossRef] [PubMed]
29. Scribner, K.B.; Pawlak, D.B.; Ludwig, D.S. Hepatic steatosis and increased adiposity in mice consuming rapidly vs. slowly absorbed carbohydrate. *Obesity* **2007**, *15*, 2190–2199. [CrossRef]
30. So, P.W.; Yu, W.S.; Kuo, Y.T.; Wasserfall, C.; Goldstone, A.P.; Bell, J.D.; Frost, G. Impact of resistant starch on body fat patterning and central appetite regulation. *PLoS ONE* **2007**, *2*, e1309. [CrossRef] [PubMed]
31. Scribner, K.B.; Pawlak, D.B.; Aubin, C.M.; Majzoub, J.A.; Ludwig, D.S. Long-term effects of dietary glycemic index on adiposity, energy metabolism, and physical activity in mice. *Am. J. Physiol. Endocrinol. Metab.* **2008**, *295*, E1126–E1131. [CrossRef] [PubMed]

32. Isken, F.; Weickert, M.O.; Tschöp, M.H.; Nogueiras, R.; Möhlig, M.; Abdelrahman, A.; Klaus, S.; Thorens, B.; Pfeiffer, A.F. Metabolic effects of diets differing in glycaemic index depend on age and endogenous glucose-dependent insulinotrophic polypeptide in mice. *Diabetologia* **2009**, *52*, 2159–2168. [CrossRef]
33. Van Schothorst, E.M.; Bunschoten, A.; Schrauwen, P.; Mensink, R.P.; Keijer, J. Effects of a high-fat, low- versus high-glycemic index diet: Retardation of insulin resistance involves adipose tissue modulation. *FASEB J.* **2009**, *23*, 1092–1101. [CrossRef]
34. Andersson, U.; Rosén, L.; Wierup, N.; Östman, E.; Björck, I.; Holm, C. A low glycaemic diet improves oral glucose tolerance but has no effect on β-cell function in C57BL/6J mice. *Diabetes Obes. Metab.* **2010**, *12*, 976–982. [CrossRef] [PubMed]
35. Isken, F.; Klaus, S.; Petzke, K.J.; Loddenkemper, C.; Pfeiffer, A.F.H.; Weickert, M.O. Impairment of fat oxidation under high- vs. Low-glycemic index diet occurs before the development of an obese phenotype. *Am. J. Physiol. Endocrinol. Metab.* **2010**, *298*, E287–E295. [CrossRef] [PubMed]
36. Colbert Coate, K.; Huggins, K.W. Consumption of a high glycemic index diet increases abdominal adiposity but does not influence adipose tissue pro-oxidant and antioxidant gene expression in C57BL/6 mice. *Nutr. Res.* **2010**, *30*, 141–150. [CrossRef] [PubMed]
37. Van Schothorst, E.M.; Bunschoten, A.; Verlinde, E.; Schrauwen, P.; Keijer, J. Glycemic index differences of high-fat diets modulate primarily lipid metabolism in murine adipose tissue. *Physiol. Genom.* **2011**, *43*, 942–949. [CrossRef] [PubMed]
38. Uchiki, T.; Weikel, K.A.; Jiao, W.; Shang, F.; Caceres, A.; Pawlak, D.; Handa, J.T.; Brownlee, M.; Nagaraj, R.; Taylor, A. Glycation-altered proteolysis as a pathobiologic mechanism that links dietary glycemic index, aging, and age-related disease (in nondiabetics). *Aging Cell* **2012**, *11*, 1–13. [CrossRef] [PubMed]
39. Weikel, K.A.; FitzGerald, P.; Shang, F.; Andrea Caceres, M.; Bian, Q.; Handa, J.T.; Stitt, A.W.; Taylor, A. Natural history of age-related retinal lesions that precede amd in mice fed high or low glycemic index diets. *Investig. Ophthalmol. Vis. Sci.* **2012**, *53*, 622–632. [CrossRef] [PubMed]
40. Birarda, G.; Holman, E.A.; Fu, S.; Weikel, K.; Hu, P.; Blankenberg, F.G.; Holman, H.Y.; Taylor, A. Synchrotron infrared imaging of advanced glycation endproducts (AGEs) in cardiac tissue from mice fed high glycemic diets. *Biomed. Spectrosc. Imaging* **2013**, *2*, 301–315. [PubMed]
41. Rowan, S.; Weikel, K.; Chang, M.L.; Nagel, B.A.; Thinschmidt, J.S.; Carey, A.; Grant, M.B.; Fliesler, S.J.; Smith, D.; Taylor, A. Cfh genotype interacts with dietary glycemic index to modulate age-related macular degeneration-like features in mice. *Investig. Ophthalmol. Vis. Sci.* **2014**, *55*, 492–501. [CrossRef] [PubMed]
42. Kleckner, A.S.; Wong, S.; Corkey, B.E. The intra- or extracellular redox state was not affected by a high vs. Low glycemic response diet in mice. *PLoS ONE* **2015**, *10*, e0128380. [CrossRef] [PubMed]
43. Byrnes, S.E.; Miller, J.C.B.; Denyer, G.S. Amylopectin starch promotes the development of insulin resistance in rats. *J. Nutr.* **1995**, *125*, 1430–1437. [PubMed]
44. Higgins, J.A.; Brand Miller, J.C.; Denyer, G.S. Development of insulin resistance in the rat is dependent on the rate of glucose absorption from the diet. *J. Nutr.* **1996**, *126*, 596–602. [PubMed]
45. Lerer-Metzger, M.; Rizkalla, S.W.; Luo, J.; Champ, M.; Kabir, M.; Bruzzo, F.; Bornet, F.; Slama, G. Effects of long-term low-glycaemic index starchy food on plasma glucose and lipid concentrations and adipose tissue cellularity in normal and diabetic rats. *Br. J. Nutr.* **1996**, *75*, 723–732. [CrossRef] [PubMed]
46. Suga, A.; Hirano, T.; Kageyama, H.; Osaka, T.; Namba, Y.; Tsuji, M.; Miura, M.; Adachi, M.; Inoue, S. Effects of fructose and glucose on plasma leptin, insulin, and insulin resistance in lean and VMH-lesioned obese rats. *Am. J. Physiol. Endocrinol. Metab.* **2000**, *278*, E677–E683. [PubMed]
47. Widdup, G.; Bryson, J.M.; Pawlak, D.; Phuyal, J.L.; Denyer, G.S.; Caterson, I.D. In vivo and in vitro suppression by leptin of glucose-stimulated insulin hypersecretion in high glucose-fed rats. *Eur. J. Endocrinol.* **2000**, *143*, 431–437. [CrossRef] [PubMed]
48. Pawlak, D.B.; Bryson, J.M.; Denyer, G.S.; Brand-Miller, J.C. High glycemic index starch promotes hypersecretion of insulin and higher body fat in rats without affecting insulin sensitivity. *J. Nutr.* **2001**, *131*, 99–104. [PubMed]
49. Kopilas, M.A.; Dang, L.N.T.; Anderson, H.D.I. Effect of dietary chromium on resistance artery function and nitric oxide signaling in the sucrose-fed spontaneously hypertensive rat. *J. Vasc. Res.* **2007**, *44*, 110–118. [CrossRef] [PubMed]
50. Aziz, A.A.; Kenney, L.S.; Goulet, B.; Abdel-Aal, E.S. Dietary starch type affects body weight and glycemic control in freely fed but not energy-restricted obese rats. *J. Nutr.* **2009**, *139*, 1881–1889. [CrossRef] [PubMed]

51. Belobrajdic, D.P.; King, R.A.; Christophersen, C.T.; Bird, A.R. Dietary resistant starch dose-dependently reduces adiposity in obesity-prone and obesity-resistant male rats. *Nutr. Metab.* **2012**, *9*, 93. [CrossRef] [PubMed]
52. Ble-Castillo, J.L.; Aparicio-Trapala, M.A.; Juárez-Rojop, I.E.; Torres-Lopez, J.E.; Mendez, J.D.; Aguilar-Mariscal, H.; Olvera-Hernández, V.; Palma-Cordova, L.C.; Diaz-Zagoya, J.C. Differential effects of high-carbohydrate and high-fat diet composition on metabolic control and insulin resistance in normal rats. *Int. J. Environ. Res. Public Health* **2012**, *9*, 1663–1676. [CrossRef] [PubMed]
53. Stavrovskaya, I.G.; Bird, S.S.; Marur, V.R.; Sniatynski, M.J.; Baranov, S.V.; Greenberg, H.K.; Porter, C.L.; Kristal, B.S. Dietary macronutrients modulate the fatty acyl composition of rat liver mitochondrial cardiolipins. *J. Lipid Res.* **2013**, *54*, 2623–2635. [CrossRef] [PubMed]
54. Gugusheff, J.; Sim, P.; Kheng, A.; Gentili, S.; Al-Nussairawi, M.; Brand-Miller, J.; Muhlhausler, B. The effect of maternal and post-weaning low and high glycaemic index diets on glucose tolerance, fat deposition and hepatic function in rat offspring. *J. Dev. Orig. Health Dis.* **2015**, *7*, 320–329. [CrossRef] [PubMed]
55. Thompson, H.J.; Neuhouser, M.L.; Lampe, J.W.; McGinley, J.N.; Neil, E.S.; Schwartz, Y.; McTiernan, A. Effect of low or high glycemic load diets on experimentally induced mammary carcinogenesis in rats. *Mol. Nutr. Food Res.* **2016**, *60*, 1416–1426. [CrossRef] [PubMed]
56. Pawlak, D.B.; Kushner, J.A.; Ludwig, D.S. Effects of dietary glycaemic index on adiposity, glucose homoeostasis, and plasma lipids in animals. *Lancet* **2004**, *364*, 778–785. [CrossRef]
57. Zhou, J.; Martin, R.J.; Tulley, R.T.; Raggio, A.M.; McCutcheon, K.L.; Shen, L.; Danna, S.C.; Tripathy, S.; Hegsted, M.; Keenan, M.J. Dietary resistant starch upregulates total GLP-1 and PYY in a sustained day-long manner through fermentation in rodents. *Am. J. Physiol. Endocrinol. Metab.* **2008**, *295*, E1160–E1166. [CrossRef] [PubMed]
58. Reeves, P.G.; Nielsen, F.H.; Fahey, G.C., Jr. AIN-93 purified diets for laboratory rodents: Final report of the American institute of nutrition ad hoc writing committee on the reformulation of the AIN-76A rodent diet. *J. Nutr.* **1993**, *123*, 1939–1951. [PubMed]
59. Le Leu, R.K.; Hu, Y.; Brown, I.L.; Young, G.P. Effect of high amylose maize starches on colonic fermentation and apoptotic response to DNA-damage in the colon of rats. *Nutr. Metab.* **2009**, *6*, 11. [CrossRef] [PubMed]
60. Wolever, T.M.; Jenkins, D.J.; Jenkins, A.L.; Josse, R.G. The glycemic index: Methodology and clinical implications. *Am. J. Clin. Nutr.* **1991**, *54*, 846–854. [CrossRef] [PubMed]
61. Campbell, G.J.; Bell-Anderson, K.S. GI testing of standard and high sugar rodent diets in vivo in C57BL/6 mice. Unpublished work, **2017**.
62. Hedrington, M.S.; Davis, S.N. Sexual dimorphism in glucose and lipid metabolism during fasting, hypoglycemia, and exercise. *Front. Endocrinol.* **2015**, *6*, 61. [CrossRef] [PubMed]
63. Ter Horst, K.W.; Gilijamse, P.W.; de Weijer, B.A.; Kilicarslan, M.; Ackermans, M.T.; Nederveen, A.J.; Nieuwdorp, M.; Romijn, J.A.; Serlie, M.J. Sexual dimorphism in hepatic, adipose tissue, and peripheral tissue insulin sensitivity in obese humans. *Front. Endocrinol.* **2015**, *6*, 182. [CrossRef] [PubMed]
64. Passonneau, J.V.; Brunner, E.A.; Molstad, C.; Passonneau, R. The effects of altered endocrine states and of ether anaesthesia on mouse brain. *J. Neurochem.* **1971**, *18*, 2317–2328. [CrossRef] [PubMed]
65. Gauna, C.; Uitterlinden, P.; Kramer, P.; Kiewiet, R.M.; Janssen, J.A.; Delhanty, P.J.; van Aken, M.O.; Ghigo, E.; Hofland, L.J.; Themmen, A.P.; et al. Intravenous glucose administration in fasting rats has differential effects on acylated and unacylated ghrelin in the portal and systemic circulation: A comparison between portal and peripheral concentrations in anesthetized rats. *Endocrinology* **2007**, *148*, 5278–5287. [CrossRef] [PubMed]
66. Kassis, N.; Bernard, C.; Pusterla, A.; Casteilla, L.; Penicaud, L.; Richard, D.; Ricquier, D.; Ktorza, A. Correlation between pancreatic islet uncoupling protein-2 (UCP2) mRNA concentration and insulin status in rats. *Int. J. Exp. Diabetes Res.* **2000**, *1*, 185–193. [CrossRef] [PubMed]
67. McArthur, M.D.; You, D.; Klapstein, K.; Finegood, D.T. Glucose effectiveness is the major determinant of intravenous glucose tolerance in the rat. *Am. J. Physiol.* **1999**, *276*, E739–E746. [PubMed]

8

Efficacy of a Moderately Low Carbohydrate Diet in a 36-Month Observational Study of Japanese Patients with Type 2 Diabetes

Mariko Sanada [1], Chinatsu Kabe [1], Hisa Hata [1], Junichi Uchida [1], Gaku Inoue [1], Yoko Tsukamoto [1], Yoshifumi Yamada [2], Junichiro Irie [3], Shogo Tabata [1], Mitsuhisa Tabata [1] and Satoru Yamada [1,*]

1 Kitasato Institute Hospital, Diabetes Center, 5-9-1 Shirokane, Minato-ku, Tokyo 108-0072, Japan; mrksmd@insti.kitasato-u.ac.jp (M.S.); kabe@insti.kitasato-u.ac.jp (C.K.); h-izumi@insti.kitasato-u.ac.jp (H.H.); uchida-j@insti.kitasato-u.ac.jp (J.U.); inoueg@pharm.kitasato-u.ac.jp (G.I.); tsuka-y@insti.kitasato-u.ac.jp (Y.T.); sky_walker_718@a6.keio.jp (S.T.); mitsutabata@gmail.com (M.T.)

2 Boei Ika Daigakko Boei Igagku Kenkyu Center, 3-2 Namiki, Tokorozawa, Saitama 359-0042, Japan; yamayoshi0718@yahoo.co.jp

3 School of Medicine, Keio University, Internal Medicine, 35 Shinanomachi, Shinjuku, Tokyo 160-8582, Japan; j-irie@z8.keio.jp

* Correspondence: yamada-s@insti.kitasato-u.ac.jp

Abstract: We previously showed that a non-calorie-restricted, moderately low-carbohydrate diet (mLCD) is more effective than caloric restriction for glycemic and lipid profile control in patients with type 2 diabetes. To determine whether mLCD intervention is sustainable, effective, and safe over a long period, we performed a 36-month observational study. We sequentially enrolled 200 patients with type 2 diabetes and taught them how to follow the mLCD. We compared the following parameters pre- and post-dietary intervention in an outpatient setting: glycated hemoglobin (HbA1c), body weight, lipid profile (total cholesterol, low and high-density lipoprotein cholesterol, triglycerides), systolic and diastolic blood pressure, liver enzymes (aspartate aminotransferase, alanine aminotransferase), and renal function (urea nitrogen, creatinine, estimated glomerular filtration rate). Data from 157 participants were analyzed (43 were lost to follow-up). The following parameters decreased over the period of study: HbA1c (from 8.0 ± 1.5% to 7.5 ± 1.3%, $p < 0.0001$) and alanine aminotransferase (from 29.9 ± 23.6 to 26.2 ± 18.4 IL/L, $p = 0.009$). Parameters that increased were high-density lipoprotein cholesterol (from 58.9 ± 15.9 to 61.2 ± 17.4 mg/dL, $p = 0.001$) and urea nitrogen (from 15.9 ± 5.2 to 17.0 ± 5.4 mg/dL, $p = 0.003$). Over 36 months, the mLCD intervention showed sustained effectiveness (without safety concerns) in improving HbA1c, lipid profile, and liver enzymes in Japanese patients with type 2 diabetes.

Keywords: low-carbohydrate diet; type 2 diabetes mellitus; observational study

1. Introduction

The most recent dietary guidelines of the American Diabetes Association (ADA) emphasize that no single diet is suitable for all people with diabetes, and likewise there is no ideal macronutrient balance [1]. Several dietary approaches have been proposed in Western countries for people with diabetes [1,2], with guidelines recommending that individuals discuss with health professionals (physicians and dietitians) which approach would be preferable, most effective, and sustainable for them.

Recently, the Japanese Diabetes Society relaxed their dietary approach, recommending a caloric restriction of 25–35 kcal/kg ideal body weight with carbohydrates composing 50–60% of total energy consumption. No other dietary approach is currently approved by the Japanese Diabetes Society guidelines [3]. In an endeavor to make dietary approaches more flexible and sustainable for diabetes patients in Japan, in August 2009 we adopted a non-calorie restricted, moderately low-carbohydrate diet (mLCD) with the approval of the Institutional Ethical Review Board of our hospital in Tokyo, Japan. In a randomized clinical trial, we found this mLCD to be more effective than caloric restriction for glycemic and lipid profile control in patients with type 2 diabetes [4]. However, this trial was limited to six months in duration. To evaluate the long-term efficacy and safety of mLCD as a sustainable dietary therapy and to check for rebound effects (which are common in dietary studies [5]), we conducted a 36-month observational study of patients with diabetes following our mLCD.

2. Materials and Methods

We retrospectively enrolled 200 patients with type 2 diabetes who received outpatient treatment in Kitasato Institute Hospital, Tokyo, Japan between August 2009 and October 2016. Participants were instructed to restrict their carbohydrate intake to 20–40 g per meal and 70–130 g per day, with 10 g of carbohydrates consumed as a snack or drink at least once daily. Although we did not recommend any percentage of carbohydrate, fat, and protein to total caloric intake, it was 30:45:20 in our previous study [4]. A dietary salt restriction intervention was also performed on patients for whom it was deemed appropriate. Patients who injected insulin were recommended to monitor their capillary glucose levels frequently after mLCD was initiated.

At the first nutritional intervention and at six-month intervals thereafter, we measured the following: glycated hemoglobin (HbA1c), body weight, lipid profile (total cholesterol (TC), low-density lipoprotein cholesterol (LDL-C), high-density lipoprotein cholesterol (HDL-C), triglyceride (TG)), blood pressure (systolic blood pressure (SBP), diastolic blood pressure (DBP)), liver enzymes (aspartate aminotransferase (AST), alanine aminotransferase (ALT)), and renal function (urea nitrogen (UN), uric acid (UA), creatinine (Cr), estimated glomerular filtration rate (eGFR)). We also recorded the incidence of hypoglycemia (defined as self-monitored blood glucose levels less than 70 mg/dL, with or without hypoglycemic symptoms) for 2 months before the first intervention and for 2-month intervals during the intervention, and calculated the corresponding before/after ratios. Missing values were replaced with values obtained during the previous or following two months.

To investigate the interactions between response to the mLCD and participant baseline HbA1c level or body mass index (BMI, kg/m^2), we conducted post hoc analyses. In one analysis, we classified participants according to their change in HbA1c during the 36 months of dietary intervention as follows: responder (decrease in HbA1c), unchanged (no change in HbA1c), or worsened (increase in HbA1c). In other analyses, we classified participants according to their baseline HbA1c (HbA1c $< 7\%$, $7\% \leq$ HbA1c $< 8\%$, $8\% \leq$ HbA1c $< 9\%$, or $9\% \leq$ HbA1c) or BMI (BMI < 25, $25 \leq$ BMI < 30, or $30 \leq$ BMI).

Values are presented as the mean $\pm$ standard deviation (SD). Statistical analyses were performed using IBM SPSS 19 software (IBM Japan, Tokyo, Japan). We compared baseline and 36-month parameter values using the Wilcoxon signed-rank test. Multiple comparisons were made as appropriate using two-way analysis of variance (ANOVA).

This study was approved by the institutional review board of Kitasato Institution Hospital and performed in accordance with the Declaration of Helsinki. Informed consent was obtained in the form of an opt-out, by posting notices requesting that diabetes patients who had received guidance about low carbohydrate diets inform us if they did not want their records to be used for research purposes. This consent process was approved by the ethical review board at Kitasato Institution Hospital. All participants' anonymity is preserved. This study was registered as clinical trial ID UMIN000022910.

3. Results

The characteristics of the 200 patients enrolled are shown in Table 1. Of these, 43 participants were lost to follow-up during the 36-month study period. The most common reasons for drop-out were a discontinuation of visits to our hospital (n = 24) and referral to general physicians (n = 15). The other four participants lost to follow-up died (two from myocardial infarction, one from cardiac arrest, and one from a head injury). There were no differences in the baseline characteristics between the 43 patients who dropped out and the remaining 157.

Table 1. Baseline characteristics of the study participants

	All Participants	Retained	Lost to Follow-Up
n	200	157	43
Female/Male	71/129	51/106	20/23
Age	59.7 ± 12.9	59.5 ± 12.4	60.5 ± 13.9
BMI (kg/m^2)	26.4 ± 4.9	26.6 ± 4.7	25.4 ± 5.1
FPG (mg/dL)	151 ± 57	153 ± 58	145 ± 50
HbA1c (%)	8.0 ± 1.5	8.0 ± 1.5	8.0 ± 1.5
TG (mg/dL)	147 ± 120	147 ± 121	144 ± 106
LDL-C (mg/dL)	116 ± 33	116 ± 33	121 ± 45
HDL-C (mg/dL)	60 ± 17	59 ± 16	62 ± 21
BP (mmHg)	128 ± 15/76 ± 12	128 ± 15/77 ± 12	127 ± 16/72 ± 12

Values are the mean ± standard deviation. BMI, body mass index; FPG, fasting plasma glucose; HbA1c, glycated hemoglobin; TG, triglyceride; LDL-C, low-density lipoprotein cholesterol; HDL-C, high-density lipoprotein cholesterol; BP, blood pressure.

Among the 157 patients, HbA1c levels had improved (decreased) in 104 participants (i.e., the responder rate was 66.2%), remained unchanged in 10 participants, and worsened (increased) in 43 patients at 36 months after first mLCD intervention. From baseline to 36 months, there were statistically significant improvements in HbA1c (decrease), DBP (decrease), TC (decrease), LDL-C (increase), and ALT (decrease) (Table 2). For HbA1c levels, the improvement occurred during the first 6 months and was maintained through 36 months (Figures 1 and 2). The UN level increased significantly over 36 months, while Cr and eGFR showed no change. No significant changes were observed during the study period for body weight, HDL-C, TG, SBP, AST, or UA (Table 2). The record of hypoglycemic agents showed that the number of participants taking insulin injections and/or sulfonylureas did not change during the study period. As for dosage, the mean total daily dose of insulin per person decreased from 29.9 units at the start of the intervention to 23.6 units at 36 months post-intervention. The mean dose of glimepiride (which all sulfonylurea users were prescribed) per person also decreased, from 1.39 mg at the start of the intervention to 1.11 mg at 36 months. Participants who reduced their insulin and/or glimepiride dosage started taking metformin and/or dipeptidyl peptidase-4 inhibitors instead. Thus, the number of participants taking metformin and dipeptidyl peptidase-4 inhibitors increased during the 36 months (from 71 to 89 and 48 to 93, respectively).

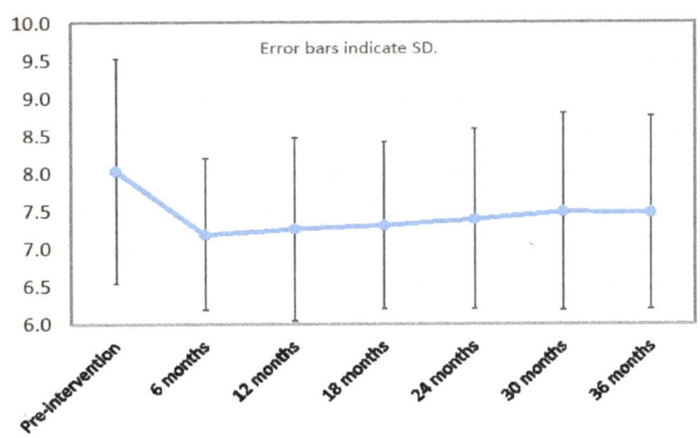

Figure 1. HbA1c level (%). Error bars indicate standard deviation (n = 157).

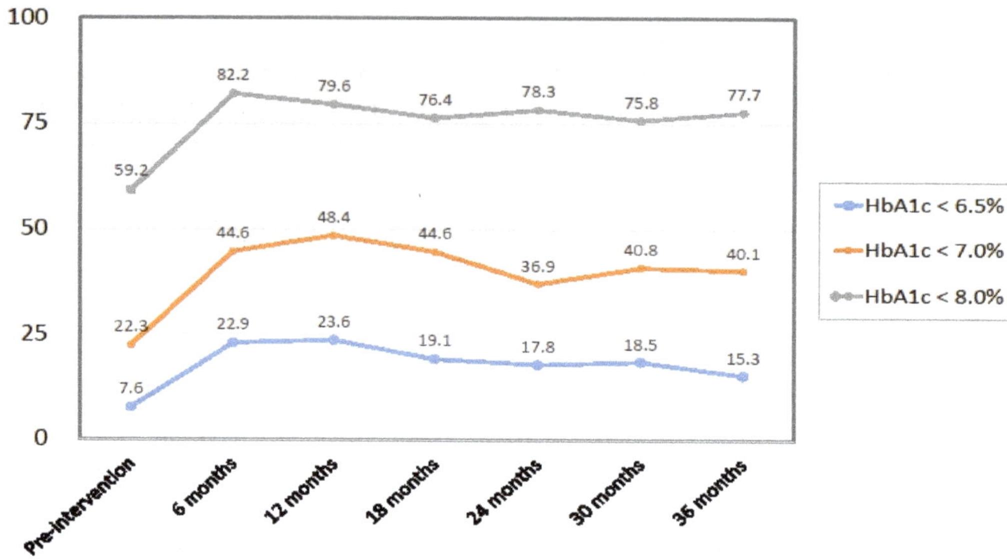

Figure 2. Percentage of patients who reached target HbA1c levels (%).

During the 36 months, there was also an increase in the prescription of anti-hyperlipidemic agents. Thus, we performed a last-observation carried forward (LOCF) analysis on lipid profiles using the values when anti-hyperlipidemic agents were started or when their dosages increased. This analysis showed that LOCF TC improved, and LOCF TG worsened (Table 2).

Table 2. Changes in the outcome measures of study participants on a moderately low-carbohydrate diet over 36 months.

	Pre-Intervention		12 Months	24 Months	36 Months	*p* Value
Body weight (kg)	72.5 ± 15.2		71.6 ± 14.9	72.0 ± 15.0	71.9 ± 15.1	n.s.
FBS (mg)	153.1 ± 58.0		143.3 ± 47.2	144.4 ± 48.6	140.6 ± 43.5	n.s.
SBP (mmHg)	127.7 ± 15.4		125.8 ± 13.3	127.1 ± 13.1	125.0 ± 13.1	n.s.
DBP (mmHg)	76.8 ± 11.8		74.8 ± 10.9	75.4 ± 9.5	74.5 ± 10.6	0.029
HbA1c (%)	8.0 ± 1.5		7.3 ± 1.2	7.4 ± 1.2	7.5 ± 1.3	<0.0001
TC (mg/dL)	200.7 ± 44.1		194.0 ± 39.0	192.8 ± 32.9	189.9 ± 33.3	0.003
LDL-C (mg/dL)	116.1 ± 33.0		107.2 ± 28.2	108.1 ± 26.7	106.7 ± 26.9	<0.0001
HDL-C (mg/dL)	59.0 ± 15.9		61.7 ± 16.7	61.2 ± 16.9	59.8 ± 18.3	n.s.
TG (mg/dL)	146.6 ± 120.7		142.7 ± 137.4	141.2 ± 102.9	152.5 ± 122.2	n.s.
LOCF TC (mg/dL)	200.8 ± 44.1		196.2 ± 40.3	196.2 ± 35.9	189.9 ± 33.3	0.0007
LOCF LDL-C (mg/dL)	116.1 ± 33.0		109.0 ± 29.7	110.6 ± 29.7	106.7 ± 26.9	n.s.
LOCF HDL-C (mg/dL)	59.1 ± 15.9		61.4 ± 16.4	61.3 ± 16.7	59.8 ± 18.3	n.s.
LOCF TG (mg/dL)	146.5 ± 120.7		147.7 ± 139.6	144.7 ± 113.6	152.5 ± 122.2	0.02
AST (IU/L)	26.6 ± 13.3		24.2 ± 10.8	25.1 ± 11.7	26.4 ± 13.6	n.s.
ALT (IU/L)	29.9 ± 23.6		23.4 ± 15.3	25.1 ± 18.5	26.2 ± 18.4	0.009
Cr (mg/dL)	0.8 ± 0.2		0.8 ± 0.2	0.8 ± 0.2	0.8 ± 0.2	0.046
eGFR (mL/(min·1.73 m^2))	74.4 ± 18.8		73.6 ± 19.2	73.1 ± 19.0	72.1 ± 20.8	0.007
UA (mg/dL)	5.8 ± 1.4		5.9 ± 1.4	5.9 ± 1.4	6.0 ± 1.7	n.s.
UN (mg/dL)	15.8 ± 5.0		17.5 ± 6.2	16.8 ± 5.0	17.0 ± 5.5	0.002
ACR (mg/g Cr)	196.6 ± 828.0		123.6 ± 517.1	166.4 ± 515.1	123.3 ± 287.4	n.s.
Urinary protein	(−)*	91 (58%)	102 (65%)	92 (59%)	99 (63%)	n.s. †
	(+/−)*	38 (24%)	38 (24%)	40 (25%)	31 (20%)	
	(1+) *	20 (13%)	14 (9%)	17 (11%)	23 (15%)	
	(2+) *	8 (5%)	3 (2%)	8 (5%)	4 (2%)	

† Result of a chi-square test. Values are the mean ± standard deviation or number (percentage) of participants. * Although urinary protein test is qualitative, these content were similar with below; (−) 10 mg/dL, (+/−) 10–20 mg/dL, (1+) 100 mg/dL, (2+) 300 mg/dL. FBS, fasting blood sugar; SBP, systolic blood pressure; DBP, diastolic blood pressure; HbA1c, glycated hemoglobin; TC, total cholesterol; LDL-C, low-density lipoprotein cholesterol; HDL-C, high-density lipoprotein cholesterol; TG, triglyceride; LOCF, last-observation carried forward; AST, aspartate aminotransferase; ALT, alanine aminotransferase; Cr, creatinine; eGFR, estimated glomerular filtration rate; UA, uric acid; UN, urea nitrogen; ACR, albumin to creatinine ratio (from random spot urine sampling); n.s., not significant.

Of the 43 participants receiving insulin, 31 maintained blood glucose self-monitoring records. Among these 31 participants, the incidence of hypoglycemia was 1.46% before the introduction of mLCD, which then increased to a maximum of 2.43% for 1–2 months after the first intervention. Several months later, the incidence of hypoglycemia stabilized at approximately 1.0% (Table 3).

Table 3. Incidence of hypoglycemia in the 31 participants who received insulin and maintained blood glucose self-monitoring records while on a moderately low-carbohydrate diet for 36 months.

2-Month Pre-Intervention Period	1 to 2 Months	3 to 4 Months	5 to 6 Months	7 to 8 Months	9 to 10 Months	11 to 12 Months
31/2121 (1.46%)	73/3010 (2.43%)	60/2887 (2.08%)	39/2387 (1.63%)	49/2709 (1.81%)	53/2367 (2.24%)	17/2098 (0.81%)
	13 to 14 months	15 to 16 months	17 to 18 months	19 to 20 months	21 to 22 months	23 to 24 months
	44/2698 (1.63%)	26/2634 (0.99%)	26/2544 (1.02%)	12/2347 (0.51%)	30/2430 (1.23%)	20/2562 (0.78%)
	25 to 26 months	27 to 28 months	29 to 30 months	31 to 32 months	33 to 34 months	35 to 36 months
	19/2361 (0.80%)	26/2657 (0.98%)	23/2609 (0.88%)	33/2711 (1.22%)	44/2748 (1.60%)	31/3066 (1.01%)

Values are the number of hypoglycemic readings/total number of readings (percent incidence of hypoglycemia).

To identify characteristics of participants who responded to the mLCD, we classified the 157 participants according to their change in HbA1c levels from baseline to 36 months as either responders, unchanged non-responders, or worsened non-responders. At baseline, the responders were younger and had higher HbA1c levels than the other two groups (Table 4). We also classified participants according to their baseline HbA1c levels and found that the HbA1c $\geq$ 9% group had the greatest improvement in HbA1c (Figure 3). On the other hand, the ALT $\geq$ 9% group had the greatest improvement in ALT. Change in body weight was independent of baseline HbA1c.

Table 4. Baseline characteristics of participants classified as responders or non-responders according to their change in HbA1c levels over the 36-month study period.

Characteristic	All (n = 157)	Responders (n = 109)	Non-Responders	
			Worsened (n = 41)	Unchanged (n = 7)
Age (years)	59.5	57.7	63.8	62.6
BMI (kg/m^2)	26.6	26.9	26.2	25.3
FPG (mg/dL)	153	159	144	116
HbA1c (%)	8.0	8.3	7.4	7.0
TG (mg/dL)	147	159	119	112
LDL-C (mg/dL)	116	118	112	115
HDL-C (mg/dL)	59.0	56.9	61.8	76.6
BP (mmHg)	128/77	128/78	128/74	122/72
Dietary education sessions	2.2	2.3	2.2	2.1
Disease duration (years)	10.0	9.7	10.6	11.3

Values are the means. BMI, body mass index; FPG, fasting plasma glucose; HbA1c, glycated hemoglobin; TG, triglyceride; LDL-C, low-density lipoprotein cholesterol; HDL-C, high-density lipoprotein cholesterol; BP, blood pressure.

We then classified the participants according to baseline BMI. While HbA1c decreased independently of baseline BMI level, the change in body weight across the study period differed between BMI groups. While participants with a baseline BMI < 25 showed sustained body weight, and those with BMI $\geq$ 25 showed a decrease in body weight (Figure 4).

Although two participants experienced myocardial infarction and died, there was no incidence of stroke, peripheral artery disease, renal dysfunction, or liver dysfunction among the participants in this study. The two patients who died from myocardial infarction had a 10+ year history of diabetes and presented multiple risk factors including hypertension, type IIb dyslipidemia, obesity, and a history of smoking.

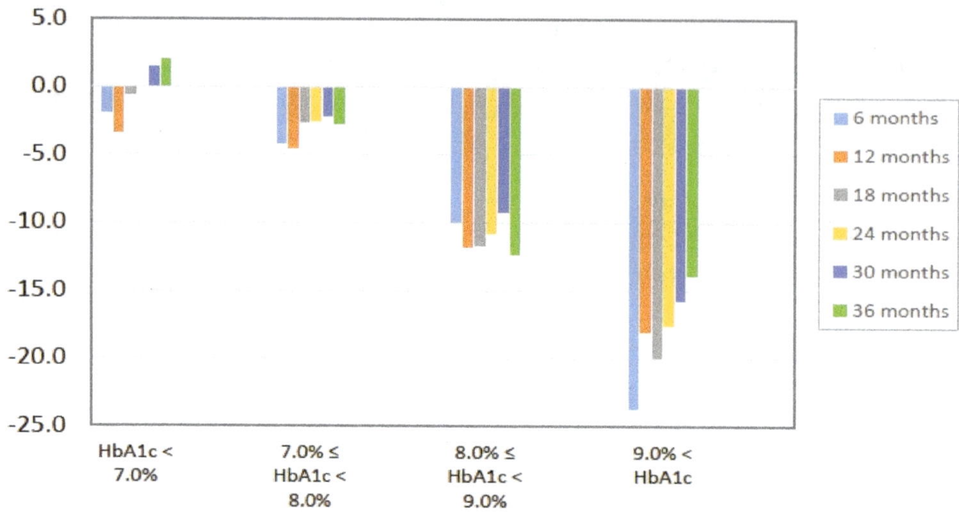

Figure 3. Percent changes in HbA1c stratified by baseline HbA1c (%).

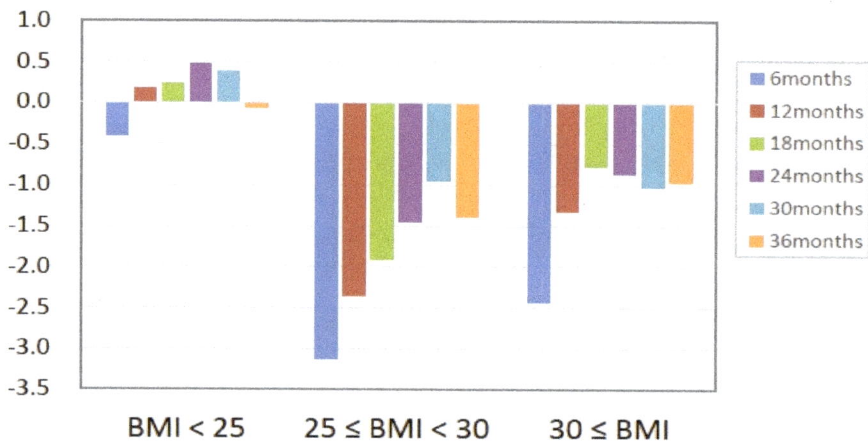

Figure 4. Absolute changes in body weight stratified by baseline BMI (kg).

4. Discussion

This study has three noteworthy aspects. First, this study is a long-term (36 months) observational study on a dietary approach for diabetes. To the best of our knowledge, this is the first long-term observational study on such a diet in East Asians. This moderately low-carbohydrate diet improved HbA1c levels within the first 6 months and then maintained that improvement for 36 months. According to the recently published ADA Standards of Medical Care [6], the effects of low-carbohydrate diets remain unclear because any improvements by such a diet tend to occur on a short-term basis and are not maintained. As described by the ADA, the wide range of definitions for a low-carbohydrate diet have created confusion. According to our current data, the improvements caused by a moderately low-carbohydrate diet can be maintained. Furthermore, the fact that East Asians have traditionally consumed a high-carbohydrate diet may explain the finding that a moderately low-carbohydrate diet is effective in reducing HbA1c in this population.

Second, we found that a moderately low-carbohydrate diet improved HbA1c levels without causing undernutrition in non-obese patients with diabetes. Previous dietary approaches for diabetes have been considered successful if they result in weight loss. While this may be acceptable for white and black patients with type 2 diabetes, almost all of whom are obese [7,8], such diets might cause undernutrition in East Asians who develop diabetes in the absence of obesity [9]. In fact, there have been almost no studies of East Asians consuming a Mediterranean diet or the DASH diet. The CALERIE trial indicated that caloric restrictions cause loss of muscle and bone mineral density in non-obese individuals [10,11]. Thus, a moderately low-carbohydrate diet might be a safe dietary approach for East Asians or diabetics who are not obese.

Third, our findings indicate the safety of a moderately low-carbohydrate diet. Diminished kidney function and a worse lipid profile are common concerns with a restricted carbohydrate diet [12]. In the current study, there were statistically significant changes in kidney function (eGFR; from 74.4 ± 18.8 to 72.1 ± 20.8 (mL/(min·1.73 m^2)) during 36 months) and lipid profiles, but those changes were either not clinically significant. As for kidney function it may represent improvements compared with previous data, which have shown an annual eGFR decline of 0.7–2.0 mL/(min·1.73 m^2) in diabetic patients [13,14]. In addition, the frequency of hypoglycemia increased in our patients using a sulfonylurea or insulin, but those patients recovered once the dose of that medication was adjusted. We therefore conclude that a moderately low-carbohydrate diet is a highly safe diet.

As for low-carbohydrate diets, there is a controversy whether high fat or high protein is more beneficial. Most of previous studies of low-carbohydrate diets were high fat and Feinman et al. described high fat as being recommended in general [15]. However, meta-analysis of Clifton et al. showed the importance of protein [16]. Our current study did not provide any information to this controversy.

This study has several limitations. Because this was an observational study and it did not compare subjects to a control group, bias, and confounding factors cannot be ruled out. In addition, the sample size of 200 patients precluded any examination of the effects of the low-carbohydrate diet on cancer or dementia.

In conclusion, we have shown that a moderately low-carbohydrate diet is highly effective, safe, and sustainable. To address the study's limitations, large-scale long-term randomized controlled trials should be conducted in the future.

Acknowledgments: This study was funded by a Kitasato Institute Hospital Research Grant (Grant No. 8125).

Author Contributions: M.S. analyzed the data and wrote the manuscript. J.U., H.H. and C.K. conceived and designed the experiments. Y.Y., J.I., S.T. and M.T. performed the experiments. G.I. and Y.T. analyzed the data. S.Y. conceived and designed the experiments, performed the experiments, and analyzed the data.

References

1. Evert, A.B.; Boucher, J.L.; Cypress, M.; Dunbar, S.A.; Franz, M.J.; Mayer-Davis, E.J.; Neumiller, J.J.; Nwankwo, R.; Verdi, C.L.; Urbanski, P.; et al. Nutrition therapy recommendations for the management of adults with diabetes. *Diabetes Care* **2013**, *36*, 3821–3842. [CrossRef] [PubMed]
2. Ley, S.H.; Hamdy, O.; Mohan, V.; Hu, F.B. Prevention and management of type 2 diabetes: Dietary components and nutritional strategies. *Lancet* **2014**, *383*, 1999–2007. [CrossRef]
3. Tajima, N.; Noda, M.; Origasa, H.; Noto, H.; Yabe, D.; Fujita, Y.; Goto, A.; Fujimoto, K.; Sakamoto, M.; Haneda, M. Evidence-based practice guideline for the treatment for diabetes in Japan 2013. *Diabetol. Int.* **2015**, *6*, 151–187. [CrossRef]
4. Yamada, Y.; Uchida, J.; Izumi, H.; Tsukamoto, Y.; Inoue, G.; Watanabe, Y.; Irie, J.; Yamada, S. A non-calorie-restricted low-carbohydrate diet is effective as an alternative therapy for patients with type 2 diabetes. *Intern. Med.* **2014**, *53*, 13–19. [CrossRef] [PubMed]
5. Banasik, J.L.; Walker, M.K.; Randall, J.M.; Netjes, R.B.; Foutz, M.S. Low-calorie diet induced weight loss may alter regulatory hormones and contribute to rebound visceral adiposity in obese persons with a family history of type-2 diabetes. *J. Am. Assoc. Nurse Pract.* **2013**, *25*, 440–448. [CrossRef] [PubMed]
6. American Diabetes Association. Lifestyle management: Standards of medical care in diabetes-2018. *Diabetes Care* **2018**, *41*, S38–S50. [CrossRef]
7. Looker, H.C.; Knowler, W.C.; Hanson, R.L. Changes in BMI and weight before and after the development of type 2 diabetes. *Diabetes Care* **2001**, *24*, 1917–1922. [CrossRef] [PubMed]
8. De Fine Olivarius, N.; Richelsen, B.; Siersma, V.; Andreasen, A.H.; Beck-Nielsen, H. Weight history of patients with newly diagnosed Type 2 diabetes. *Diabet. Med.* **2008**, *25*, 933–941. [CrossRef] [PubMed]

9. Heianza, Y.; Arase, Y.; Kodama, S.; Tsuji, H.; Saito, K.; Hara, S.; Sone, H. Trajectory of body mass index before the development of type 2 diabetes in Japanese men: Toranomon Hospital Health Management Center Study 15. *J. Diabetes Investig.* **2015**, *6*, 289–294. [CrossRef] [PubMed]
10. Villareal, D.T.; Fontana, L.; Das, S.K.; Redman, L.; Smith, S.R.; Saltzman, E.; Bales, C.; Rochon, J.; Pieper, C.; Huang, M.; et al. Effect of two-year caloric restriction on bone metabolism and bone mineral density in non-obese younger adults: A randomized clinical trial. *J. Bone Miner. Res.* **2016**, *31*, 40–51. [CrossRef] [PubMed]
11. Das, S.K.; Roberts, S.B.; Bhapkar, M.V.; Villareal, D.T.; Fontana, L.; Martin, C.K.; Racette, S.B.; Fuss, P.J.; Kraus, W.E.; Wong, W.W.; et al. Body-composition changes in the Comprehensive Assessment of Long-term Effects of Reducing Intake of Energy (CALERIE)-2 study: A 2-y randomized controlled trial of calorie restriction in nonobese humans. *Am. J. Clin. Nutr.* **2017**, *105*, 913–927. [CrossRef] [PubMed]
12. American Diabetes Association; Bantle, J.P.; Wylie-Rosett, J.; Albright, A.L.; Apovian, C.M.; Clark, N.G.; Franz, M.J.; Hoogwerf, B.J.; Lichtenstein, A.H.; Mayer-Davis, E.; et al. Nutrition recommendations and interventions for diabetes: A position statement of the American Diabetes Association. *Diabetes Care* **2008**, *31*, S61–S78. [CrossRef] [PubMed]
13. Araki, S.; Haneda, M.; Koya, D.; Isshiki, K.; Kume, S.; Sugimoto, T.; Kawai, H.; Nishio, Y.; Kashiwagi, A.; Uzu, T. Association between urinary type IV collagen level and deterioration of renal function in type 2 diabetic patients without overt proteinuria. *Diabetes Care* **2010**, *33*, 1805–1810. [CrossRef] [PubMed]
14. Araki, S.; Haneda, M.; Koya, D.; Sugaya, T.; Isshiki, K.; Kume, S.; Kashiwagi, A.; Uzu, T.; Maegawa, H. Predictive effects of urinary liver-type fatty acid-binding protein for deteriorating renal function and incidence of cardiovascular disease in type 2 diabetic patients without advanced nephropathy. *Diabetes Care* **2013**, *36*, 1248–1253. [CrossRef] [PubMed]
15. Feinman, R.D.; Pogozelski, W.K.; Astrup, A.; Bernstein, R.K.; Fine, E.J.; Westman, E.C.; Accurso, A.; Frassetto, L.; Gower, B.A.; McFarlane, S.I.; et al. Dietary carbohydrate restriction as the first approach in diabetes management. *Nutrition* **2015**, *31*, 1–13. [CrossRef] [PubMed]
16. Clifton, P.M.; Condo, D.; Keogh, J.B. Long term weight maintenance after advice to consume low carbohydrate, higher protein diets. *Nutr. Metab. Cardiovasc. Dis.* **2014**, *24*, 224–235. [CrossRef] [PubMed]

9

Prebiotic Dietary Fiber and Gut Health: Comparing the in Vitro Fermentations of Beta-Glucan, Inulin and Xylooligosaccharide

Justin L. Carlson [1,†], Jennifer M. Erickson [1,†], Julie M. Hess [1], Trevor J. Gould [2] and Joanne L. Slavin [1,*]

1 Department of Food Science and Nutrition, University of Minnesota, 1334 Eckles Ave, St. Paul, MN 55108, USA; carl2814@umn.edu (J.L.C.); eric2472@umn.edu (J.M.E.); jmhess@umn.edu (J.M.H.)

2 Informatics Institute, University of Minnesota, 101 Pleasant St., Minneapolis, MN 55455, USA; goul0109@umn.edu

* Correspondence: jslavin@umn.edu

† Authors contributed equally to this work.

Abstract: Prebiotic dietary fiber supplements are commonly consumed to help meet fiber recommendations and improve gastrointestinal health by stimulating beneficial bacteria and the production of short-chain fatty acids (SCFAs), molecules beneficial to host health. The objective of this research project was to compare potential prebiotic effects and fermentability of five commonly consumed fibers using an in vitro fermentation system measuring changes in fecal microbiota, total gas production and formation of common SCFAs. Fecal donations were collected from three healthy volunteers. Materials analyzed included: pure beta-glucan, Oatwell (commercially available oat-bran containing 22% oat β-glucan), xylooligosaccharides (XOS), WholeFiber (dried chicory root containing inulin, pectin, and hemi/celluloses), and pure inulin. Oatwell had the highest production of propionate at 12 h (4.76 μmol/mL) compared to inulin, WholeFiber and XOS samples ($p < 0.03$). Oatwell's effect was similar to those of the pure beta-glucan samples, both samples promoted the highest mean propionate production at 24 h. XOS resulted in a significant increase in the genus *Bifidobacterium* after 24 h of fermentation (0 h:0.67 OTUs (operational taxonomic unit); 24 h:5.22 OTUs; $p = 0.038$). Inulin and WholeFiber increased the beneficial genus *Collinsella*, consistent with findings in clinical studies. All analyzed compounds were fermentable and promoted the formation of beneficial SCFAs.

Keywords: prebiotic; microbiota; fermentation; dietary fiber; microbiome

---

1. Introduction

Prebiotic definitions vary among different scientific and political arenas across the world [1]. Depending on the local definition, nearly all prebiotics can be classified as dietary fiber, but not all fibers are considered prebiotics [2]. The most recent definition describes a prebiotic as "a substrate that is selectively utilized by host microorganisms conferring a health benefit" [3]. Functional characteristics of prebiotics include the ability to: resist the low pH of the stomach, resist hydrolysis by mammalian enzymes, resist absorption in the upper gastrointestinal tract, the ability to be fermented by intestinal microbiota and selectively stimulate the growth and/or activity of intestinal bacteria associated with host health and overall well-being [4,5]. Inulin, beta-glucans, and xylooligosaccharides all provide health benefits to consumers that are related to the fermentation of these compounds in the distal gastrointestinal tract, and are also considered functional fibers with many other benefits [6]. As the definition of "prebiotic" broadens to include the overall impact from the metabolism from these compounds, the category of prebiotics will expand [7]. The importance of displaying direct health benefits due to bacterial fermentation is still the driving mechanism for all prebiotics.

As our awareness and understanding of the importance of the gut microbiome and gut microbiota increases, it is imperative for consumers to understand the key differences between different forms of prebiotics, and where they can be found in various foods and food products. XOS is an emerging prebiotic with well-displayed, consistent health benefits [8] and is composed of sugar oligomers composed of xylose units [9], found naturally in fruits, vegetables, milk, honey and bamboo shoots. XOS is commonly produced from xylan containing lignocellulosic materials through various chemical methods, direct enzymatic hydrolysis, or a combination of both treatments [10–14]. Inulin is a heterogeneous blend of fructose polymers (degree of polymerization, DP < 10) [15] which occurs naturally in thousands of plant species, including wheat, onion, bananas, garlic and chicory [16]. Beta-glucan is a polysaccharide composed of D-glucose monomers with beta-glycosidic linkages, present in either linear chains in grains, such as oat and barley (up to 7%), or in branched structures in fungi, yeast and certain bacteria [17]. These prebiotics, or prebiotic mixtures, each provide a unique carbon source for selective stimulation of different bacterial taxa and are important microbiota-shaping compounds.

Because no analytical method currently exists to measure the prebiotic capacity of foods in terms of their influence on gastrointestinal taxa, this field relies heavily on fecalbiotics (living or once living fecal microbial populations) to quantify the effects of these compounds. In vitro fermentation models allow for quantitative analysis of specific materials and are semi-representative models of colonic fermentation [18]. Although not a complete substitute for human studies, when paired with in vivo models, in vitro analysis can be an accurate systematic approach to analyzing different parameters and end points in colonic fermentation [19].

With the recent release of the International Scientific Association for Probiotics and Prebiotics consensus statement, XOS has been categorized as a prebiotic or prebiotic candidate [3]. The prebiotic effects of XOS have previously been summarized by Broekaert et al. [20]. While there is less evidence supporting the prebiotic effects of XOS compared to other types of prebiotics, studies have shown that XOS supplementation in humans can increase SCFA and bifidobacteria, as well as improve stool consistency and frequency [21–23]. This paper compares the fermentation effects of XOS to previously established prebiotics (inulin and beta-glucans) in a controlled in vitro model. To the authors' knowledge, this is the first controlled in vitro study comparing the effects of XOS to these known prebiotics. The objective of this project was to compare currently available prebiotics by their ability to change specific taxa as well as compare differences in the production of gas and common short chain fatty acids (SCFA) between these products. Inulin, XOS and beta-glucan based products were chosen for this experiment because they are established and emerging prebiotics that are commonly consumed, and offer well-demonstrated health benefits to their consumers.

2. Materials and Methods

2.1. Prebiotic Dietary Fibers Analyzed

Five common prebiotic dietary fibers were chosen for this study (Table 1), including different types of beta-glucans, inulin and xylooligosaccharide supplements.

Table 1. Comparison Prebiotic Dietary Fibers Analyzed with in vitro Fermentation System.

Prebiotic Dietary Fibers	Supplier Information
OatWell (Oatbran containing 28% beta-glucan)	DSM Nutritional Products, Ltd. (Kaiseraugust, Switzerland)
WholeFiber (A dried chicory root blend containing: inulin, pectin, hemi/cellulose)	WholeFiber, Inc. (Pennington, NJ, USA)
Xylooligosaccharide (XOS)	AIDP, Inc. (Industry, CA, USA)
Pure Inulin	Cargill, Inc. (Wayzata, MN, USA)
Pure Beta-glucan	Megazyme, Inc. (Bray, Wicklow, Ireland)

2.2. Donor Information

Fecal samples were collected from three healthy volunteers (2 males, 1 female) under anaerobic conditions. Donors included individuals (ages 22–28) consuming non-specific Western diets, who do not consume any supplements, including fiber supplements. Donors were non-smokers, did not receive any antibiotic treatments in the last year, and were not affected by any known gastrointestinal diseases (Table 2).

Table 2. Demographic Characteristics of Three Fecal Donors.

Demographic characteristics	Donor 1	Donor 2	Donor 3
Age	26	25	22
Sex	Female	Male	Male
Body Mass Index (kg/m^2)	28.1	26.3	23.0

2.3. Fecal Collection

Fecal samples were anaerobically collected within 5 min of the start of the fermentation (Medline Specimen Collection Kit, Medline, Inc., Rogers, MN, USA), and homogenized immediately upon collection. All data and samples collected were done in accordance with University of Minnesota policies and procedures.

2.4. Fermentation

The fiber samples were fermented using in vitro methods to mimic the environment of the distal colon. These methods have been used in previous in vitro studies, including Koecher et al., who found complementary results between these in vitro methods and a human intervention study of the same fibers [24]. Fiber samples (0.5 g) were hydrated in 40 mL of prepared sterile trypticase peptone fermentation media in 100 mL serum bottles, capped, and incubated for 12 h at 4 °C to limit possibility of microbial growth [25]. Following incubation, serum bottles were transferred to a circulating water bath at 37 °C for 2 h to allow the samples to reach body temperature. Post-collection, fecal samples were mixed using a 6:1 ratio of phosphate buffer solution to fecal sample. After mixing, obtained fecal slurry was combined with prepared reducing solution (2.52 g cysteine hydrochloride, 16 mL 1 N NaOH, 2.56 g sodium sulfide nonanhydride, 380 mL DD H_2O) at a 2:15 ratio. 10 mL of the prepared fecal inoculum was added to each of the serum bottles, 0.8 mL Oxyrase® was added, flushed with CO_2, sealed, and then immediately placed in a 37 °C circulating water bath. Fecal inoculum control samples with no fiber added were prepared for SCFA and gas production comparison. Baseline pH of the fermentation media was measured, with a mean of 6.83 ± 0.04, to mimic the environment of the distal colon. Samples were prepared in triplicate and analyzed at 0, 12 and 24 h. Upon removal at each time point, total gas volume was measured. Then samples were divided into aliquots for analysis and 1 mL of copper sulfate (200 g/L) was added to cease fermentation. All samples were immediately frozen and stored at −80 °C for further analysis.

2.5. SCFA Analysis

SCFA samples were extracted according to Schneider et al. [26] with minor modifications, and analyzed with previously described methods [27].

2.6. DNA Extractions

Fecal bacteria DNA from the in vitro system were extracted using a PowerSoil DNA Isolation Kit (Mo Bio Laboratories, Inc., Carlsbad, CA, USA) following the provided operating instruction, including bead beating for 20 min.

2.6.1. Primary/Secondary Amplification

The V1-V3 region of the 16S rRNA was amplified using a two-step PCR protocol. The primary amplification was done using an ABI7900 qPCR machine (Applied Biosystems, Foster City, CA, USA). The following recipe was used: 3 μL template DNA, 0.48 μL nuclease-free water, 1.2 μL 5× KAPA HiFi buffer (Kapa Biosystems, Woburn, MA, USA), 0.18 μL 10 mM dNTPs (Kapa Biosystems, Woburn, MA, USA), 0.3 μL DMSO (Fisher Scientific, Waltham, MA, USA), 0.12 μL ROX (25 μM) (Life Technologies, Carlsbad, CA, USA), 0.003 μL 1000× SYBR Green, 0.12 μL KAPA HiFi Polymerase (Kapa Biosystems, Woburn, MA, USA), 0.3 μL forward primer (10 μM), 0.3 μL reverse primer (10 μM). Cycling conditions were: 95 °C for 5 min, followed by 20 cycles of 98 °C for 20 s, 55 °C for 15 s, and 72 °C for 1 min. The primers for the primary amplification contained both 16S-specific primers (V1_27F and V3_V34R), as well as adapter tails for adding indices and Illumina flow cell adapters in a secondary amplification. The following primers were used (16S-specific sequences in bold): Meta_V1_27F (TCGTCGGCAGCGTCAGATGTGTATAAGAGACAGAGAGTTTGATCMTGGCTCAG) and Meta_V3_534R (GTCTCGTGGGCTCGGAGATGTGTATAAGAGACAGATTACCGCGGCTGCTGG).

The amplicons from the primary PCR were diluted 1:100 in sterile, nuclease-free water, and a second PCR reaction was set up to add the Illumina flow cell adapters (Illumina Inc., San Diego, CA, USA) and indices. The secondary amplification was done on a fixed block BioRad Tetrad PCR machine (Bio-Rad Laboratories, Inc., Hercules, CA, USA) using the following recipe: 5 μL template DNA, 1 μL nuclease-free water, 2 μL 5× KAPA HiFi buffer (Kapa Biosystems, Woburn, MA, USA), 0.3 μL 10 mM dNTPs (Kapa Biosystems, Woburn, MA, USA), 0.5 μL DMSO (Fisher Scientific, Waltham, MA, USA) 0.2 μL KAPA HiFi Polymerase (Kapa Biosystems, Woburn, MA, USA), 0.5 μL forward primer (10 μM), 0.5 μL reverse primer (10 μM). Cycling conditions were: 95 °C for 5 min, followed by 10 cycles of 98 °C for 20 s, 55 °C for 15 s, 72 °C for 1 min, followed by a final extension at 72 °C for 10 min. The following indexing primers were used (X indicates the positions of the 8 bp indices): Forward indexing primer: AATGATACGGCGACCACCGAGATCTACACXXXXXXXXTCGTCGGCAGCGTC and Reverse indexing primer: CAAGCAGAAGACGGCATACGAGATXXXXXXXXGTCTCGTGGGCTCGG.

2.6.2. Normalization and Sequencing

The samples were normalized using a SequalPrep capture-resin bead plate (Life Technologies, Carlsbad, CA, USA) and pooled using equal volume. The final pools were quantified via PicoGreen dsDNA assay (Life Technologies, Carlsbad, CA, USA) and diluted to 2 nM. 10 μL of the 2 nM pool was denatured with 10 μL of 0.2 N NaOH, diluted to 8 pM in Illumina's HT1 buffer, spiked with 15% phiX, heat denatured at 96 °C for 2 min, and sequenced using a MiSeq 600 cycle v3 kit (Illumina, San Diego, CA, USA).

2.6.3. Sequence Processing and Analysis

Generated sequence data was processed and analyzed using QIIME [28]. Fastq sequence data was processed with the University of Minnesota's gopher-pipeline for metagenomics [29]. Sequence data had adapters removed and sliding quality trimming window by Trimmomatic [30]; primers removed and overlapping reads merged by Pandaseq [31]. Within QIIME, chimera checking done by chimera slayer, Open reference OTU picking completed with Usearch61, taxonomic identification using GreenGenes (Version 13.8) reference database, rarefied to 14,393 sequences per sample. Analysis was performed using *R* (*R* Development Core Team, Vienna, Austria, 2012).

2.7. Statistical Analysis

All statistical analysis was performed using *R* software (Version 3.2.2, *R* Development Core Team, Vienna, Austria, 2012). Differences in means were determined using the Kruskal-Wallis ANOVA test, testing the null hypothesis that the location parameter of the groups of abundancies for a given OTU is the same. Multiple comparisons were corrected using the Benjamini-Hochberg

FDR (false discovery rate) procedure for multiple comparisons. For gas and SCFA data, ANOVA with Tukey HSD was used to compare means. Significance was set for p-values < 0.05 for all statistical tests.

2.8. Consent Ethics Approval Code

Voluntary informed consent was obtained from all fecal donors prior to this study according to University of Minnesota policies and procedures.

3. Results

3.1. Gas Production

At 12 h, the OatWell and the pure beta-glucan samples produced similar amounts of total gas (Figure 1). The XOS samples produced significantly more gas than the pure beta glucan samples ($p < 0.01$) or the OatWell samples ($p < 0.01$). The WholeFiber and pure inulin samples produced similar amounts of total gas ($p = 0.102$), and the total gas production for both of these prebiotic dietary fibers was significantly higher than the XOS samples, ($p < 0.01$ and $p = 0.045$), respectively. At 24 h, the OatWell samples had the lowest gas production (46.2 mL) and were similar to the pure beta-glucan samples (63.7 mL; $p = 0.498$). The 24 h XOS samples (74.0 mL) were also similar to the beta-glucan samples ($p = 0.926$). However, the 24 h WholeFiber (109.6 mL) and pure inulin (107.1 mL) samples produced significantly more gas than XOS, beta-glucan and Oatwell samples ($p < 0.01$). Individual variation in gas production can be seen in Table S1.

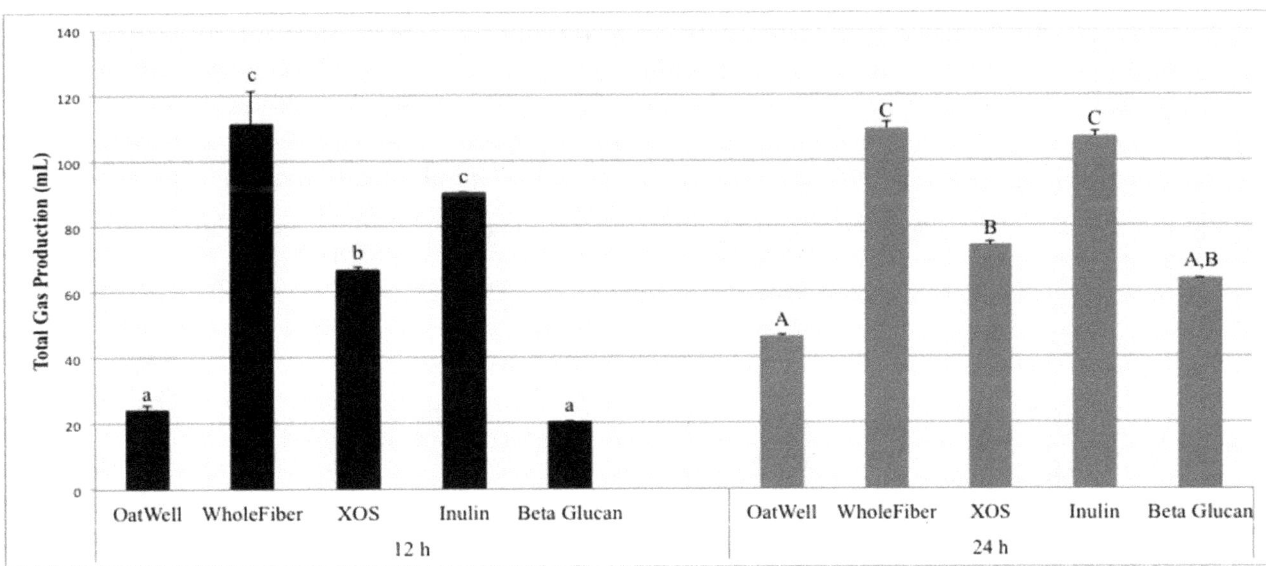

Figure 1. Total gas production comparing fermentation differences among five prebiotic dietary fibers for three individuals at 12 h and 24 h post-exposure to fecal microbiota in an in vitro fermentation system. Data displayed are means (3 donors × 3 replicates = 9) for each prebiotic dietary fiber ± SD. Columns with different letters are significantly different from one another within each time measurement (lowercase: 12 h; uppercase: 24 h). Data were analyzed using ANOVA with Tukey HSD ($p < 0.05$).

3.2. SCFA Production

For all SCFA analysis, analysis at 12 and 24 h shows production only, from baseline corrected samples. Acetate, propionate and butyrate production is shown as μmol/mL of fermentation media. Individual variation in SCFA production can be seen in Table S1.

Acetate production at 12 h was similar for the Oatwell, WholeFiber and beta-glucan samples (Figure 2). The XOS samples produced significantly more acetate at 12 h than the Oatwell, WholeFiber or beta-glucan samples ($p < 0.05$). The inulin samples had similar amounts of acetate compared to the WholeFiber and XOS samples, and significantly more than the Oatwell ($p = 0.024$) and beta-glucan ($p = 0.013$) samples at 12 h. After 24 h, the inulin samples contained less acetate than the XOS samples ($p = 0.038$), while the Oatwell, WholeFiber and beta-glucan samples were similar to both the XOS and inulin samples.

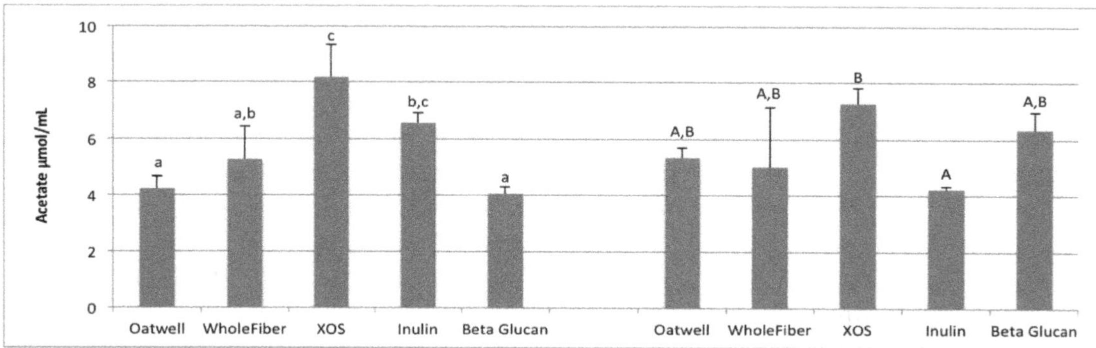

Figure 2. Acetate production at 12 h and 24 h of fermentation for five prebiotic dietary fibers displayed as µmol/mL of fermentation inoculum. Data displayed are means (3 donors × 3 replicates = 9) for each prebiotic dietary fiber ± SD. Columns with different letters are significantly different from one another (lowercase: 12 h; uppercase: 24 h). Data were analyzed using ANOVA with Tukey HSD ($p < 0.05$).

Propionate production at 12 h of fermentation was highest for the OatWell samples (4.76 µmol/mL) and was significantly greater than the WholeFiber ($p = 0.029$), XOS ($p = 0.005$) and inulin samples ($p = 0.004$), and similar to the beta-glucan samples (Figure 3). At 24 h of fermentation, the Oatwell samples had the highest mean production 5.05 µmol/mL, which was significantly greater than the XOS samples (2.58 µmol/mL; $p = 0.021$), and similar to WholeFiber, inulin and beta-glucan samples.

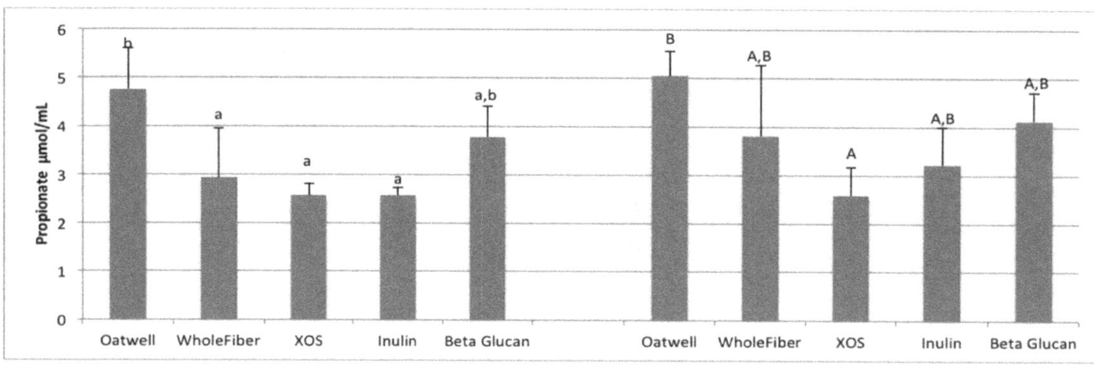

Figure 3. Propionate production at 12 h and 24 h of fermentation for five prebiotic dietary fibers displayed as µmol/mL of fermentation inoculum. Data displayed are means (3 donors × 3 replicates = 9) for each prebiotic dietary fiber ± SD. Columns with different letters are significantly different from one another (lowercase: 12 h; uppercase: 24 h). Data were analyzed using ANOVA with Tukey HSD ($p < 0.05$).

Butyrate production after 12 h of fermentation ranged from 7.30 µmol/mL for the beta-glucan samples to 16.76 µmol/mL for the inulin samples (Figure 4). The inulin samples had the highest average production, and were similar to the XOS (16.38 µmol/mL) and WholeFiber samples (12.89 µmol/mL). The XOS samples were significantly higher than the Oatwell ($p = 0.035$) and beta-glucan samples ($p = 0.014$). At 24 h of fermentation, all five prebiotic dietary fibers were statistically similar to one another, ranging from 7.93–14.08 µmol/mL due to a wide ranges in response differences between the three fecal donors used in this study.

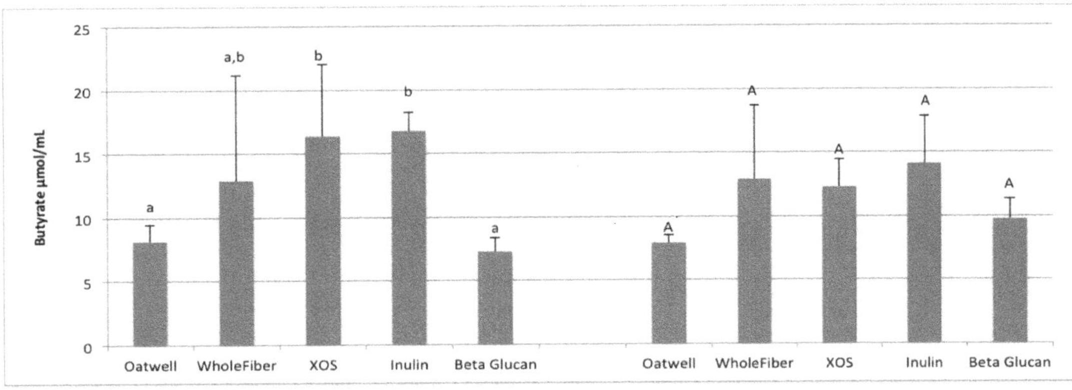

Figure 4. Butyrate production at 12 h and 24 h of fermentation for five prebiotic dietary fibers displayed as µmol/mL of fermentation inoculum. Data displayed are means (3 donors × 3 replicates = 9) for each prebiotic dietary fiber ± SD. Columns with different letters are significantly different from one another (lowercase: 24 h; uppercase: 24 h). Data were analyzed using ANOVA with Tukey HSD ($p < 0.05$).

3.3. Microbiota Analysis

Extracted DNA from in vitro samples were sequenced using the MiSeq Illumina platforms (Illumina Inc., San Diego, CA, USA) generating a total of 31,591,899 sequence reads. Sequencing parameters identified reads belonging to 11 bacterial phyla, 61 families and 97 genera.

For all three donors, the phyla Bacteroidetes and Firmicutes represented > 80% of all sequence reads (Figure S1) across 24 h of fermentation. At the family level, 13 families represented 85% of all sequence reads (Figure S2), while 11 genera represented >75% of all sequence reads (Figure S3). Six metrics measuring α-diversity for all donors showed various degrees of similarity by donors (Figure S4), and by treatment (Figure S5). Both Unifrac and Bray-Curtis β-diversity metrics (measuring pairwise dissimilarity between samples), showed similarity among technical replicates of treatment groups for each donor (Figure S6) as well as for all treatment groups for each respective donor (Figure S7).

After 24 h of fermentation, the Oatwell samples significantly decreased the population of SMB53 (0 h:9.11 OTUs; 24 h:2.11 OTUs; $p = 0.008$), Lachnospira and Faecalibacterium (0 h:26.56 OTUs; 24 h:4.44 OTUs; $p = 0.008$ and 0 h 136.44 OTUs; 24 h:66 OTUs; $p = 0.022$, respectively) (Table 3). No genera analyzed showed significant increases in 24 h for the Oatwell samples measured for the three fecal donors in this study. The WholeFiber samples (Table 4) significantly increased the genus Collinsella at 24 h compared to 0 h (0 h:68 OTUs; 24 h:299.78 OTUs; $p = 0.011$). Bifidobacterium populations were only significantly increased at 24 h compared to 0 h for the XOS samples (0 h:0.67 OTUs; 24 h:5.22 OTUs; $p = 0.038$), while the same samples showed a significant decrease in Lachnospira and Faecalibacterium ($p = 0.038$ and $p = 0.03$) (Table 5). The inulin samples (Table 6) increased Collinsella (0 h:55.11 OTUs; 24 h:291.44 OTUs; $p = 0.016$). The pure beta glucan samples significantly decreased Lachnospira and Faecalibacterium ($p = 0.008$) (Table 7).

Table 3. Combined changes across 24 h of fermentation for Oatwell samples of identified genera [1].

Genera	0 h	24 h	*p*-Value
Actinobacteria			
Bifidobacterium	1.22	0.89	0.660
Adlercreutzia	1.44	3.00	0.470
Collinsella	48.44	140.56	0.089
Bacteroidetes			
Alistipes	2.56	1.33	0.674
Parabacteroides	135.00	155.89	0.952
Bacteroides	755.67	865.00	0.192

Table 3. *Cont.*

Genera	0 h	24 h	*p*-Value
Firmicutes			
Eubacterium	0.44	0.56	0.817
Veillonella	1.11	1.22	0.980
Dorea	2.33	3.56	0.516
Acidaminococcus	3.22	10.44	0.817
Clostridium	7.67	8.33	0.769
Anaerostipes	8.11	6.00	0.674
Turicibacter	8.67	1.22	0.286
SMB53	9.11	2.11	0.008 *
Ruminococcus	11.22	23.22	0.263
Lactococcus	11.67	10.67	0.980
Streptococcus	15.22	8.11	0.511
Roseburia	20.22	22.33	0.980
Oscillospira	21.78	36.67	0.121
Lachnospira	26.56	4.44	0.008 *
Phascolarctobacterium	27.78	173.33	0.263
Dialister	39.56	43.00	0.560
Blautia	41.89	53.11	0.470
Coprococcus	49.89	39.00	0.396
Ruminococcus	61.33	40.67	0.289
Faecalibacterium	136.44	66.00	0.022 *
Proteobacteria			
Escherichia	0.44	1.44	0.325
Haemophilus	10.22	0.67	0.286
Sutterella	10.78	14.44	0.980
Bilophila	13.67	14.78	0.788
Verrucomicrobia			
Akkermansia	5.00	12.00	0.980

[1] Replicate samples were pooled among donor at each respective time point (3 donors × 3 replicated = 9). Samples were analyzed between differentially represented OTUs for significant changes after 24 h of fermentation compared to 0 h samples. Values are the number of OTUs after rarefaction to 3668 sequences per sample. Data were analyzed using the Kruskal-Wallis ANOVA test, with the FDR (false discovery rate) multiple comparisons correction. * Indicates significance at $p \leq 0.05$.

Table 4. Combined changes across 24 h of fermentation for WholeFiber samples of identified genera [1].

Genera	0 h	24 h	*p*-Value
Actinobacteria			
Adlercreutzia	0.89	3.89	0.239
Bifidobacterium	1.11	1.11	0.785
Collinsella	68.00	299.78	0.011 *
Bacteroidetes			
Alistipes	1.11	0.56	0.894
Parabacteroides	131.44	142.00	0.913
Bacteroides	743.56	776.56	0.785
Firmicutes			
Eubacterium	1.11	0.78	0.799
Veillonella	1.22	1.00	0.960
Dorea	2.00	5.00	0.785
Acidaminococcus	2.67	11.33	0.894
SMB53	5.67	4.00	0.239
Clostridium	7.33	13.22	0.896
Anaerostipes	10.22	1.22	0.239
Ruminococcus	10.89	19.67	0.943

Table 4. *Cont.*

Genera	0 h	24 h	*p*-Value
Firmicutes			
Streptococcus	12.67	8.78	0.785
Turicibacter	14.22	2.44	0.960
Lachnospira	14.78	72.00	0.237
Oscillospira	17.22	14.89	0.647
Lactococcus	20.44	9.22	0.896
Phascolarctobacterium	24.67	60.44	0.501
Dialister	26.11	58.22	0.943
Roseburia	28.56	6.00	0.674
Blautia	32.44	49.44	0.156
Coprococcus	45.78	66.44	0.501
Ruminococcus	54.22	39.33	0.261
Faecalibacterium	154.89	93.11	0.080
Proteobacteria			
Escherichia	0.78	1.44	0.960
Sutterella	4.00	32.44	0.894
Haemophilus	10.67	0.56	0.107
Bilophila	10.67	7.67	0.896
Verrucomicrobia			
Akkermansia	17.00	3.33	0.501

[1] Replicate samples were pooled among donor at each respective time point (3 donors × 3 replicated = 9). Samples were analyzed between differentially represented OTUs for significant changes after 24 h of fermentation compared to 0 h samples. Values are the number of OTUs after rarefaction to 3668 sequences per sample. Data were analyzed using the Kruskal-Wallis ANOVA test, with the FDR multiple comparisons correction. * Indicates significance at $p \leq 0.05$.

Table 5. Combined changes across 24 h of fermentation for xylooligosaccharide samples of identified genera [1].

Genera	0 h	24 h	*p*-Value
Actinobacteria			
Bifidobacterium	0.67	5.22	0.038 *
Adlercreutzia	1.33	1.78	0.972
Collinsella	58.44	154.00	0.413
Bacteroidetes			
Alistipes	1.44	0.56	0.413
Parabacteroides	147.33	133.33	0.972
Bacteroides	770.89	870.44	0.189
Firmicutes			
Eubacterium	0.33	1.67	0.364
Veillonella	0.67	0.00	0.162
Acidaminococcus	1.33	2.33	0.972
Dorea	2.11	3.67	0.423
SMB53	7.33	5.44	0.558
Anaerostipes	7.44	3.44	0.447
Turicibacter	8.00	8.56	0.972
Clostridium	8.44	4.00	0.087
Ruminococcus	12.78	26.11	0.087
Streptococcus	14.11	4.67	0.367
Lachnospira	21.11	5.33	0.038 *
Oscillospira	21.33	21.78	0.972
Phascolarctobacterium	23.44	16.33	0.972
Lactococcus	23.89	21.00	0.982
Roseburia	28.89	35.33	0.972
Dialister	33.89	41.56	0.831

Table 5. *Cont.*

Genera	0 h	24 h	*p*-Value
Firmicutes			
Blautia	39.22	65.00	0.087
Ruminococcus	45.11	37.33	0.385
Coprococcus	47.11	48.67	0.705
Faecalibacterium	148.56	79.56	0.030 *
Proteobacteria			
Escherichia	0.89	0.44	0.972
Haemophilus	6.44	3.11	0.972
Bilophila	17.78	6.22	0.107
Sutterella	25.78	40.89	0.831
Verrucomicrobia			
Akkermansia	2.78	5.00	0.841

[1] Replicate samples were pooled among donor at each respective time point (3 donors × 3 replicated = 9). Samples were analyzed between differentially represented OTUs for significant changes after 24 h of fermentation compared to 0 h samples. Values are the number of OTUs after rarefaction to 3668 sequences per sample. Data were analyzed using the Kruskal-Wallis ANOVA test, with the FDR multiple comparisons correction. * Indicates significance at $p \leq 0.05$.

Table 6. Combined changes across 24 h of fermentation for pure inulin samples of identified genera [1].

Genera	0 h	24 h	*p*-Value
Actinobacteria			
Bifidobacterium	1.33	5.44	0.304
Adlercreutzia	1.33	2.00	0.845
Collinsella	55.11	291.44	0.016 *
Bacteroidetes			
Alistipes	1.56	0.89	0.878
Parabacteroides	147.44	164.78	0.887
Bacteroides	726.78	644.44	0.652
Firmicutes			
Veillonella	0.78	0.56	0.908
Eubacterium	0.89	1.56	0.908
Dorea	1.78	7.00	0.640
Acidaminococcus	3.11	18.67	0.887
SMB53	7.44	9.11	0.965
Turicibacter	7.78	4.89	0.652
Clostridium	8.22	7.11	0.845
Ruminococcus	9.56	34.11	0.309
Anaerostipes	11.22	4.67	0.652
Streptococcus	13.00	12.44	0.887
Lactococcus	19.11	9.67	0.908
Lachnospira	21.00	4.89	0.022 *
Phascolarctobacterium	26.22	21.00	0.887
Oscillospira	26.33	10.11	0.034 *
Roseburia	26.78	14.11	0.887
Dialister	32.67	95.11	0.887
Blautia	38.22	50.22	0.690
Coprococcus	48.11	60.89	0.640
Ruminococcus	52.33	43.00	0.908
Faecalibacterium	148.11	187.33	0.652
Proteobacteria			
Escherichia	1.00	1.22	0.908
Haemophilus	9.11	2.67	0.652
Sutterella	14.00	31.22	0.908
Bilophila	16.89	7.78	0.309

Table 6. *Cont.*

Genera	0 h	24 h	*p*-Value
Verrucomicrobia			
Akkermansia	7.78	7.44	0.304

[1] Replicate samples were pooled among donor at each respective time point (3 donors × 3 replicated = 9). Samples were analyzed between differentially represented OTUs for significant changes after 24 h of fermentation compared to 0 h samples. Values are the number of OTUs after rarefaction to 3668 sequences per sample. Data were analyzed using the Kruskal-Wallis ANOVA test, with the FDR multiple comparisons correction. * Indicates significance at $p \leq 0.05$.

Table 7. Combined changes across 24 h of fermentation for pure beta-glucan samples of identified genera [1].

Genera	0 h	24 h	*p*-Value
Actinobacteria			
Bifidobacterium	0.33	0.33	1.000
Adlercreutzia	2.00	1.89	0.843
Collinsella	69.22	85.11	0.723
Bacteroidetes			
Alistipes	0.78	0.89	0.778
Parabacteroides	119.56	179.78	0.778
Bacteroides	776.11	854.33	0.664
Firmicutes			
Eubacterium	0.11	0.44	0.778
Veillonella	0.56	0.22	0.778
Dorea	0.89	3.11	0.110
Acidaminococcus	2.33	15.11	0.778
SMB53	6.11	4.89	0.778
Lactococcus	6.11	0.67	0.778
Anaerostipes	7.44	5.22	0.778
Turicibacter	8.11	3.00	0.803
Ruminococcus	9.44	18.67	0.166
Clostridium	10.11	3.33	0.110
Streptococcus	14.89	6.44	0.256
Roseburia	16.11	54.33	0.510
Lachnospira	21.22	3.89	0.008 *
Oscillospira	24.33	35.11	0.389
Phascolarctobacterium	29.00	125.33	0.283
Dialister	30.56	43.67	0.819
Coprococcus	44.11	20.78	0.211
Blautia	45.11	68.11	0.408
Ruminococcus	59.67	44.44	0.500
Faecalibacterium	152.11	62.67	0.008 *
Proteobacteria			
Escherichia	0.89	0.56	0.778
Haemophilus	11.00	0.78	0.110
Sutterella	14.00	35.44	0.778
Bilophila	14.44	13.89	0.778
Verrucomicrobia			
Akkermansia	9.11	15.89	0.778

[1] Replicate samples were pooled among donor at each respective time point (3 donors × 3 replicated = 9). Samples were analyzed between differentially represented OTUs for significant changes after 24 h of fermentation compared to 0 h samples. Values are the number of OTUs after rarefaction to 3668 sequences per sample. Data were analyzed using the Kruskal-Wallis ANOVA test, with the FDR multiple comparisons correction. * Indicates significance at $p \leq 0.05$.

4. Discussion

The aim of this study was to investigate the beneficial effects of commonly consumed prebiotic dietary fibers, including their ability to influence the growth of identified bacterial populations, form beneficial SCFAs, and the amount of gas they produce due to fermentation. Total gas production due to fiber fermentation depends on a wide range of factors. The inulin samples and the WholeFiber samples (mixture of dried chicory root inulin, pectin and hemi/cellulose) resulted in the highest gas production at both 12 and 24 h. These results are consistent with results from both clinical feeding studies and other in vitro experiments, in which fermentation of inulin products resulted in high amounts of gas production, sometimes resulting in mild negative gastrointestinal symptoms, depending on the dosage [32,33]. Similar in vitro studies have found inulin to be much more fermentable than beta-glucan products, for both barley and oat-derived beta-glucans [34]. XOS fermentation results in less gas production than the inulin products, and more gas than beta-glucan products. Because of these findings, previous studies based on digestive tolerance and parameters have established a tolerated daily dosage for XOS of approximately 12 g/day [35].

SCFA production due to the fermentation of prebiotic dietary fibers promotes many beneficial health outcomes to the host. SCFA production may contribute to up to 10% of the host's metabolizable energy daily, with production of total SCFAs usually between 100–200 mmol/day, but is highly dependent on the donor and availability of substrates for fermentation [36,37]. At 12 h of fermentation, the OatWell and beta-glucan samples had significantly higher concentrations of propionate, and the highest mean concentration at 24 h, compared to the other prebiotic dietary fibers analyzed. Similar in vitro studies with beta-glucan based products have also shown similar preference for these products to result in propionate formation [34]. Although no mechanism has been identified, and studies show conflicting results [38], elevated serum propionate concentrations have been shown to have a hypocholesterolaemic effect [39]. Propionate may also play an influential role in satiety, although mechanisms still remain unclear [40,41]. Cholesterol-lowering properties of beta-glucans may be limited to effects from the upper-GI, although many propionate-producing bacteria have a preference to fermenting various types of beta-glucans (*Bacteroides, Prevotella, Clostridium*) based on the presence of genes responsible for endo-β-glucanase enzyme production [42].

Microbial diversity among fecal donors complicates the identification of trends among the five treatment groups (Supplemental Figures S8 and S9). In terms of taxonomic shift, the inulin-based products were fermented nearly identically by all three fecal donors. Both pure inulin and WholeFiber promoted the growth of *Collinsella* comparing the 24 h samples to the 0 h samples. Inulin-type fructans have been shown in clinical studies to promote substantial growth of *Collinsella*, paralleled with increased urinary hippurate levels [43]. Hippurate is a metabolite derived from various fermentation processes in the gut that has been found in decreased concentrations in obese individuals compared to lean individuals, and also between diabetics and non-diabetics [44–46]. The genus *Collinsella* has been found in lower concentrations in individuals with IBD compared to healthy controls [47], while *Collinsella aerofaciens* has been associated with low risk of colorectal cancer [48]. Increases in *Collinsella* and increased urinary hippurate levels are considered a beneficial effect of inulin consumption due to its prebiotic capacity [43]. In vivo studies with inulin, scFOS and resistant starch supplementation have found decreases in the SMB53 genus, consistent with the OatWell treatment in the present study [30,31].

A significant increase in the genus *Bifidobacterium* was observed only with the XOS treatment. Rycroft et al. found a similar affinity of *Bifidobacterium* toward XOS [49]. However, previous studies have shown inulin to also stimulate the growth of *Bifidobacterium* [49–52]. While there was an overall rise in *Bifidobacterium* with the inulin treatment group between 0 h and 24 h (1.33, 5.44 OTUs respectively), this study did not find that increase to be significant ($p = 0.304$). The small sample size and individual microbiome variability likely played a role in this result. Increases in *Bifidobacterium* have been heavily studied and reviewed, and are considered a beneficial effect due to their correlation with many positive health outcomes [1]. *Bifidobacteria* reside naturally in the gastrointestinal tract of healthy human adults and have a strong affinity to ferment oligosaccharides, making them a common marker for prebiotic capacity. *Bifidobacterium* is a unique genus of bacteria in that no gas is formed as an end product of metabolism [53]. Like *Lactobacillus*, these bacteria are saccharolytic, often considered a beneficial trait [54]. *Bifidobacteria* also do not produce any known carcinogenic substances in vivo. *Bifidobacteria* concentrations have been negatively associated with obesity and weight gain [55–58]. Increases in *Bifidobacteria* have also been correlated with a decrease in blood lipopolysaccharides (LPS), inflammatory reagents that play a role in the development of inflammatory metabolic disorders and conditions, and are primarily found in gram-negative bacteria [59]. LPS induce the activation of Toll-like receptor 4 (TLR4), which leads to inflammation due to release of pro-inflammatory cytokines and chemokines [60].

In vitro fermentations are semi-representative models of colonic fermentation, but have limitations [18]. This study did not include an in vitro digestion process, which would remove digestible contents from the samples prior to fermentation, and would be a more representative model. However, because the test substrates are primarily fiber, which is non-digestible, this should have minimal impact on the results of this study. In vivo, formed gases are continually absorbed and colonic absorption is rapid. Because SCFAs are rapidly absorbed and difficult to measure, in vitro models help to understand the kinetics of colonic fermentation. However, in vitro models must be paired with similar in vivo models to better understand the full mechanisms of action resulting from colonic fermentation of prebiotic dietary fibers. Because the SCFA are not absorbed in in vitro models, the SCFA produced can alter the pH of the fermentation media. While the fermentation media was designed to mimic the pH of the distal colon at baseline, the pH of the media in this study was not further controlled throughout the experiment. This is another limitation of this in vitro model. An additional limitation of this study was the small sample size. The present study was conducted using fecal inoculum from only three donors. Due to the individual variability between the donor's microbiota (Figure S7), a larger sample size may be needed to achieve a more representative view of the effects of each of the fibers.

5. Conclusions

All five prebiotics measured in this study display fermentability and SCFA production that could have potential health benefits. Depending on their structure, each compound offers a specific carbon source for fermentation by different bacterial populations, yielding changes in beneficial taxa and production of various amounts of SCFAs and gas in vitro. For instance, while OatWell and beta-glucans promoted propionate production, XOS increased concentrations of *Bifodobacterium*, and WholeFiber and pure inulin promoted *Collinsella* growth. Findings in this study are consistent with other in vitro studies with similar prebiotic dietary fibers, as well as clinical feeding studies [34,43,49,61–63].

Supplementary Materials:
Table S1: Gas and SCFA Production Comparing Fermentation Differences of Five Prebiotic Dietary Fibers at 12 h and 24 h Post-Exposure to Fecal Microbiota from Three Individual Donors in an In Vitro Fermentation System, Figure S1: Identified phyla from three fecal donors microbiota at 0, 12 and 24 h of fermentation for five prebiotic dietary fibers analyzed based on percent of sequence reads, Figure S2: Identified abundant families for three fecal donors at 0, 12 and 24 h of fermentation for five prebiotic dietary fibers analyzed based on percent of sequence reads, Figure S3: Identified abundant genera for three fecal donors at 0, 12 and 24 h of fermentation for five prebiotic dietary fibers analyzed based on percent of sequence reads, Figure S4: Six metrics of analysis for alpha-diversity among samples at 0, 12 and 24 h of analysis, grouped by donor for all five prebiotic dietary fibers analyzed, Figure S5: Six metrics of analysis for alpha-diversity among samples at 0, 12 and 24 h of analysis, grouped by treatment for all three fecal donors, Figure S6: Bray-Curtis β-diversity principal component analysis of technical replicates among each treatment group between microbiota analysis of three fecal donors, Figure S7: Bray-Curtis β-diversity principal component analysis among microbiota of three fecal donors at 0, 12 and 24 h of analysis, Figure S8: Variations in abundant phyla among three donors analyzed, Figure S9: Variations in treatment groups and pooled donors analyzed.

Acknowledgments: This study was funded by DSM. The authors would like to thank Hannah Paruzynski for the laboratory assistance, the University of Minnesota Genomics Center for the analysis of the samples, The University of Minnesota Doctoral Dissertation Fellowship for financial research support, and the companies who donated time and resources to this project.

Author Contributions: Joanne L. Slavin and Justin L. Carlson conceived and designed the experiment; Justin L. Carlson, Jennifer M. Erickson and Julie M. Hess performed the experiments. Justin L. Carlson analyzed the data, Trevor J. Gould was responsible for analysis of sequencing data. Manuscript was prepared by Justin L. Carlson and Jennifer M. Erickson, and read and approved by all authors.

References

1. Carlson, J.; Slavin, J. Health benefits of fibre, prebiotics and probiotics: A review of intestinal health and related health claims. *Qual. Assur. Saf. Crop. Foods* **2016**, *6*, 1–16. [CrossRef]
2. Brownawell, A.M.; Caers, W.; Gibson, G.R.; Kendall, C.W.C.; Lewis, K.D.; Ringel, Y.; Slavin, J.L. Prebiotics and the Health Benefits of Fiber: Current Regulatory Status, Future Research, and Goals. *J. Nutr.* **2012**, *142*, 962–974. [CrossRef] [PubMed]
3. Gibson, G.R.; Hutkins, R.; Sanders, M.E.; Prescott, S.L.; Reimer, R.A.; Salminen, S.J.; Scott, K.; Stanton, C.; Swanson, K.S.; Cani, P.D.; et al. Expert consensus document: The International Scientific Association for Probiotics and Prebiotics (ISAPP) consensus statement on the definition and scope of prebiotics. *Nat. Rev. Gastroenterol. Hepatol.* **2017**. [CrossRef] [PubMed]
4. Gibson, G.R.; Roberfroid, M.B. Dietary modulation of the human colonic microbiota: Introducing the concept of prebiotics. *J. Nutr.* **1995**, *125*, 1401–1412. [CrossRef] [PubMed]
5. Gibson, G.R.; Probert, H.M.; Van Loo, J.; Rastall, R.A.; Roberfroid, M.B. Dietary modulation of the human colonic microbiota: Updating the concept of prebiotics. *Nutr. Res. Rev.* **2004**, *17*, 259–275. [CrossRef] [PubMed]
6. Slavin, J. Fiber and prebiotics: Mechanisms and health benefits. *Nutrients* **2013**, *5*, 1417–1435. [CrossRef] [PubMed]
7. Bindels, L.B.; Delzenne, N.M.; Cani, P.D.; Walter, J. Towards a more comprehensive concept for prebiotics. *Nat. Rev. Gastroenterol. Hepatol.* **2015**. [CrossRef] [PubMed]
8. Aachary, A.A.; Prapulla, S.G. Xylooligosaccharides (XOS) as an Emerging Prebiotic: Microbial Synthesis, Utilization, Structural Characterization, Bioactive Properties, and Applications. *Compr. Rev. Food Sci. Food Saf.* **2011**, *10*, 2–16. [CrossRef]
9. Vázquez, M.; Alonso, J.; Domıínguez, H.; Parajó, J. Xylooligosaccharides: Manufacture and applications. *Trends Food Sci. Technol.* **2000**, *11*, 387–393. [CrossRef]
10. Christakopoulos, P.; Katapodis, P. Antimicrobial activity of acidic xylo-oligosaccharides produced by family 10 and 11 endoxylanases. *Int. J. Biol. Macromol.* **2003**, *31*, 171–175. [CrossRef]
11. Katapodis, P.; Kavarnou, A.; Kintzios, S. Production of acidic xylo-oligosaccharides by a family 10 endoxylanase from thermoascus aurantiacus and use as plant growth regulators. *Biotechnol. Lett.* **2002**, *24*, 1413–1416. [CrossRef]
12. Vardakou, M.; Katapodis, P.; Topakas, E.; Kekos, D.; Macris, B.J.; Christakopoulos, P. Synergy between enzymes involved in the degradation of insoluble wheat flour arabinoxylan. *Innov. Food Sci. Emerg. Technol.* **2004**, *5*, 107–112. [CrossRef]
13. Yang, R.; Xu, S.; Wang, Z.; Yang, W. Aqueous extraction of corncob xylan and production of xylooligosaccharides. *LWT-Food Sci. Technol.* **2005**, *38*, 677–682. [CrossRef]
14. Yuan, Q.; Zhang, H. Pilot-plant production of xylo-oligosaccharides from corncob by steaming, enzymatic hydrolysis and nanofiltration. *J. Chem. Technol. Biotechnol.* **2004**, *78*, 1073–1079. [CrossRef]
15. Niness, K.R. Inulin and Oligofructose: What Are They? *J. Nutr.* **1999**, *129*, 1402S–1406S. [PubMed]
16. Carpita, N.C.; Kanabus, J.; Housley, T.L. Linkage Structure of Fructans and Fructan Oligomers from Triticum aestivum and Festuca arundinacea Leaves. *J. Plant Physiol.* **1989**, *134*, 162–168. [CrossRef]
17. Lam, K.L.; Chi-Keung Cheung, P. Non-digestible long chain beta-glucans as novel prebiotics. *Bioact. Carbohydr. Diet. Fibre* **2013**, *2*, 45–64. [CrossRef]
18. Wisker, E.; Daniel, M. Fermentation of non-starch polysaccharides in mixed diets and single fibre sources: Comparative studies in human subjects and in vitro. *Br. J. Nutr.* **1998**, *80*, 253–261. [PubMed]

19. Payne, A.N.; Zihler, A.; Chassard, C.; Lacroix, C. Advances and perspectives in in vitro human gut fermentation modeling. *Trends Biotechnol.* **2012**, *30*, 17–25. [CrossRef] [PubMed]
20. Broekaert, W.F.; Courtin, C.M.; Verbeke, K.; Van de Wiele, T.; Verstraete, W.; Delcour, J.A. Prebiotic and Other Health-Related Effects of Cereal-Derived Arabinoxylans, Arabinoxylan-Oligosaccharides, and Xylooligosaccharides. *Crit. Rev. Food Sci. Nutr.* **2011**, *51*, 178–194. [CrossRef] [PubMed]
21. Okazaki, M.; Fufikawa, S.; Matsumoto, N. Effect of xylooligosaccharides on the growth of bifidobacteria. *Bifidobact. Microflora* **1990**, *9*, 77–86. [CrossRef]
22. Na, M.H.; Kim, W.K. Effects of Xyooligosaccharide Intake on Fecal Bifidobacteria, Lactic acid and Lipid Concentration in Korean Young Women. *Korean J. Nutr.* **2004**, *37*, 662–668.
23. Tateyama, I.; Hashii, K.; Johno, I.; Iino, T.; Hirai, K.; Suwa, Y.; Kiso, Y. Effect of xylooligosaccharide intake on severe constipation in pregnant women. *J. Nutr. Sci. Vitaminol. (Tokyo)* **2005**, *51*, 445–448. [CrossRef] [PubMed]
24. Koecher, K.J.; Noack, J.A.; Timm, D.A.; Klosterbuer, A.S.; Thomas, W.; Slavin, J.L. Estimation and Interpretation of Fermentation in the Gut: Coupling Results from a 24 h Batch in Vitro System with Fecal Measurements from a Human Intervention Feeding Study Using Fructo-oligosaccharides, Inulin, Gum Acacia, and Pea Fiber. *J. Agric. Food Chem.* **2014**, *62*, 1332–1337. [CrossRef] [PubMed]
25. McBurney, M.I.; Thompson, L.U. Effect of human faecal inoculum on in vitro fermentation variables. *Br. J. Nutr.* **1987**, *58*, 233. [CrossRef] [PubMed]
26. Schneider, S.M.; Girard-Pipau, F.; Anty, R.; van der Linde, E.G.M.; Philipsen-Geerling, B.J.; Knol, J.; Filippi, J.; Arab, K.; Hébuterne, X. Effects of total enteral nutrition supplemented with a multi-fibre mix on faecal short-chain fatty acids and microbiota. *Clin. Nutr.* **2006**, *25*, 82–90. [CrossRef] [PubMed]
27. Carlson, J.; Hospattankar, A.; Deng, P.; Swanson, K.; Slavin, J. Prebiotic Effects and Fermentation Kinetics of Wheat Dextrin and Partially Hydrolyzed Guar Gum in an In Vitro Batch ermentation System. *Foods* **2015**, *4*, 349–358. [CrossRef] [PubMed]
28. Caporaso, J.G.; Kuczynski, J.; Stombaugh, J.; Bittinger, K.; Bushman, F.D.; Costello, E.K.; Fierer, N.; Peña, A.G.; Goodrich, J.K.; Gordon, J.I.; et al. QIIME allows analysis of high-throughput community sequencing data. *Nat. Methods* **2010**, *7*, 335–336. [CrossRef] [PubMed]
29. Garbe, J.; Gould, T.; Gohl, D.; Knights, D.; Beckman, K. *Metagenomics Pipeline*, version 1; Gopher-Pipelines: Minneapolis, MN, USA, 2016.
30. Bolger, A.M.; Lohse, M.; Usadel, B. Trimmomatic: A flexible trimmer for Illumina sequence data. *Bioinformatics* **2014**, *30*, 2114–2120. [CrossRef] [PubMed]
31. Masella, A.P.; Bartram, A.K.; Truszkowski, J.M.; Brown, D.G.; Neufeld, J.D. PANDAseq: Paired-end assembler for illumina sequences. *BMC Bioinform.* **2012**, *13*, 31. [CrossRef] [PubMed]
32. Bonnema, A.L.; Kolberg, L.W.; Thomas, W.; Slavin, J.L. Gastrointestinal tolerance of chicory inulin products. *J. Am. Diet. Assoc.* **2010**, *110*, 865–868. [CrossRef] [PubMed]
33. Timm, D.A.; Stewart, M.L.; Hospattankar, A.; Slavin, J.L. Wheat Dextrin, Psyllium, and Inulin Produce Distinct Fermentation Patterns, Gas Volumes, and Short-Chain Fatty Acid Profiles In Vitro. *J. Med. Food* **2010**, *13*, 961–966. [CrossRef] [PubMed]
34. Hughes, S.A.; Shewry, P.R.; Gibson, G.R.; Mccleary, B.V.; Rastall, R.A. In vitro fermentation of oat and barley derived b-glucans by human faecal microbiota. *FEMS Microbiol. Ecol.* **2008**, *64*, 482–493. [CrossRef] [PubMed]
35. Xiao, L.; Ning, J.; Xu, G. Application of Xylo-oligosaccharide in modifying human intestinal function. *Afr. J. Microbiol. Res.* **2012**, *6*, 2116–2119. [CrossRef]
36. Livesey, G. Energy values of unavailable carbohydrate and diets: An inquiry and analysis. *Am. J. Clin. Nutr.* **1990**, *51*, 617–637. [PubMed]
37. Cook, S.I.; Sellin, J.H. Review article: Short chain fatty acids in health and disease. *Aliment. Pharmacol. Ther.* **1998**, *12*, 499–507. [CrossRef] [PubMed]
38. Malkki, Y.; Autio, K.; Hanninen, O.; Myllymaki, O.; Pelkonen, K.; Suortti, T.; Torronen, R. *Oat Bran Concentrates:* Physical Properties of Beta-Glucan and Hypocholesterolemic Effects in Rats; FAO: Rome, Italy, 1992.
39. Chen, W.-J.L.; Anderson, J.W.; Jennings, D. Propionate May Mediate the Hypocholesterolemic Effects of Certain Soluble Plant Fibers in Cholesterol-Fed Rats. *Exp. Biol. Med.* **1984**, *175*, 215–218. [CrossRef]
40. Chambers, E.S.; Morrison, D.J.; Frost, G.; Mozaffarian, D. Control of appetite and energy intake by SCFA: What are the potential underlying mechanisms? *Proc. Nutr. Soc.* **2015**, *74*, 328–336. [CrossRef] [PubMed]

41. Chambers, E.; Viardot, A.; Psichas, A.; Morrison, D. Effects of targeted delivery of propionate to the human colon on appetite regulation, body weight maintenance and adiposity in overweight adults. *Gut* **2015**, *64*, 1744–1754. [CrossRef] [PubMed]
42. Zappe, H.; Jones, W.A.; Jones, D.T.; Woods, D.R. Structure of an endo-beta-1,4-glucanase gene from *Clostridium acetobutylicum* P262 showing homology with endoglucanase genes from *Bacillus* spp. *Appl. Environ. Microbiol.* **1988**, *54*, 1289–1292. [PubMed]
43. Dewulf, E.M.; Cani, P.D.; Claus, S.P.; Fuentes, S.; Puylaert, P.G.; Neyrinck, A.M.; Bindels, L.B.; de Vos, W.M.; Gibson, G.R.; Thissen, J.-P.; et al. Insight into the prebiotic concept: Lessons from an exploratory, double blind intervention study with inulin-type fructans in obese women. *Gut* **2013**, *62*, 1112–1121. [CrossRef] [PubMed]
44. Calvani, R.; Miccheli, A.; Capuani, G.; Tomassini Miccheli, A.; Puccetti, C.; Delfini, M.; Iaconelli, A.; Nanni, G.; Mingrone, G. Gut microbiome-derived metabolites characterize a peculiar obese urinary metabotype. *Int. J. Obes.* **2010**, *34*, 1095–1098. [CrossRef] [PubMed]
45. Salek, R.M.; Maguire, M.L.; Bentley, E.; Rubtsov, D.V.; Hough, T.; Cheeseman, M.; Nunez, D.; Sweatman, B.C.; Haselden, J.N.; Cox, R.D.; et al. A metabolomic comparison of urinary changes in type 2 diabetes in mouse, rat, and human. *Physiol. Genom.* **2007**, *29*, 99–108. [CrossRef] [PubMed]
46. Waldram, A.; Holmes, E.; Wang, Y.; Rantalainen, M.; Wilson, I.D.; Tuohy, K.M.; McCartney, A.L.; Gibson, G.R.; Nicholson, J.K. Top-Down Systems Biology Modeling of Host Metabotype—Microbiome Associations in Obese Rodents. *J. Proteome Res.* **2009**, *8*, 2361–2375. [CrossRef] [PubMed]
47. Kassinen, A.; Krogius-Kurikka, L.; Mäkivuokko, H.; Rinttilä, T.; Paulin, L.; Corander, J.; Malinen, E.; Apajalahti, J.; Palva, A. The Fecal Microbiota of Irritable Bowel Syndrome Patients Differs Significantly From That of Healthy Subjects. *Gastroenterology* **2007**, *133*, 24–33. [CrossRef] [PubMed]
48. Moore, W.E.; Moore, L.H. Intestinal floras of populations that have a high risk of colon cancer. *Appl. Environ. Microbiol.* **1995**, *61*, 3202–3207. [PubMed]
49. Rycroft, C.E.; Jones, M.R.; Gibson, G.R.; Rastall, R.A. A comparative in vitro evaluation of the fermentation properties of prebiotic oligosaccharides. *J. Appl. Microbiol.* **2001**, *91*, 878–887. [CrossRef] [PubMed]
50. Wang, X.; Gibson, G.R. Effects of the in vitro fermentation of oligofructose and inulin by bacteria growing in the human large intestine. *J. Appl. Bacteriol.* **1993**, *75*, 373–380. [CrossRef] [PubMed]
51. Gibson, G.R.; Beatty, E.R.; Wang, X.; Cummings, J.H. Selective stimulation of bifidobacteria in the human colon by oligofructose and inulin. *Gastroenterology* **1995**, *108*, 975–982. [CrossRef]
52. Ramirez-Farias, C.; Slezak, K.; Fuller, Z.; Duncan, A.; Holtrop, G.; Louis, P. Effect of inulin on the human gut microbiota: Stimulation of Bifidobacterium adolescentis and Faecalibacterium prausnitzii. *Br. J. Nutr.* **2009**, *101*, 533. [CrossRef] [PubMed]
53. Buchanan, R.; Gibbons, N. *Bergey's Manual of Determinative Bacteriology*; Williams & Wilkins Co.: Baltimore, MD, USA, 1974.
54. Salyers, A. Energy sources of major intestinal fermentative anaerobes. *Am. J. Clin. Nutr.* **1979**, *32*, 158–163. [PubMed]
55. Collado, M.; Isolauri, E. Distinct composition of gut microbiota during pregnancy in overweight and normal-weight women. *Am. J. Clin. Nutr.* **2008**, *55*, 894–899.
56. Kalliomäki, M.; Collado, M. Early differences in fecal microbiota composition in children may predict overweight. *Am. J. Clin. Nutr.* **2008**, *87*, 534–538. [PubMed]
57. Santacruz, A. Gut microbiota composition is associated with body weight, weight gain and biochemical parameters in pregnant women. *Br. J. Nutr.* **2010**, *104*, 83–84. [CrossRef] [PubMed]
58. Schwiertz, A.; Taras, D.; Schäfer, K.; Beijer, S. Microbiota and SCFA in lean and overweight healthy subjects. *Obesity* **2010**, *18*, 190–195. [CrossRef] [PubMed]
59. Knaapen, M.; Kootte, R.S.; Zoetendal, E.G.; de Vos, W.M.; Dallinga-Thie, G.M.; Levi, M.; Stroes, E.S.; Nieuwdorp, M. Obesity, non-alcoholic fatty liver disease, and atherothrombosis: A role for the intestinal microbiota? *Clin. Microbiol. Infect.* **2013**, *19*, 331–337. [CrossRef] [PubMed]
60. Nakamura, Y.; Omaye, S. Metabolic diseases and pro-and prebiotics: Mechanistic insights. *Nutr. Metab. (Lond.)* **2012**, *9*, 1–11. [CrossRef] [PubMed]
61. Kedia, G.; Vázquez, J.A.; Charalampopoulos, D.; Pandiella, S.S. In Vitro Fermentation of Oat Bran Obtained by Debranning with a Mixed Culture of Human Fecal Bacteria. *Curr. Microbiol.* **2009**, *58*, 338–342. [CrossRef] [PubMed]

62. Kim, H.J.; White, P.J. In Vitro Fermentation of Oat Flours from Typical and High β-Glucan Oat Lines. *J. Agric. Food Chem.* **2009**, *57*, 7529–7536. [CrossRef] [PubMed]
63. Finegold, S.M.; Li, Z.; Summanen, P.H.; Downes, J.; Thames, G.; Corbett, K.; Dowd, S.; Krak, M.; Heber, D. Xylooligosaccharide increases bifidobacteria but not lactobacilli in human gut microbiota. *Food Funct.* **2014**, *5*, 436. [CrossRef] [PubMed]

10

Post-Exercise Carbohydrate-Energy Replacement Attenuates Insulin Sensitivity and Glucose Tolerance the Following Morning in Healthy Adults

Harry L. Taylor [1], Ching-Lin Wu [2], Yung-Chih Chen [1], Pin-Ging Wang [2], Javier T. Gonzalez [1,*] and James A. Betts [1,*]

[1] Department for Health, University of Bath, Bath BA2 7AY, UK; taylor210@googlemail.com (H.L.T.); y.chen2@bath.ac.uk (Y.-C.C.)

[2] Graduate Institute of Sports and Health Management, National Chung Hsing University, Taichung 402, Taiwan; wuchinglin@icloud.com (C.-L.W.); pspgw@dragon.nchu.edu.tw (P.-G.W.)

* Correspondence: j.t.gonzalez@bath.ac.uk (J.T.G.); j.betts@bath.ac.uk (J.A.B.)

Abstract: The carbohydrate deficit induced by exercise is thought to play a key role in increased post-exercise insulin action. However, the effects of replacing carbohydrate utilized during exercise on postprandial glycaemia and insulin sensitivity are yet to be determined. This study therefore isolated the extent to which the insulin-sensitizing effects of exercise are dependent on the carbohydrate deficit induced by exercise, relative to other exercise-mediated mechanisms. Fourteen healthy adults performed a 90-min run at 70% $\dot{V}O_2max$ starting at 1600–1700 h before ingesting either a non-caloric artificially-sweetened placebo solution (CHO-DEFICIT) or a 15% carbohydrate solution (CHO-REPLACE; 221.4 $\pm$ 59.3 g maltodextrin) to precisely replace the measured quantity of carbohydrate oxidized during exercise. The alternate treatment was then applied one week later in a randomized, placebo-controlled, and double-blinded crossover design. A standardized low-carbohydrate evening meal was consumed in both trials before overnight recovery ahead of a two-hour oral glucose tolerance test (OGTT) the following morning to assess glycemic and insulinemic responses to feeding. Compared to the CHO-DEFICIT condition, CHO-REPLACE increased the incremental area under the plasma glucose curve by a mean difference of 68 mmol·L^{-1} (95% CI: 4 to 132 mmol·L^{-1}; $p = 0.040$) and decreased the Matsuda insulin sensitivity index by a mean difference of -2 au (95% CI: -1 to -3 au; $p = 0.001$). This is the first study to demonstrate that post-exercise feeding to replaceme the carbohydrate expended during exercise can attenuate glucose tolerance and insulin sensitivity the following morning. The mechanism through which exercise improves insulin sensitivity is therefore (at least in part) dependent on carbohydrate availability and so the day-to-day metabolic health benefits of exercise might be best attained by maintaining a carbohydrate deficit overnight.

Keywords: insulin sensitivity; exercise; carbohydrate metabolism; oral glucose tolerance test

---

1. Introduction

Physical activity is a powerful tool to improve insulin sensitivity and glycemic control [1]. Accordingly, increasing physical activity is a crucial counter-measure in reducing T2D prevalence [2,3]. On an acute level, single bouts of exercise consistently enhance insulin sensitivity and muscle glucose uptake in both insulin-resistant [4] and healthy individuals [5], although the acute effects of exercise on glucose *tolerance* are less clear [6,7].

Metabolic flexibility is a key aspect of insulin sensitivity and reflects the ability to switch between substrate sources for oxidation according to availability. Individuals with robust metabolic flexibility display high rates of fat oxidation in the fasted state, switching to high rates of carbohydrate oxidation in the fed (or insulin-stimulated) state. It has been suggested that impaired metabolic flexibility may be an early cause of insulin resistance via lipid accumulation [8,9], although the direction of the relationship between metabolic flexibility and insulin sensitivity remains unclear. Notwithstanding this, substrate selection in the fasted and fed state may be an important mechanism by which exercise alters insulin sensitivity and postprandial glycemia.

The beneficial effects of exercise on glycemic control and insulin sensitivity are thought to be mediated, at least partly, by whole-body carbohydrate status. The increased insulin action after a single bout of exercise, or during the early phases (6 d) of moderate-intensity exercise training (walking), are attenuated when the energy and/or carbohydrate utilized by exercise is replaced by dietary intake [10–12]. These responses appear to be largely driven by carbohydrate status rather than energy status, since an exercise-induced carbohydrate deficit increases insulin sensitivity even in the presence of energy balance, whereas an exercise-induced energy deficit in the presence of high muscle glycogen does not [13]. Furthermore, in rodents, adrenaline-induced muscle glycogen depletion enhances insulin sensitivity of the muscle to glucose transport [14], highlighting the role of muscle carbohydrate status in insulin sensitivity, independent of exercise.

Whilst a number of studies have assessed post-exercise glucose metabolism and/or insulin action under conditions of carbohydrate and/or energy replacement, these studies have all employed intravenous tests of glucose metabolism and insulin sensitivity. Notwithstanding the strengths of tightly-controlled intravenous tests, there is a need to understand postprandial responses with the oral ingestion of glucose. This is particularly important since the acute exercise-induced increases in glucose disposal can be offset by increases in glucose appearance rates, thereby altering glucose tolerance [6,15]. Furthermore, it has been suggested that carbohydrate status around the exercise period may be a further mediator of glucose tolerance post-exercise [16]. Therefore, to translate these mechanistic findings for application, an understanding of metabolic responses to food ingestion is needed.

The purpose of this study was to investigate the role of replacing post-exercise carbohydrate on glucose tolerance and insulin sensitivity using an oral glucose tolerance test (OGTT). It was hypothesized that post-exercise replacement of the carbohydrate utilized during 90 min of treadmill running at ~70% $\dot{V}O_2max$ exercise would impair glucose tolerance and insulin sensitivity the following morning during an OGTT, compared to when the exercise-induced carbohydrate deficit is maintained overnight.

2. Materials and Methods

This study was approved by the University of Bath Research Ethics Approval Committee for Health (REACH—EP 15/16 182). Fourteen healthy participants (11 men and 3 women) were recruited for the study (Table 1). Written informed consent was obtained from participants after confirming their understanding of the study design and possible risks. Nine participants (6 men and 3 women) were tested in the United Kingdom and were native to the UK, and five participants (all men) were tested in Taiwan and were native to Taiwan. None of the participants self-reported as smokers. The insulin sensitivity responses to the intervention did not differ between locations (data not shown).

Table 1. Summary of participant characteristics, $n = 14$.

	Mean ± SD
Age (years)	24 ± 5
Height (m)	1.76 ± 0.06
Mass (kg)	71.1 ± 9.0
BMI (kg/m^2)	23.6 ± 4.5
$\dot{V}O_2max$ (mL·kg^{-1}·min^{-1})	56 ± 10

2.1. Experimental Design

This study was a dual-center (University of Bath and National Chung Hsing University), randomized, double-blind crossover design with two treatment arms. All participants underwent two 2-day experimental trials with a 7-day washout period between trials. On day 1, between 1600–1700 h, participants were asked to run on a treadmill at 70% $\dot{V}O_2max$ for 90 min. After exercise, subjects were immediately given either a carbohydrate replacement drink (CHO-REPLACE) or placebo drink (CHO-DEFICIT). A low carbohydrate pack-dinner was provided in both trials. The following morning after an overnight fast, participants were asked to perform an oral glucose tolerance test (OGTT; Figure 1). In order to standardize metabolic parameters prior to trials, participants were asked to record their diet 3 days before the first trial and repeated the same diet before the next trial. In addition, they were asked to refrain from smoking and ingesting alcohol- and caffeine-containing beverages for 24 h before the OGTT. All participants reported successful replication of lifestyle prior to trials.

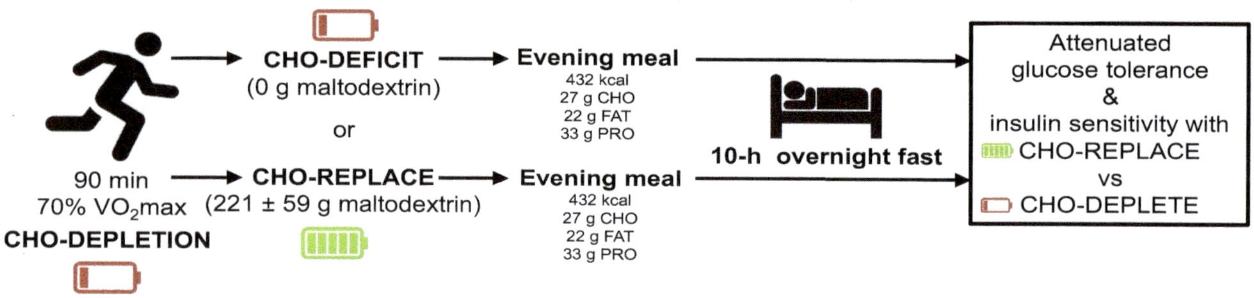

Figure 1. Schematic of the study design. CHO, carbohydrate; FAT, fat, PRO, protein; OGTT, oral glucose tolerance test.

2.2. Preliminary Tests

Subjects completed two preliminary tests: a maximal oxygen uptake test ($\dot{V}O_2max$) and a familiarization test, at least 1 week before the main trial. The $\dot{V}O_2max$ test protocol has been described previously [17]. At least 3 days prior to the first main trial, a 60-min familiarization run was performed to accustom participants to an extended period of treadmill-running. The session was also used to re-affirm the appropriate treadmill speed required to achieve an exercise intensity of 70% $\dot{V}O_2max$. Accordingly, heart-rate, RPE, and expired air samples were collected and analyzed at 15 min intervals.

2.3. Main Trials

Day 1—90-min run: Participants were asked to arrive at the laboratory between 15:30–15:45, and body-mass and stature were recorded. Participants were then fitted with a heart-rate monitor and the 90-min run at 70% $\dot{V}O_2max$ initiated at ~16:00. After the run, a test drink containing either carbohydrate or placebo was ingested immediately post-exercise and participants were asked to ingest the drink within one hour. Finally, a standardized dinner (432 kcal; 27 g carbohydrate (23 g of which sugars), 22 g fat, 33 g protein) was also provided, to be consumed between 19:30 and 20:00. Participants were then asked to abstain from consuming any further food or drink other than water.

Day 2—Oral Glucose Tolerance Test (OGTT): Participants attended the laboratory between 07:30–07:45, to perform a two-hour OGTT having completed an overnight fast (>10 h) and refrained from further exercise.

Upon arrival, participants rested for 15-min in a semi-recumbent position with their hand placed in a hot-box set to 55 °C [17], with a subsequent five-minute (baseline) expired air sample collected from a subgroup (n = 7). Following this, a cannula was inserted into an antecubital vein of the participant's forearm and a 5-mL (baseline) blood sample drawn. A 75 g glucose load was then administered orally (113 mL Polycal: Nutricia, UK (mixed with 87 mL water)) and blood samples were collected at 30 min intervals over 2-h. 5-min expired air samples were also collected at 25 to 30, 55 to 60, 85 to 90, and 115 to 120-min from a subgroup ($n = 7$). Since there were some slight differences in protocols between University of Bath and the National Chung Hsing University (namely, Bath protocols included a hot-box for blood sampling and expired breath analysis), the data from both institutions were initially analyzed separately to check that responses were similar. Since both protocols produced similar overall responses for glycaemia, insulinemia, and insulin sensitivity indices, the data were combined for the present manuscript ($n = 14$).

2.4. Test Drink

During the CHO-REPLACE trial, a 15% Maltodextrin solution (MyProtein, Cheshire, UK; Batch No.: L626929168) was ingested to precisely replace carbohydrate oxidized during the preceding run. The total amount of carbohydrate utilized during exercise were determined via indirect calorimetry from expired gases collected every 15-min during exercise. The amount of carbohydrate replacement for the CHO-REPLACE trial was 221.4 ± 59.3 g. Conversely, a (0 g carbohydrate) 1.5% artificially-sweetened placebo solution (Truvia, Silver Spoon, Peterborough, UK) was ingested during the CHO-DEFICIT trial.

2.5. Blood and Expired Air Samples Collection and Analysis

2.5.1. Blood Sample Collection and Analysis

The arterialized blood samples were obtained via a cannula inserted into antecubital vein of each subject's forearm [17]. A non-heparinized tube was used to collect 2 mL of blood sample, and it was allowed to stand for 1 h to wait for the blood to coagulate. Another tube containing ethylenediaminetetraacetic acid (EDTA; BD, Oxford, UK) was used to collect 3 mL of blood sample. The collected sample was then centrifuged (Eppendorf 5810, Hamburg, Germany) in 4 °C at 2500 g for 10 min. The extracted serum and plasma samples were stored at −80 °C before later analysis. Serum insulin concentrations were analyzed using enzyme-linked immunosorbent assays (ELISA, Mercodia AB, Uppsala, Sweden), following the manufacturer's instructions. Minimal detectable concentrations for serum insulin were set at 18 pmol·L^{-1} and intra-plate coefficients of variation were <4.4%. Plasma glucose concentrations were analyzed using a spectrophotometric analyzer (Randox Daytona, Randox Laboratories Ltd., Crumlin, UK). Due to a cannula blockage on one trial for one participant, data for blood-based variables are ($n = 13$).

2.5.2. Expired Gas Samples Collection and Analysis

The Douglas bag method was used to assess substrate metabolism at rest and during exercise. For all samples, participants were provided the mouthpiece before gas collections for a stabilization period. At rest, the stabilization and gas collection periods were each 5 min, whereas during exercise the stabilization and gas collection periods were each 1 min. Samples were collected in 200 L Douglas bags (Hans Rudolph, Kansas City, MO, USA) through falconia tubing (Baxter, Woodhouse and Taylor Ltd., Macclesfield, UK). Expired O_2 and CO_2 concentrations were measured in a known volume of each sample, using paramagnetic and infrared transducers, respectively (Mini HF 5200, Servomex Group Ltd., Crowborough, East Sussex, UK). The sensor was calibrated using known concentrations of low (99.998% Nitrogen, 0% O_2 and CO_2) and high (balance nitrogen mix, 16.04% O_2, 5.06% CO_2) calibration gases (both BOC Industrial Gases, Linde AG, Munich, Germany). Substrate utilization was determined during exercise using the equations of Jeukendrup and Wallis (2005) [18], whilst Frayn's (1983) [19] equations were used for samples collected at rest as follows (where $\dot{V}O_2$ and $\dot{V}CO_2$ are expressed in L/min):

$$\text{Fat utilisation at rest and during exercise (g/min)} = \left(1.695 \times \dot{V}O_2\right) - \left(1.701 \times \dot{V}CO_2\right) \quad (1)$$

$$\text{Carbohydrate utilisation at rest (g/min)} = \left(4.585 \times \dot{V}CO_2\right) - \left(3.226 \times \dot{V}O_2\right) \quad (2)$$

$$\text{Carbohydrate utilisation during exercise (g/min)} = \left(4.210 \times \dot{V}CO_2\right) - \left(2.962 \times \dot{V}O_2\right) \quad (3)$$

2.6. Sample Size Estimation

The sample size estimation was performed using data on insulin concentrations during steady-state intravenous glucose infusion following exercise training with, or without, carbohydrate and energy replacement. In the absence of carbohydrate replacement, insulin concentrations were ~225 $\pm$ 141 pmol·L^{-1}, compared to ~345 $\pm$ 85 pmol·L^{-1} when the carbohydrate and energy utilized during exercise was replaced. Based on this effect size (d = 1.03), 12 participants should provide more than a 90% chance of detecting such an effect with an alpha level of 0.05.

2.7. Statistical Analysis

Incremental area under the curve (iAUC; divided by 120 min to provide time average values) and Matsuda Insulin sensitivity index (Matsuda index; [18]) were calculated from plasma glucose and serum insulin data using Microsoft Excel (Version 15.26, Microsoft, Redmond, WA, USA). The updated homeostasis assessment model of insulin resistance (HOMA2-IR; [19]) was calculated using freely available online software (https://www.dtu.ox.ac.uk/homacalculator/). Statistical analyses were performed using GraphPad Prism v7 (GraphPad Software, San Diego, CA, USA). Differences between trials in time-dependent variables (glucose and insulin concentrations, and carbohydrate and fat oxidation rates) were analyzed by a two-way ANOVA with repeated measures. For non-time dependent variables, paired t-tests were applied. A p-value of $\leq$0.05 was considered statistically significant. Data are presented in the body of the text as mean $\pm$ SD, whereas error bars on figures are confidence intervals normalized to remove between subject variance, consistent with this within-subject design [20]. With this approach, any error bars that do not overlap the mean of their respective comparison can be considered to have a significance level of <0.05.

3. Results

3.1. Indirect Calorimetry during the Treadmill Run

The mean rates of oxygen consumption and carbon dioxide production were 2.65 $\pm$ 0.43 L·min^{-1} and 2.65 $\pm$ 0.48 L·min^{-1}, respectively. This resulted in a respiratory exchange ratio of 1.00 $\pm$ 0.12 ($\dot{V}O_2$:$\dot{V}CO_2$). Based on data collected at Bath, the total amount of carbohydrate oxidized during the run in CHO-DEPLETE was 205 $\pm$ 58 g vs. 220 $\pm$ 52 g in the CHO-REPLACE trial.

3.2. Glycemia, Insulinemia and Insulin Sensitivity

Pre-OGTT glucose concentrations were 4.56 $\pm$ 0.55 mmol·L^{-1} during the CHO-REPLACE trial and 4.36 $\pm$ 0.51 mmol·L^{-1} during the CHO-DEFICIT trial (p = 0.149). Following ingestion of the OGTT, plasma glucose concentrations rose to a greater extent in CHO-REPLACE versus CHO-DEFICIT (Figure 2A,B; p = 0.040), whereby peak glucose concentrations were 9.74 $\pm$ 1.22 mmol·L^{-1} on the CHO-REPLACE and 8.33 $\pm$ 1.76 mmol·L^{-1} on the CHO-DEFICIT trial. Repeated measures ANOVA revealed main effects of time (p < 0.001) and treatment (p = 0.007), but no time–treatment interaction effect (p = 0.170).

Pre-OGTT insulin concentrations were higher during the CHO-REPLACE trial compared to the CHO-DEFICIT trial (36 $\pm$ 31 pmol·L^{-1} compared to 30 $\pm$ 20 pmol·L^{-1}, respectively p = 0.023). Following ingestion of the OGTT, the increase in serum insulin concentrations was greater with CHO-REPLACE versus CHO-DEFICIT (Figure 2C,D), whereby peak insulin concentrations were 337 $\pm$ 107 pmol·L^{-1} during CHO-REPLACE, compared to 260 $\pm$ 101 pmol·L^{-1} during CHO-DEFICIT

($p = 0.012$). Repeated measures ANOVA revealed main effects of time ($p < 0.001$) and treatment ($p = 0.028$), but no time—treatment interaction effect ($p = 0.158$).

The HOMA2-IR was ~16% higher with CHO-REPLACE versus CHO-DEFICIT (Figure 3A; $p = 0.015$), whereas the Matsuda insulin sensitivity index was ~25% lower with CHO-REPLACE vs. CHO-DEFICIT (Figure 3B; $p = 0.001$).

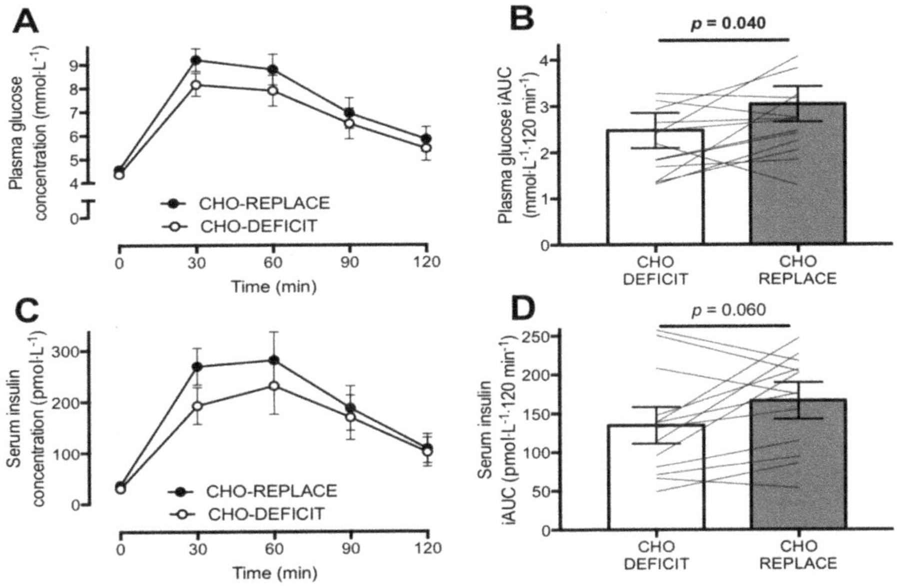

Figure 2. Postprandial glycaemia (**A**,**B**) and insulinemia (**C**,**D**) expressed as absolute concentrations (**A**,**C**) or as the incremental time-averaged area under the curve (iAUC; **B**,**D**) during the oral glucose tolerance test conducted ~16 h after exercise with either carbohydrate replacement (CHO-REPLACE) or a maintenance of the exercise-induced carbohydrate deficit (CHO-DEFICIT). $n = 13$. Data are means ± normalized 95% CI.

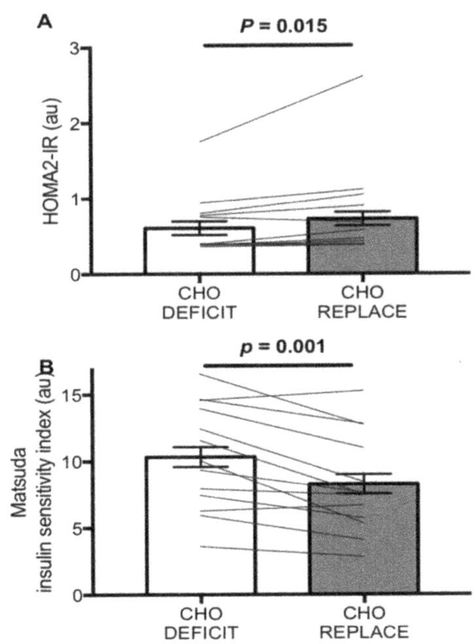

Figure 3. Homeostasis model of insulin resistance (HOMA2-IR) (**A**) and the Matsuda insulin sensitivity index (**B**) during the oral glucose tolerance test conducted ~16 h after exercise with either carbohydrate replacement (CHO-REPLACE) or a maintenance of the exercise-induced carbohydrate deficit (CHO-DEFICIT). $n = 13$. Data are means ± normalized 95% CI.

3.3. Whole-Body Substrate Utilisation

Pre-OGTT, whole-body carbohydrate utilization was 0.08 ± 0.05 g·min^{-1} during the CHO-REPLACE trial and 0.06 ± 0.05 g·min^{-1} during the CHO-DEFICIT trial (p = 0.639). Following ingestion of the OGTT, carbohydrate utilization increased ~2-fold in both trials (Figure 4A; time effect: $p < 0.001$), with no differences between trials (treatment effect: $p = 0.378$; time–treatment interaction effect: $p = 0.099$).

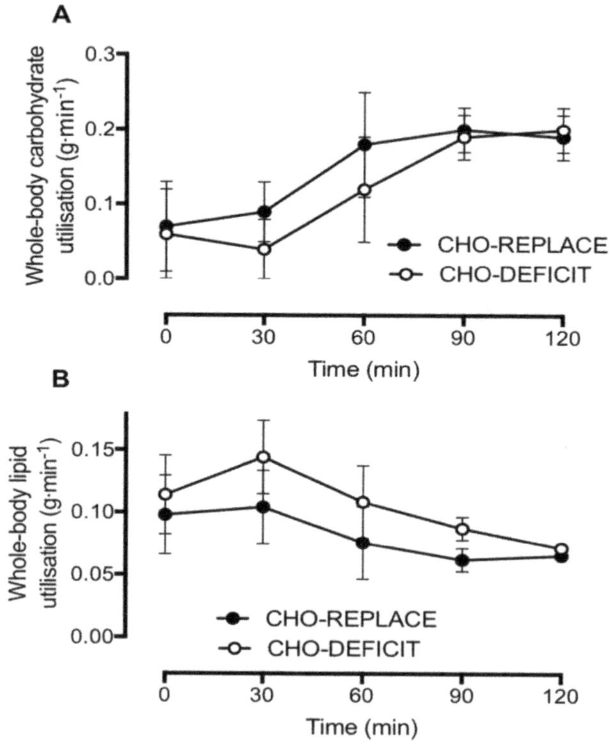

Figure 4. Whole-body carbohydrate (**A**) and lipid utilization (**B**) during an oral glucose tolerance test conducted ~16 h after exercise with either carbohydrate replacement (CHO-REPLACE) or a maintenance of the exercise-induced carbohydrate deficit (CHO-DEFICIT). n = 7. Data are means ± normalized 95% CI.

Pre-OGTT, whole-body lipid utilization was 0.10 ± 0.03 g·min^{-1} during the CHO-REPLACE trial and 0.11 ± 0.03 g·min^{-1} during the CHO-DEFICIT trial (p = 0.350). Following ingestion of the OGTT, lipid utilization was suppressed in both trials (Figure 4B; time effect: $p < 0.001$), but to a greater extent in CHO-REPLACE vs. CHO-DEFICIT (Figure 4B; treatment effect: $p = 0.033$; time–treatment interaction effect: $p = 0.048$).

4. Discussion

The present study demonstrates that replacement of the carbohydrate utilized during a single bout of exercise impairs both insulin sensitivity and glucose tolerance by ~20–25% the following morning, relative to when the exercise-induced carbohydrate deficit is maintained. Importantly, these changes were most clearly apparent in the postprandial state. Furthermore, postprandial fat oxidation was suppressed by post-exercise replacement of carbohydrate use.

Previous work has demonstrated that, whilst exercise is a potent method of stimulating muscle glucose uptake and insulin sensitivity, the carbohydrate deficit induced by exercise is key factor that mediates these responses. However, previous work has primarily used intravenous methods of assessing insulin sensitivity and/or action, which do not necessarily translate into the tolerance of ingested nutrients.

It has been suggested that the degree of whole-body carbohydrate depletion is a key mediator of exercise induced-increases in insulin action. Indeed, a positive relationship has been reported between post-exercise carbohydrate depletion and the change in insulin action assessed during intravenous glucose infusion, whereby a carbohydrate deficit of greater than 90 g was associated with an increase in insulin action [21]. In the present study, the mean carbohydrate deficit was 221 $\pm$ 59 g; all participants had a carbohydrate deficit of at least 99 g and there was a clear ~25% increase in insulin sensitivity as assessed by the Matsuda index, which was apparent in 12 of 14 individuals. Furthermore, whilst we did not have an energy-matched, low-carbohydrate condition to isolate the effect of carbohydrate versus energy-replacement, it has previously been demonstrated that re-feeding fat post-exercise does not influence glucose tolerance or insulin sensitivity the following morning [22]. Therefore, our data extend those findings demonstrating that post-exercise carbohydrate re-feeding does influence glucose tolerance and insulin sensitivity the following morning. Taken together, the evidence suggests that whole-body carbohydrate depletion induced by exercise is a key mediator of the enhanced insulin sensitivity and glucose control induced by exercise.

We report that both HOMA2-IR and the Matsuda insulin sensitivity index indicated an impairment in insulin sensitivity with post-exercise carbohydrate replacement, by ~16% and ~25%, respectively. Fasting concentrations of insulin and glucose primarily reflect changes in hepatic insulin sensitivity, whereas at postprandial concentrations, hepatic glucose production is negligible [18,23]. On this basis, it has been suggested that HOMA2-IR is primarily reflective of hepatic insulin sensitivity, whereas the Matsuda insulin sensitivity index is more heavily influenced by peripheral insulin sensitivity [24]. The finding that postprandial metabolic responses are more clearly altered than fasted measures by post-exercise carbohydrate replacement suggests that peripheral insulin sensitivity was more heavily influenced by replacement of carbohydrate compared to hepatic insulin sensitivity. It should be acknowledged that the present data does not allow for interpretation of insulin secretion to be assessed. Therefore, the reduction in glucose tolerance with carbohydrate replacement compared to the maintenance of the carbohydrate deficit could be due, in part, to an inability of the pancreas to secrete sufficient insulin to compensate for the change in insulin sensitivity. Furthermore, it has previously been shown that the timing of carbohydrate re-feeding post-exercise can alter insulin action the following day [11]. Delaying the re-feeding of carbohydrate by 3 h results in lower insulin action compared to immediate post-exercise carbohydrate refeeding. Therefore, the immediate re-feeding in the present study may result in a lower-bound estimate of the impairment in insulin sensitivity with carbohydrate replacement in the hours following exercise.

During a prolonged bout (90 min) of moderate-to-high intensity exercise (70% VO_2peak), both muscle and liver glycogen concentrations can be expected to be depleted by ~60% [25–27]. In the absence of meaningful quantities of carbohydrate or glycogenic amino acid ingestion, only negligible net quantities of muscle and liver glycogen will be synthesized. Therefore, prior to the OGTT we can be confident that both muscle and liver glycogen stores would have been depleted with the carbohydrate restriction trial, compared to the carbohydrate replacement trial. Accordignly, the observed suppression of insulin sensitivity with replacement of carbohydrate is likely to represent depletion of all major glycogen stores. This is important, since hepatic and muscle insulin sensitivity appear to respond differentially to carbohydrate status during acute (3-d) overfeeding [28].

Increased insulin sensitivity after exercise does not always translate into changes in glucose control after the ingestion of nutrients. Post-exercise increases in glucose disposal can be offset by changes in the rate of appearance of glucose from both endogenous and exogenous sources [6], leading to either no change or even a worsening of glucose tolerance after a single bout of exercise [7]. This highlights the importance of complementing mechanistic studies of insulin sensitivity that involve intravenous infusion methods, with oral ingestion of nutrients. In the present study, we employed an oral glucose tolerance test and demonstrated that restoring carbohydrate balance via post-exercise feeding increases postprandial glycaemia compared to a maintenance of the exercise-induced carbohydrate deficit.

We also observed a difference in postprandial substrate metabolism, whereby whole-body lipid utilization was suppressed when the carbohydrate deficit of prior exercise had been replaced. This suppression of postprandial lipid utilization is consistent with findings from others in which the energy utilized by exercise was replaced [12] and further highlights the role of carbohydrate balance in the regulation of whole-body lipid utilization. Furthermore, the greater suppression of postprandial lipid utilization with carbohydrate replacement is consistent with the high fasting and postprandial insulinemia that we observed, since insulin is a potent inhibitor of adipose tissue lipolysis in vivo [29].

The present study design does not allow for inferences to be drawn about the effects of exercise on insulin sensitivity and glycemic control, since there was no non-exercise trial. Therefore, the carbohydrate replacement in this study could be either: (1) partly attenuating the effects of exercise; (2) completely reversing the effects of exercise; or (3) superseding the effects of exercise. However, the effects of exercise on glycemia and insulin sensitivity are well-characterized, and the aim of the present investigation was specifically to establish the degree to which the carbohydrate deficit of exercise alters glycemia and insulin sensitivity. By comparing the carbohydrate replacement trial with the maintenance of the exercise-induced carbohydrate deficit, we are able to establish the extent to which the whole-body carbohydrate deficit alters postprandial glycaemia and insulin sensitivity. Furthermore, the findings of this study will need further work to provide greater generalizability and to further characterize the underlying mechanisms. In order to be able to generalize the findings to people at risk of metabolic disease, this work should be repeated in overweight/obese people, and at lower exercise intensities. Some disease states and lower exercise intensities would reduce the reliance on glycogen use during exercise, thereby altering the nutrition interaction with exercise. Furthermore, to firmly establish the underlying mechanisms, isotopic tracers and euglycemic hyperinsulinemic clamps could establish rates of appearance and disappearance of glucose, and peripheral insulin sensitivity, respectively. Nonetheless, the present study provides the first evidence, as proof of principle, that replacing the carbohydrate deficit induced by exercise has the capacity to reduce postprandial glycemic control and insulin sensitivity the following morning.

5. Conclusions

This study is the first to show that feeding carbohydrate to replace that utilized during exercise can reduce insulin sensitivity and glucose tolerance the next morning in healthy adults, when compared to a preservation of the exercise-induced carbohydrate deficit. Furthermore, carbohydrate replacement suppresses subsequent postprandial fat utilization. The mechanism through which exercise improves insulin sensitivity and glucose control is therefore (at least partly) dependent on carbohydrate availability, and so the day-to-day metabolic health benefits of exercise might be best attained by maintaining a carbohydrate deficit overnight.

Acknowledgments: The study was partially funded by Ministry of Science and Technology in Taiwan (MOST 105-2918-I-005-004). We appreciate the technical support provided by the Sport Science Research Center of National Taiwan University of Sport.

Author Contributions: C.-L.W., J.A.B. and J.T.G. conceived and designed the experiments and wrote the manuscript; H.L.T. and P.-G.W. performed the experiments; Y.-C.C. ran assays and analyzed the data; C.-L.W., H.L.T., J.A.B. and J.T.G analyzed the data. All authors contributed to editing the manuscript.

References

1. Edinburgh, R.M.; Betts, J.A.; Burns, S.F.; Gonzalez, J.T. Concordant and divergent strategies to improve postprandial glucose and lipid metabolism. *Nutr. Bull.* **2017**, *42*, 113–122. [CrossRef]
2. Maarbjerg, S.J.; Sylow, L.; Richter, E.A. Current understanding of increased insulin sensitivity after exercise—Emerging candidates. *Acta Physiol.* **2011**, *202*, 323–335. [CrossRef] [PubMed]

3. Pan, X.R.; Li, G.W.; Hu, Y.H.; Wang, J.X.; Yang, W.Y.; An, Z.X.; Hu, Z.X.; Lin, J.; Xiao, J.Z.; Cao, H.B.; et al. Effects of diet and exercise in preventing NIDDM in people with impaired glucose tolerance. The Da Qing IGT and diabetes study. *Diabetes Care* **1997**, *20*, 537–544. [CrossRef] [PubMed]
4. Rabol, R.; Petersen, K.F.; Dufour, S.; Flannery, C.; Shulman, G.I. Reversal of muscle insulin resistance with exercise reduces postprandial hepatic de novo lipogenesis in insulin resistant individuals. *Proc. Natl. Acad. Sci. USA* **2011**, *108*, 13705–13709. [CrossRef] [PubMed]
5. Mikines, K.J.; Sonne, B.; Farrell, P.A.; Tronier, B.; Galbo, H. Effect of physical exercise on sensitivity and responsiveness to insulin in humans. *Am. J. Physiol.* **1988**, *254*, E248–E259. [CrossRef] [PubMed]
6. Rose, A.J.; Howlett, K.; King, D.S.; Hargreaves, M. Effect of prior exercise on glucose metabolism in trained men. *Am. J. Physiol. Endocrinol. Metab.* **2001**, *281*, E766–E771. [CrossRef] [PubMed]
7. Gonzalez, J.T.; Veasey, R.C.; Rumbold, P.L.; Stevenson, E.J. Breakfast and exercise contingently affect postprandial metabolism and energy balance in physically active males. *Br. J. Nutr.* **2013**, *110*, 721–732. [CrossRef] [PubMed]
8. Kelley, D.E.; Mandarino, L.J. Fuel selection in human skeletal muscle in insulin resistance: A reexamination. *Diabetes* **2000**, *49*, 677–683. [CrossRef] [PubMed]
9. Galgani, J.E.; Moro, C.; Ravussin, E. Metabolic flexibility and insulin resistance. *Am. J. Physiol. Endocrinol. Metab.* **2008**, *295*, E1009–E1017. [CrossRef] [PubMed]
10. Black, S.E.; Mitchell, E.; Freedson, P.S.; Chipkin, S.R.; Braun, B. Improved insulin action following short-term exercise training: Role of energy and carbohydrate balance. *J. Appl. Physiol.* **2005**, *99*, 2285–2293. [CrossRef] [PubMed]
11. Stephens, B.R.; Sautter, J.M.; Holtz, K.A.; Sharoff, C.G.; Chipkin, S.R.; Braun, B. Effect of timing of energy and carbohydrate replacement on post-exercise insulin action. *Appl. Physiol. Nutr. Metab.* **2007**, *32*, 1139–1147. [CrossRef] [PubMed]
12. Burton, F.L.; Malkova, D.; Caslake, M.J.; Gill, J.M. Energy replacement attenuates the effects of prior moderate exercise on postprandial metabolism in overweight/obese men. *Int. J. Obes.* **2008**, *32*, 481–489. [CrossRef] [PubMed]
13. Newsom, S.A.; Schenk, S.; Thomas, K.M.; Harber, M.P.; Knuth, N.D.; Goldenberg, N.; Horowitz, J.F. Energy deficit after exercise augments lipid mobilization but does not contribute to the exercise-induced increase in insulin sensitivity. *J. Appl. Physiol.* **2010**, *108*, 554–560. [CrossRef] [PubMed]
14. Nolte, L.A.; Gulve, E.A.; Holloszy, J.O. Epinephrine-induced in vivo muscle glycogen depletion enhances insulin sensitivity of glucose transport. *J. Appl. Physiol.* **1994**, *76*, 2054–2058. [CrossRef] [PubMed]
15. Gonzalez, J.T. Paradoxical second-meal phenomenon in the acute post-exercise period. *Nutrition* **2014**, *30*, 961–967. [CrossRef] [PubMed]
16. Gonzalez, J.T.; Stevenson, E.J. Assessment of the post-exercise glycemic response to food: Considering prior nutritional status. *Nutrition* **2014**, *30*, 122–123. [CrossRef] [PubMed]
17. Edinburgh, R.M.; Hengist, A.; Smith, H.A.; Betts, J.A.; Thompson, D.; Walhin, J.P.; Gonzalez, J.T. Prior exercise alters the difference between arterialised and venous glycaemia: Implications for blood sampling procedures. *Br. J. Nutr.* **2017**, *117*, 1414–1421. [CrossRef] [PubMed]
18. Matsuda, M.; DeFronzo, R.A. Insulin sensitivity indices obtained from oral glucose tolerance testing: Comparison with the euglycemic insulin clamp. *Diabetes Care* **1999**, *22*, 1462–1470. [CrossRef] [PubMed]
19. Levy, J.C.; Matthews, D.R.; Hermans, M.P. Correct homeostasis model assessment (HOMA) evaluation uses the computer program. *Diabetes Care* **1998**, *21*, 2191–2192. [CrossRef] [PubMed]
20. Loftus, G.R.; Masson, M.E. Using confidence intervals in within-subject designs. *Psychon. Bull. Rev.* **1994**, *1*, 476–490. [CrossRef] [PubMed]
21. Holtz, K.A.; Stephens, B.R.; Sharoff, C.G.; Chipkin, S.R.; Braun, B. The effect of carbohydrate availability following exercise on whole-body insulin action. *Appl. Physiol. Nutr. Metab.* **2008**, *33*, 946–956. [CrossRef] [PubMed]
22. Fox, A.K.; Kaufman, A.E.; Horowitz, J.F. Adding fat calories to meals after exercise does not alter glucose tolerance. *J. Appl. Physiol.* **2004**, *97*, 11–16. [CrossRef] [PubMed]
23. Radziuk, J. Homeostatic model assessment and insulin sensitivity/resistance. *Diabetes* **2014**, *63*, 1850–1854. [CrossRef] [PubMed]

24. Gonzalez, J.T.; Barwood, M.J.; Goodall, S.; Thomas, K.; Howatson, G. Alterations in whole-body insulin sensitivity resulting from repeated eccentric exercise of a single muscle group: A pilot investigation. *Int. J. Sport Nutr. Exerc. Metab.* **2015**, *25*, 405–410. [CrossRef] [PubMed]
25. Gonzalez, J.T.; Fuchs, C.J.; Betts, J.A.; van Loon, L.J. Liver glycogen metabolism during and after prolonged endurance-type exercise. *Am. J. Physiol. Endocrinol. Metab.* **2016**, *311*, E543–E553. [CrossRef] [PubMed]
26. Gonzalez, J.T.; Fuchs, C.J.; Smith, F.E.; Thelwall, P.E.; Taylor, R.; Stevenson, E.J.; Trenell, M.I.; Cermak, N.M.; van Loon, L.J. Ingestion of glucose or sucrose prevents liver but not muscle glycogen depletion during prolonged endurance-type exercise in trained cyclists. *Am. J. Physiol. Endocrinol. Metab.* **2015**, *309*, E1032–E1039. [CrossRef] [PubMed]
27. Alghannam, A.F.; Jedrzejewski, D.; Tweddle, M.G.; Gribble, H.; Bilzon, J.; Thompson, D.; Tsintzas, K.; Betts, J.A. Impact of muscle glycogen availability on the capacity for repeated exercise in man. *Med. Sci. Sports Exerc.* **2016**, *48*, 123–131. [CrossRef] [PubMed]
28. Lundsgaard, A.M.; Sjoberg, K.A.; Hoeg, L.D.; Jeppesen, J.; Jordy, A.B.; Serup, A.K.; Fritzen, A.M.; Pilegaard, H.; Myrmel, L.S.; Madsen, L.; et al. Opposite regulation of insulin sensitivity by dietary lipid versus carbohydrate excess. *Diabetes* **2017**, *66*, 2583–2595. [CrossRef] [PubMed]
29. Jensen, M.D.; Caruso, M.; Heiling, V.; Miles, J.M. Insulin regulation of lipolysis in nondiabetic and IDDM subjects. *Diabetes* **1989**, *38*, 1595–1601. [CrossRef] [PubMed]

11

Carbohydrate Knowledge and Expectations of Nutritional Support among Five Ethnic Groups Living in New Zealand with Pre- and Type 2 Diabetes

Zhuoshi Zhang [1], John Monro [2] and Bernard J. Venn [1,*]

[1] Department of Human Nutrition, University of Otago, PO Box 56, Dunedin 9054, New Zealand; zhuoshi.zhang@gmail.com

[2] New Zealand Institute for Plant & Food Research Ltd., Private Bag 11600, Palmerston North 4442, New Zealand; John.Monro@plantandfood.co.nz

* Correspondence: bernard.venn@otago.ac.nz

Abstract: Despite availability of diabetes and nutrition information for people with pre- and type 2 diabetes, the uptake and understanding of these resources may differ among ethnic groups. Our objective was to explore dietary knowledge and diabetes experiences amongst Māori, European, Pacific Island, Indian and East Asian people living in New Zealand with a focus on carbohydrate-containing foods. A registered diabetes dietitian led ethnic-specific discussions in groups involving 29 people with pre- or type 2 diabetes. Discussions were audio-recorded, fully transcribed and coded independently by two investigators. Themes were developed using deductive and inductive techniques. Five themes emerged: knowledge, concerns, achievements, simplicity and self-determination. Nutritional knowledge was lacking and a greater awareness of trustworthy dietary resources was needed. There were concerns about diabetes complications and appropriate carbohydrate-containing foods and portions. Contrary to this, people felt proud when achieving dietary goals and grateful for support from health care providers and family. Participants were willing to engage in self-care if advice from health professionals was given in plain language, and in a culturally appropriate manner. Given the desire to take an active role in diabetes self-management and willingness to use electronic devices, an ethnic-specific nutrition education resource could be a valuable tool.

Keywords: diabetes; ethnicity; knowledge; discussion groups; qualitative

---

1. Introduction

Diabetes is one of the fastest growing chronic conditions in the world [1–3]. In 2014, an estimated 422 million adults were living with diabetes compared to 108 million in 1980 [4]. To provide the best diabetes care, a structured multidisciplinary team input is required [5,6]. However, the reality for many countries is a general lack of resources to cater for the growing number of people with diabetes, resulting in a knowledge gap for people both recently diagnosed and for those with a longstanding diagnosis [7,8]. To fill the knowledge gap, people with pre- and type 2 diabetes can obtain information on their condition from healthcare professionals and also from less regulated sources such as the internet or from other people [9]. However, information obtained from unregulated sources can lead to misunderstanding, frustration and anxiety [10–12], poor compliance in treatment [12–15] and unnecessary food avoidance [12,16,17]. In questioning people with diabetes, there was confusion about the effect of macronutrients on glucose metabolism with carbohydrates being particularly misunderstood to the extent that some people were avoiding fruit due to the sugar content [17].

Psychological stresses for people with diabetes including fear, worry and perceived discrimination have been found in the second Diabetes Attitudes, Wishes and Needs (DAWN2) study [10].

Negative emotions and lack of knowledge could be even more pronounced in ethnic minorities living in Caucasian counties, who tend to receive less diabetes education [18], have less diabetes and nutritional knowledge [19], are less engaged with diabetes services [20,21], and have higher emotional distress [22,23] compared with the ethnic majority. Compounding these inequalities is a tendency for ethnic minority groups to have a higher prevalence of type 2 diabetes and to have poorer health outcomes compared with the ethnic majority group [18,24,25].

Identifying barriers and expectations to diabetes care and nutrition education is important if ethnic inequalities are to be addressed. Little work has been carried out comparing differences among ethnicities regarding diabetes nutrition management [10,12,13,17]. New Zealand is a country in which ethnic experiences can be explored because it has indigenous and immigrant minority groups living in a predominantly Caucasian population, reflecting ethnic diversity in many other countries [26]. The research described herein was aimed at exploring experiences and emotions among Māori, European, Pacific Island, Indian, and East Asian people living with diabetes or pre-diabetes using ethnic-specific discussion groups. The purpose was to ascertain participants knowledge and beliefs pertaining to diabetes and nutrition management with an emphasis on carbohydrate-containing foods, and expectations of diabetes care.

2. Materials and Methods

2.1. Ethics and Recruitment

Discussion groups were recruited through verbal referral from general practitioners' practices, primary health organisations and community health support services; and via advertisements in local medical centres, libraries, community centres, sports facilities and supermarkets within Auckland city, New Zealand. A Māori group was recruited in Palmerston North, New Zealand through contacts with funders of the study. Adults with pre- and type 2 diabetes who expressed interest were asked for their consent to receive a telephone call regarding the study. Eligible participants were invited to attend one discussion group based on their ethnicity. The inclusion criteria were: A diagnosis of pre-diabetes or type 2 diabetes confirmed by medical records, New Zealand residency and the ability to communicate in English. The exclusion criteria were people with severe speech or hearing difficulties, inability to speak English or over 79 years of age. The Ngāi Tahu Research Consultation Committee was consulted and the study was approved by the University of Otago Human Ethics Committee (Reference no. 14/179).

Of the 71 referrals and respondents (19 Europeans, 10 Māori, 11 Pacific Islanders, 14 East Asian and 17 Indian), 13 people could not be contacted and 22 declined. Of the remaining 36 people confirmed, seven did not show up on the day. Thus, 29 participants (six Europeans, five Māori, four Pacific Islanders, eight East Asians and six Indians) attended separate ethnic-specific discussion groups. Prior to the discussion group meetings, an information sheet was given to each participant, queries were answered and consent was obtained.

2.2. Procedures

The discussion groups were designed and conducted in accordance with a published protocol [27]. The discussions were held onsite in Auckland and via Skype® in Palmerston North with Māori participants, a method of synchronous interviewing that is becoming more widely used [28]. The duration of each discussion group was approximately 1 h, and was conducted in a safe and comfortable environment with each session audio-recorded. An interviewer guide was used to facilitate each discussion.

Predefined questions were open-ended and designed to avoid wording suggestive of a 'correct' answer. All participants were encouraged to speak freely, whilst the facilitator (Z.Z.) ensured that the discussion moved at an appropriate pace and finished on time. Sentence completion exercises and brainstorming on a whiteboard were used during the discussion. At the end of the session, the purpose of the discussion was repeated and final questions from participants were answered. The predefined questions were as follows:

- What do you know about pre-diabetes and type 2 diabetes?
- What diabetes support have you received?
- What nutrition for diabetes advice have you been given by clinicians?
- Where do you seek for diabetes and nutrition information and how accurate is it?
- What do you want to know about nutrition for diabetes?
- Have you seen a dietitian for pre- and type 2 diabetes?
- What foods do you think affect your blood glucose?
- What foods do you think are healthy or unhealthy?
- Would an electronic diabetes nutritional education resource be useful for you?

2.3. Data Analysis

A published thematic approach involving deductive and inductive techniques was used [29]. A priori, the broad code categories of knowledge, experience and desire were selected. All audio recordings were transcribed verbatim by the facilitator (Z.Z.) and checked by a second investigator (B.J.V.). Photographs were taken to record notes written on a whiteboard during discussions. Two researchers (Z.Z. and B.J.V.) independently coded the transcript. Potentially important words and phrases were identified through both inductive and deductive analysis. These two sets of coding phrases were compared. Any discrepancies were discussed through reviewing of the transcript and the meaning of a code until consensus was reached. Coding phrases were further developed into themes through creating a coding manual.

3. Results

Participant characteristics are given in Table 1. The average time since diagnosis for the nine people with pre-diabetes was 2.6 years and for those with type 2 diabetes, 13.7 years. Of the 29 participants, six participants were not on any diabetes medication. Of those on medication; 19 were prescribed metformin; eight sulfonylureas; one dipeptidyl peptidase-4 inhibitor and four used insulin with or without oral medications.

Table 1. Characteristics of the study participants.

	Total	**European**	**Māori**	**PI**	**East Asian**	**Indian**
	(*n* = 29)	(*n* = 6)	(*n* = 5)	(*n* = 4)	(*n* = 8)	(*n* = 6)
N, pre-diabetes	9	3	1		4	1
N, type 2 diabetes	20	3	4	4	4	5
Mean years of pre-diabetes	2.6	4.3	2.0		2.0	0.5
Mean years of type 2 diabetes	13.7	3.3	27.3	10.8	14.0	11.2
Sex, *n* (Male, Female)	11M, 18F	1M, 5F	3M, 2F	1M, 3F	2M, 6F	4M, 2F
		Age, *n*				
45–54 year	3		1		2	
55–64 year	10	2	1	2	3	2
65–74 year	15	4	3	2	3	3
74–79 year	1					1
		Diabetes medication, *n*				
None	6	3	1		2	
Metformin	19	3	3	3	5	5
Sulfonylureas	8		2	1	2	3
Insulin	4	1	2		1	
Other	1	1				
		Education, *n*				
University	10	1			6	3
Polytechnic	7	2	2		1	2
Secondary	1	1				
Did not answer	11	2	3	4	1	1

PI, Pacific Islander.

3.1. Knowledge

General practitioners (GPs) and registered nurses (RNs) were identified as the two main sources providing diabetes dietary advice across all discussion groups. Half of the participants felt that they had not received adequate nutrition advice. Being unaware of, and having limited access to a diabetes service was emphasised within the Māori, Pacific Island and Indian discussions. All groups voiced a strong need for adequate consultation time with health professionals to discuss their queries and concerns regarding nutrition and diabetes control.

> *"You don't really have a lot time, you go in there, and you just don't have time to ask some questions."—European group*

> *"So far the lecture from diabetes centre was the only one come and discuss something (sic). We have not heard from anybody else. It will help a long way if there are more dietitian lectures."—Indian group*

Apart from three people who had recently attended diabetes education classes, participants struggled when asked to describe pre- and type 2 diabetes, what the risk factors were of developing type 2 diabetes, and the reasons for pharmaceutical and lifestyle intervention. European, Māori and East Asian groups commented on the inconsistency of medical and nutritional information obtained from the Internet, and of more concern, among health professionals. Confusion due to lack of diabetes knowledge or being exposed to conflicting information was apparent within all ethnic groups. Animated discussions on suitable food and beverage options, and how to interpret laboratory test results, occurred in all discussions.

> *"You go on to the Internet and you can find that this is good. Do this and do that, and you can also go to another parts and it says this is all wrong."—European group*

Identifying "good" and "bad" dietary choices was another key discussion point in all discussions. Most participants were restricting foods and beverages that were perceived by them to be bad for diabetes whilst increasing the intake of so-called good foods. Although all participants understood foods and drinks with added sugar increased blood glucose concentrations, the majority failed to recognise or understand that other carbohydrate in food has blood glucose raising potential.

> *"Eat less potatoes, we are not allowed to eat potatoes, only once a week."—Indian group*
> *"These three fruits are deadly for diabetes. They are very high in sugar."—Māori group*

The foods in Table 2 were identified within the groups as raising blood glucose concentration. Foods identified as raising blood sugar among all groups were sugar and rice. Bread was not specifically referred to by any group and only the Indian group mentioned potato. Some ethnic-specific starchy foods were identified; taro by the Pacific Island group and noodles by the East Asian group. Three out of four Pacific Island and half of the European and East Asian participants believed that fatty foods raised blood glucose. In conclusion, half of the participants across all ethnic groups considered that they had received inadequate nutrition information from the health system. Conflicting messages from various official, online and lay sources led to misunderstanding, confusion and unnecessary dietary restriction. Māori, Pacific Island and Indian participants were less likely to have accessed specialist diabetes and dietetic services in both primary and secondary care.

3.2. Concerns

All participants were fearful and worried about diabetes complications, medication side effects, eating unhealthy foods and having inappropriate portion sizes. Suspicion regarding the credibility of information obtained from health professionals and other sources was expressed by all except the Indian group who relied heavily upon the information provided by general practitioners and practice nurses. The Indian participants were less aware of specific diabetes education services compared with the other groups. A lack of involvement in diabetes management decision making left the majority of Māori and Pacific Island participants feeling powerless over their own health destiny. One Māori and one East Asian participant also described feelings of embarrassment in discussing their diabetes with friends and family.

Table 2. Foods thought by participants to affect blood glucose.

	Europeans	Māori	PI [1]	East Asian	Indian
Carbohydrate foods or foods containing a substantial proportion of carbohydrate	Bakery food Biscuits	Banana Corn	Chocolate Lollies	Muffins Fruit	Beetroot Cola
	Cakes	Fruit	Rice	Instant noodles	Rice
	Chocolate	Refined sugar	Sugar	Rice	Soft drinks
	Pasta	Rice	Takeaways (e.g., sweet and sour)	Rice cakes	Potato
	Rice Processed foods [2]	Sprite	Taro	Sugar	
Foods containing little carbohydrate	Bacon Butter Nuts Sausages		Fatty foods	Alcohol Cheese	Alcohol

[1] PI, Pacific Islander; [2] Processed foods may or may not contain substantial amounts of carbohydrate.

"How do you know that we got diabetes? Because I don't know I have diabetes, until I had a stroke."—Pacific Island group
"It says it affect the heart, kidneys, eyes and foot. We've told it starts with eyes, heart, kidney and sensation of the foot. Sensation of the foot starts lose, any disease on the foot is difficult to get cured."—Indian group

Participants of all ethnicities, except Indian, expressed aversion to a top-down nutrition consultation style in which health providers were viewed as judgemental. With regard to food, there was some confusion and resentment expressed in all groups with health care providers making incorrect assumptions, giving mixed messages, and imposing unexplained dietary restrictions.

"The practice nurse assumed that I drank a lot of juice and coke. And I said, No! I don't!"—Māori group

"My GP tells me the same thing, keep doing some exercise, eat these and don't eat that. But I said, the food is just food. What you just told me not to eat is not fair."—Pacific Island group

"What about apple? Red apple or granny smith? Just one apple? What about rock melon? Yoghurt?"—Indian group

"My GP asked me to go back to Korean diet like rice and soup. I am kind of confused, cause I eat so much rice."—East Asian group

"You tend to not like suddenly a whole lot of restrictions coming from middle of nowhere, telling you that you can't eat this bread roll, you can't drink this, you can't do this, you can't do that. And you rebel."—European group

Frustration was expressed that some of the nutrition advice was conflicting both among health care providers and between the advice received and what they had read or believed. One Pacific Island and one Indian participant were angry with themselves for relapsing into unhealthy eating habits and not paying enough attention to their own health.

Concern was expressed in the Māori, Pacific Island and Indian groups regarding self-adjustment of medication and treatment. The main drivers were doubt about their understanding of best practice and fear of diabetes complications.

"I started to feel shaking of my hands. Then I take some sugar or any foods. Once I okay with it, I stop. If I am outside, the best thing I do is buy bananas, two or three bananas, and one or two lollies."—Indian group

"Knowing that the insulin should have not been starting at two units. I raised it up myself to straight up to 20, 30 units. My sugar level was too high and I can sense things going wrong in the eyes. I've just started to deal with it myself."—Māori group

In summary, participants were fearful about diabetes complications. Doubt, confusion, embarrassment, powerlessness, frustration and anger were all negative emotions expressed by different ethnic groups.

3.3. Achievements

All ethnic groups stated an interest in understanding diabetes, diabetes medications, diet, lifestyle, and how to make changes. Several participants in the European, Māori and Pacific Island groups expressed strong desires to halt the progression of diabetes and to stay healthy. Several participants from each ethnic group described feeling satisfied and even delighted when achieving goals such as achieving recommended blood glucose and maintaining dietary change. Some participants described their sense of gratitude towards families, friends, healthcare professionals, and other people with diabetes for psychosocial and medical support. Although this was mentioned in all group discussions, appreciation of family involvement was specifically highlighted by the majority of the Māori and Pacific Island participants.

"Sometimes, I get frustrated. I didn't want to take any more medicine, but my wife talk me out of it. That's why I need my family, because they are the part taking care of you when you are at home."—Pacific Island group

Recognising the need for good diabetes control and the setting of life goals, such as preventing diabetes complications and spending quality time with families, served as inspiration. Many participants expressed satisfaction from having discovered ways to change diet and lifestyle, being able to sustain these changes, avoiding temptation, and ultimately improving blood glucose control. Although the Indian group expressed determination to make change, the sense of achievement conveyed by the other groups was absent from the Indian group discussion.

"I felt really good now. I said I feel I have to do something for myself, and I will see a real change, even up until now, I am a really changed person."—Pacific Island group

"You need to have a reason to want to live in a long healthy life. For me, I want to see my grandchildren."—East Asian group

"I realise in the end it is the weight. I just concentrated on the quantity that I eat, and when I eat. I stopped the night snacking. I love chocolate, but I can now go to the fridge and look at the chocolate and then just walk away."—European group

Overall, all ethnic groups showed positive attitudes such as feeling motivated and satisfied when good diabetes control was attained. Family support was a highlight for Māori and Pacific Island groups.

3.4. Simplicity

All groups wanted simple explanations regarding appropriate food choices. A pictorial or video format illustrated with 'hands' and 'plate' models were favoured over text-based advice, particularly if text incorporated scientific jargon. Some European, East Asian and Indian participants were also receptive to advice in numerical form for ease of compliance, for example, 30 min of exercise.

"Dietitian said I could have enough potatoes like 3 small eggs, so that's how I used to measure my carbohydrate portions. It's like 3 small egg size."—East Asian Group

"Plate is plate. Half, quarter, quarter simple (for vegetables, protein and carbohydrate)."—Māori Group

Participants wanted advice to be practical, especially around home cooking methods and dietary patterns. Participants discussed how simple, practical advice that they had received had increased their confidence in trying and maintaining dietary and lifestyle changes. Being culturally appropriate was also highlighted by East Asian and Pacific Island groups. Although European, Māori and Indian groups felt comfortable with English-language-based education, being able to receive information in their own language was preferred by some participants in East Asian and Pacific Island groups.

"With diabetes, I want to know how to cook from what you have in your cupboards rather than buy all these lovely things, which is not realistic for your diabetes."—Māori group

"Beans, corn, and nuts ... See we've never eaten these good foods. We weren't brought up with it." —Pacific Island group

"It will be nice if you can speak Samoan."—Pacific Island group

All ethnic groups expressed a desire for simple, visual and practical dietary advice. Some participants wanted dietary advice to include cultural foods and to be presented in their familiar language.

3.5. Self-Determination

Māori, Pacific Island and Indian participants expressed a willingness to make lifestyle changes but felt overly dependent on treatment plans assigned by health professionals. Several participants described frustration at the lack of involvement in decision-making around their own diabetes care, citing poor communication with their healthcare provider. All groups indicated reluctance in making dietary and lifestyle changes because they felt inadequately informed as to the need for change as well as perceived difficulties in avoiding temptation and fitting additional self-monitoring tasks into their life.

"It's more peace of mind, actually explaining what the medication is, instead of, go it's one of these."—Māori group

"The chemist said, Oh! You don't need this medication anymore. It is not on the prescription. You are on this. I turned around and said, what do you mean? It isn't inside of what I have been taking? They've changed that, and I never knew."—Pacific Island group

Most participants supplemented the advice of their health professionals by taking initiatives to improve their diabetes knowledge by reading books, searching online, attending diabetes classes, making dietary changes and self-monitoring blood glucose.

"You would look it on the computer, because the information is there."—Māori group

"I read all about the diabetes myself from library books."—East Asian group

All ethnic groups wanted to have ongoing support and reminders to achieve and maintain a healthy diet and to increase compliance with medication. Peer support was valued by several Māori, Pacific Island and European participants who found sharing their experiences with other people with diabetes helpful and reassuring.

"Diabetes, diet is the main issue. Required to be reminded it again and again."—Indian group

"Being around with people got the same illness as myself, it's like a support group (sic). What they said was exactly what I am going through. And I think, none of us has been perfect. We all did the same thing."—Pacific Island group

The use of new technology to search for health-related information and recipes, and to create meal plans was clearly shown in all discussions. Convenience and immediate information feedback were highly regarded attributes, although reliability of this information was a major concern. Only five out of 29 participants said they would probably not use online learning resources, with cost and age identified as barriers.

"When we went on the Internet, we have to depend on it. Sometimes there is different information on one topic."—Indian group

"You cut back on the portions of your meal and then finish with a piece of fruit. You don't really know if it is the right thing or not. If you have a website that you could look at would be quite good."—European group

4. Discussion

The main findings of the discussion groups were a recognised lack of knowledge and confusion regarding diet and medication, fear of diabetes complications, a willingness to participate in the management of their condition, the need to keep advice practical, the use of simple language, avoidance of medical jargon, and engagement with self-directed searching for information despite some level of mistrust and confusion with Internet sites. All ethnic groups expressed willingness to modify diet and carbohydrate sources given reliable and culturally appropriate guidance. Ethnic-specific issues included Māori, Pacific Island and Indian participants discussing lack of group education and access to specialist diabetes services. Explanation as to why dietary modification and medication treatment was needed would provide motivation for change in the Māori and Pacific Island groups. Some Māori, Pacific Island and East Asian participants thought it desirable that information be made available in their own language. Some participants were self-checking blood glucose and body weight but there was a general feeling among the Indian participants that this should be monitored by clinicians rather than by themselves. The Māori and Pacific Island groups discussed family support more prominently than other ethnic groups.

One theme common to all groups was dietary restriction, a topic that was discussed with some resentment. In the United States, dietary restriction has been associated with diabetes distress, in part because it affected other members of the family [30]. To what extent carbohydrate foods should be restricted by people with type 2 diabetes is questionable, as carbohydrate intake has not been associated with long-term glycaemic control [31]. Food avoidance can be restrictive, but a positive idea that emerged from our Māori group was the desire to learn about food and nutrition in order to pass that knowledge onto the next generation. However, sourcing reliable dietary information was problematic for all groups. The European group cited 'on-going referrals' from health care providers to diabetes educational classes, whilst the other ethnic groups mentioned engagements in formal education sessions only sporadically. Our data are consistent with those obtained in Australia in which non-European ethnicity was associated with a lessened likelihood of having received formal diabetes education [18], highlighting the need to promote diabetes support services to non-European ethnic communities.

Participants regarded the quality of diabetes information to be variable. The Internet was challenging as it provided instantly accessible information but conflicting messages. In other work it has been found that the quality of information is dependent on various factors including whether people are seeking factual information and advice on a course of action or subjective opinion [32]. The 'hit' rates for correct, complete or appropriate responses were low, typically around 50%, with lower scores for the advice type questions [32]. Hence, the frustration and confusion expressed by our participants is entirely consistent with other people's experiences with the Internet [33]. The quality and safety of online diabetes information has been queried, with misinformation, promotional material, poor readability, lack of evidence-based recommendations and lack of medical disclaimers of concern [34–36]. Despite drawbacks, use of the Internet as a source of information will continue for all ethnicities as it is a resource that has broad reach and ease of access [37].

In contrast, there were differences among the ethnic groups for engagement and experience with health professionals. The European group discussed on-going interactions with healthcare services whereas Pacific Island participants seemed unaware of such services. The Indian group respected and trusted clinicians' knowledge and judgment similar to British Indian patients [38,39] favouring clinicians' guidance over self-care [40]. However, diabetes management requires a considerable component of self-care and advising Indian patients of the importance of this is essential [40]. The East Asian group reported positive experiences of healthcare providers despite lack of consultation time, reflecting experiences of Vietnamese women with gestational diabetes [41]. Our Māori participants were less trusting of the advice that they had received from health professionals. It has been documented that Māori and Pacific Island people are more likely to miss hospital appointments compared with Europeans [42]. Perhaps these sentiments and behaviours partly explain the reliance that Māori and Pacific Island participants placed on family for emotional and practical support, consistent with being more likely to live in multi-generational households and taking care of family members [43]. In South Africa, black African patients were found to be frequently receiving incorrect and inappropriate dietary advice from health educators [44]. In our participants, lack of dietary knowledge, confusion and mistrust in sources of dietary information identifies a clear need for reliable dietary education and advice.

Cumulatively, the views expressed by our participants encompassed those found in Canada where limited consulting time, excessive workload and insufficient trust in physicians advice led to patients' poor motivation and compliance [45]. It has been suggested that health systems set up to deal with acute care are poorly configured to cater to the needs of people with chronic conditions and that strategies are needed within those systems to foster self-management in people with diabetes [46]. A move away from an authoritarian approach to one of an equal partnership between health professionals and those with chronic conditions has been advocated [46]. Aspirational goals of partnership in disease management are in agreement with the views expressed by our participants who objected to a 'top-down' approach. To encourage partnership, communication with patients should be designed to answer their queries and to fit in with individuals' goals and culture [46,47]. A patient-centred partnership program has facilitated patient participation and shared decision-making with health care providers [48]. Although trials designed to enhance patient-practitioner partnership may have positive outcomes in terms of patient engagement, more studies are needed to assess clinical outcomes following such intervention trials [49].

The present article describes novel research in which the experiences and expectations of diabetes management has been explored by a diabetes dietitian in participants representing five ethnic groups living in New Zealand. Sample numbers for each ethnic group were small and this poses a problem for generalisability within ethnicities as factors such as urban/rural; country of origin; cultural background; socioeconomic status; and education are underlying variables to the experiences and expectations of the individuals that participated. Nevertheless, the themes described herein were expressed in all discussion groups, suggestive that at least these themes may have commonality. In that context, the findings may have generalisability to other predominantly Caucasian countries whose population includes ethnic minority groups. In Australia, language, level of education and indigenous ethnicity were associated with lower diabetes knowledge and reduced likelihood of having received diabetes education and dietetic advice [18]. In the United States, immigrant and indigenous people experience diet-related disparities in which poorer diets are consumed by minority groups compared with the white populous [50]. Limitations to the generalizability of our study are that only participants who spoke English and who had an interest in diabetes management were involved. Potentially, our information is optimistic as people with a lesser command of the English language may struggle even more with accessing reliable information. Lack of knowledge of a country's main language has been identified as disadvantaging access to health care [51]. Another limitation may be a small sample with participant numbers ranging from four to eight, although five has been suggested as an appropriate number for conducting group discussions [52]. Nevertheless, there are still limits on the generalisability of the discussions both within New Zealand, a geographically diverse country, and among other countries. Some issues though are likely to be common around the world, particularly with regard to ethnic minority groups living in Westernised countries. In summary, for people of various ethnicities with pre-diabetes and type 2 diabetes living in New Zealand, we have found heterogeneity in dietary knowledge and experience of the health care system. An overarching sentiment expressed by all ethnic groups was a desire for reliable dietary information to assist with self-management of the disease.

Our participants expressed a need to access trustworthy sources of dietary information, a view consistent with previous work in which participants with pre- or type 2 diabetes were wary of some of the dietary information that they had accessed [53]. A general feeling was expressed that the nutrition advice of primary care providers was reliable although some reservations were expressed regarding inconsistency of messages and many participants supplemented the advice of their health professionals from other sources. Confusion around food and general dietary advice expressed by our participants is perhaps not surprising given that there is still uncertainty and controversy in the best dietary approaches for the prevention and management of type 2 diabetes [54].

It has been recommended that nutritional advice be given by a registered dietitian or by referral to a diabetes self-management education (DSME) program [55]. However, success in weight loss and diabetes remission over 1 year has been reported when participants were guided by general practitioners [56]. Nevertheless, it is unclear how well long-term nutrition goals and sustained weight loss can be maintained outside of the study setting, or whether it is feasible or necessary for continuing general practitioner involvement in dietary management. In a focus group survey of general practitioners practicing in Belgium, a sentiment expressed was that dieticians could give more adequate and more varied food advice than the general practitioners themselves [57]. Indeed, dietitian advice has been found to improve clinical outcomes in people with type 2 diabetes [58,59]. However, dietary advice is time-consuming and for many countries there are too few dietitians to adequately cater to the service demand [5].

5. Conclusions

It is telling that despite a plethora of electronic devices, websites and software applications, our participants struggled to find reliable information given in a practical and culturally appropriate manner. From the participants' perspective, dietary advice needed to be consistent and to have been derived from a solid evidence base. With the challenge of an increasing prevalence of diabetes and limited health care resources, development of a professional organisation-endorsed, evidence-based, electronic resource using lay language, in video or pictorial format and available in different languages could be a highly sought after instructional tool. Consumer acceptance and performance of such a multi-ethnic resource would need to be monitored for efficacy.

Author Contributions: Conceptualization, Z.Z., B.J.V.; Methodology, Z.Z., J.M., B.J.V.; Transcription and analysis, Z.Z., B.J.V.; Draft manuscript, Z.Z., B.J.V.; Funding acquisition, J.M.; Final draft, Z.Z., B.J.V., J.M.

References

1. Whiting, D.R.; Guariguata, L.; Weil, C.; Shaw, J. IDF diabetes atlas: Global estimates of the prevalence of diabetes for 2011 and 2030. *Diabetes Res. Clin. Pract.* **2011**, *94*, 311–321. [CrossRef] [PubMed]
2. Wild, S.; Roglic, G.; Green, A.; Sicree, R.; King, H. Global prevalence of diabetes: Estimates for the year 2000 and projections for 2030. *Diabetes Care* **2004**, *27*, 1047–1053. [CrossRef] [PubMed]
3. International Diabetes Federation. IDF Diabetes Atlas, 8th edition. Available online: http://www.diabetesatlas.org/ (accessed on 26 July 2018).
4. World Health Organization. *Global Report on Diabetes*; WHO Press: Geneva, Switzerland, 2016.
5. Segal, L.; Leach, M.J.; May, E.; Turnbull, C. Regional primary care team to deliver best-practice diabetes care: A needs-driven health workforce model reflecting a biopsychosocial construct of health. *Diabetes Care* **2013**, *36*, 1898–1907. [CrossRef] [PubMed]
6. Goenka, N.; Turner, B.; Vora, J. Commissioning specialist diabetes services for adults with diabetes: Summary of a Diabetes UK Task and Finish group report. *Diabet. Med.* **2011**, *28*, 1494–1500. [CrossRef] [PubMed]
7. Nobel, J. Bridging the knowledge-action gap in diabetes: Information technologies, physician incentives and consumer incentives converge. *Chronic Illn.* **2006**, *2*, 59–69. [PubMed]
8. Saleh, F.; Ara, F.; Afnan, F. Assessment of Gap between Knowledge and Practices among Type 2 Diabetes Mellitus Patients at a Tertiary-Care Hospital in Bangladesh. Available online: http://dx.doi.org/10.1155/2016/4928981 (accessed on 16 July 2018).
9. Cantaro, K.; Jara, J.A.; Taboada, M.; Mayta-Tristan, P. Association between information sources and level of knowledge about diabetes in patients with type 2 diabetes. *Endocrinol. Nutr.* **2016**, *63*, 202–211. [CrossRef] [PubMed]
10. Stuckey, H.L.; Mullan-Jensen, C.B.; Reach, G.; Kovacs Burns, K.; Piana, N.; Vallis, M.; Wens, J.; Willaing, I.; Skovlund, S.E.; Peyrot, M. Personal accounts of the negative and adaptive psychosocial experiences of people with diabetes in the second diabetes attitudes, wishes and needs (DAWN2) study. *Diabetes Care* **2014**, *37*, 2466–2474. [CrossRef] [PubMed]
11. Benroubi, M. Fear, guilt feelings and misconceptions: Barriers to effective insulin treatment in type 2 diabetes. *Diabetes Res. Clin. Pract.* **2011**, *93* (Suppl. 1), S97–S99. [CrossRef]
12. Badruddin, N.; Basit, A.; Hydrie, M.Z.I.; Hakeem, R. Knowledge, attitude and practices of patients visiting a diabetes care unit. *Pak. J. Nutr.* **2002**, *1*, 99–102.
13. Al-Qazaz, H.; Sulaiman, S.A.; Hassali, M.A.; Shafie, A.A.; Sundram, S.; Al-Nuri, R.; Saleem, F. Diabetes knowledge, medication adherence and glycemic control among patients with type 2 diabetes. *Int. J. Clin. Pharm.* **2011**, *33*, 1028–1035. [CrossRef] [PubMed]
14. Al-Qazaz, H.K.; Hassali, M.A.; Shafie, A.A.; Syed Sulaiman, S.A.; Sundram, S. Perception and knowledge of patients with type 2 diabetes in Malaysia about their disease and medication: A qualitative study. *Res. Soc. Adm. Pharm.* **2011**, *7*, 180–191. [CrossRef] [PubMed]
15. Puder, J.J.; Keller, U. Quality of diabetes care: Problem of patient or doctor adherence? *Swiss Med. Wkly.* **2003**, *133*, 530–534. [PubMed]
16. Spronk, I.; Kullen, C.; Burdon, C.; O'Connor, H. Relationship between nutrition knowledge and dietary intake. *Br. J. Nutr.* **2014**, *111*, 1713–1726. [CrossRef] [PubMed]
17. Breen, C.; Ryan, M.; Gibney, M.J.; O'Shea, D. Diabetes-related nutrition knowledge and dietary intake among adults with type 2 diabetes. *Br. J. Nutr.* **2015**, *114*, 439–447. [CrossRef] [PubMed]
18. Bruce, D.G.; Davis, W.A.; Cull, C.A.; Davis, T.M. Diabetes education and knowledge in patients with type 2 diabetes from the community: The fremantle diabetes study. *J. Diabetes Complicat.* **2003**, *17*, 82–89. [CrossRef]
19. Hawthorne, K.; Robles, Y.; Cannings-John, R.; Edwards, A.G. Culturally appropriate health education for type 2 diabetes mellitus in ethnic minority groups. *Cochrane Database Syst. Rev.* **2008**. [CrossRef]
20. Kristensen, J.K.; Bak, J.F.; Wittrup, I.; Lauritzen, T. Diabetes prevalence and quality of diabetes care among Lebanese or Turkish immigrants compared to a native Danish population. *Prim. Care Diabetes* **2007**, *1*, 159–165. [CrossRef] [PubMed]
21. Ferguson, W.J.; Candib, L.M. Culture, language, and the doctor-patient relationship. *Fam. Med.* **2002**, *34*, 353–361. [PubMed]

22. Delahanty, L.; Grant, R.W.; Wittenberg, E.; Bosch, J.; Wexler, D.; Cagliero, E.; Meigs, J. Association of diabetes-related emotional distress with diabetes treatment in primary care patients with Type 2 diabetes. *Diabet. Med.* **2007**, *24*, 48–54. [CrossRef] [PubMed]
23. Spencer, M.S.; Kieffer, E.C.; Sinco, B.R.; Palmisano, G.; Guzman, J.R.; James, S.A.; Graddy-Dansby, G.; Two Feathers, J.; Heisler, M. Diabetes-specific emotional distress among African Americans and Hispanics with type 2 diabetes. *J. Health Care Poor Underserved* **2006**, *17*, 88–105. [CrossRef] [PubMed]
24. Lanting, L.C.; Joung, I.M.A.; Mackenbach, J.P.; Lamberts, S.W.J.; Bootsma, A.H. Ethnic differences in mortality, end-stage complications, and quality of care among diabetic patients: A review. *Diabetes Care* **2005**, *28*, 2280–2288. [CrossRef] [PubMed]
25. Mukhopadhyay, B.; Forouhi, N.G.; Fisher, B.M.; Kesson, C.M.; Sattar, N. A comparison of glycaemic and metabolic control over time among South Asian and European patients with type 2 diabetes: Results from follow-up in a routine diabetes clinic. *Diabet. Med.* **2006**, *23*, 94–98. [CrossRef] [PubMed]
26. Fearon, J.D. Ethnic and cultural diversity by country. *J. Econ. Growth* **2003**, *8*, 195–222. [CrossRef]
27. Stewart, D.W.; Shamdasani, P.N. *Focus Groups: Theory and Practice*, 3rd ed.; SAGE Publications Inc.: Thousand Oaks, CA, USA, 2015.
28. Janghorban, R.; Latifnejad Roudsari, R.; Taghipour, A. Skype interviewing: The new generation of online synchronous interview in qualitative research. *Int. J. Qual. Stud. Health Well-Being* **2014**, *9*. [CrossRef] [PubMed]
29. Fereday, J.; Muir-Cochrane, E. Demonstrating rigor using thematic analysis: A hybrid approach of inductive and deductive coding and theme development. *Int. J. Qual. Methods* **2006**, *5*, 1–11. [CrossRef]
30. Egede, L.E.; Funnell, M.M.; Hsu, W.C.; Ruggiero, L.; Siminerio, L.M.; Stuckey, H.L. Ethnic differences in family member diabetes involvement and psychological outcomes: Results from the second Diabetes Attitudes, Wishes and Needs (DAWN2) study in the USA. *Curr. Med. Res. Opin.* **2015**, *31*, 1297–1307.
31. Snorgaard, O.; Poulsen, G.M.; Andersen, H.K.; Astrup, A. Systematic review and meta-analysis of dietary carbohydrate restriction in patients with type 2 diabetes. *BMJ Open Diabetes Res. Care* **2017**, *5*. [CrossRef] [PubMed]
32. Kanthawala, S.; Vermeesch, A.; Given, B.; Huh, J. Answers to health questions: Internet search results versus online health community responses. *J. Med. Internet Res.* **2016**, *18*. [CrossRef] [PubMed]
33. Arora, N.K.; Hesse, B.W.; Rimer, B.K.; Viswanath, K.; Clayman, M.L.; Croyle, R.T. Frustrated and confused: The American public rates its cancer-related information-seeking experiences. *J. Gen. Intern. Med.* **2008**, *23*, 223–228. [CrossRef] [PubMed]
34. Greene, J.; Choudhry, N.; Kilabuk, E.; Shrank, W. Online social networking by patients with diabetes: A qualitative evaluation of communication with facebook. *J. Gen. Intern. Med.* **2011**, *26*, 287–292. [CrossRef] [PubMed]
35. Weitzman, E.R.; Cole, E.; Kaci, L.; Mandl, K.D. Social but safe? Quality and safety of diabetes-related online social networks. *J. Am. Med. Inform. Assoc.* **2011**, *18*, 292–297. [CrossRef] [PubMed]
36. Chomutare, T.; Fernandez-Luque, L.; Årsand, E.; Hartvigsen, G. Features of mobile diabetes applications: Review of the literature and analysis of current applications compared against evidence-based guidelines. *J. Med. Internet Res.* **2011**, *13*. [CrossRef] [PubMed]
37. Fox, S.; Duggan, M. PewInternet: Health online 2013. Available online: http://www.pewinternet.org/2013/01/15/health-online-2013/ (accessed on 4 September 2018).
38. Lawton, J.; Ahmad, N.; Hanna, L.; Douglas, M.; Hallowell, N. Diabetes service provision: A qualitative study of the experiences and views of Pakistani and Indian patients with type 2 diabetes. *Diabet. Med.* **2006**, *23*, 1003–1007. [CrossRef] [PubMed]
39. Lawton, J.; Ahmad, N.; Hallowell, N.; Hanna, L.; Douglas, M. Perceptions and experiences of taking oral hypoglycaemic agents among people of Pakistani and Indian origin: Qualitative study. *BMJ* **2005**, *330*. [CrossRef] [PubMed]
40. Sohal, T.; Sohal, P.; King-Shier, K.M.; Khan, N.A. Barriers and facilitators for type-2 diabetes management in South Asians: A systematic review. *PLoS ONE* **2015**, *10*. [CrossRef] [PubMed]
41. Hirst, J.E.; Tran, T.S.; Do, M.A.; Rowena, F.; Morris, J.M.; Jeffery, H.E. Women with gestational diabetes in Vietnam: A qualitative study to determine attitudes and health behaviours. *BMC Pregnancy Childbirth* **2012**, *12*. [CrossRef] [PubMed]

42. Milne, V.; Kearns, R.; Harrison, A. Patient age, ethnicity and waiting times determine the likelihood of non-attendance at a first specialist rheumatology assessment. *Int. J. Rheum. Dis.* **2014**, *17*, 19–25. [CrossRef] [PubMed]
43. Ministry of Social Development. In *New Zealand Families Today: A Briefing for the Families Commision*; Ministry of Social Development: Wellington, New Zealand, 2004.
44. Nthangeni, G.; Steyn, N.P.; Alberts, M.; Steyn, K.; Levitt, N.S.; Laubscher, R.; Bourne, L.; Dick, J.; Temple, N. Dietary intake and barriers to dietary compliance in black type 2 diabetic patients attending primary health-care services. *Public Health Nutr.* **2002**, *5*, 329–338. [CrossRef] [PubMed]
45. Brez, S.; Rowan, M.; Malcolm, J.; Izzi, S.; Maranger, J.; Liddy, C.; Keely, E.; Ooi, T.C. Transition from specialist to primary diabetes care: A qualitative study of perspectives of primary care physicians. *BMC Fam. Pract.* **2009**, *10*. [CrossRef] [PubMed]
46. Funnell, M.M.; Anderson, R.M. Empowerment and Self-Management of Diabetes. *Clin. Diabetes* **2004**, *22*, 123–127. [CrossRef]
47. Bains, S.S.; Egede, L.E. Associations between health literacy, diabetes knowledge, self-care behaviors, and glycemic control in a low income population with type 2 diabetes. *Diabetes Technol. Ther.* **2011**, *13*, 335–341. [CrossRef] [PubMed]
48. Varming, A.R.; Hansen, U.M.; Andresdottir, G.; Husted, G.R.; Willaing, I. Empowerment, motivation, and medical adherence (EMMA): The feasibility of a program for patient-centered consultations to support medication adherence and blood glucose control in adults with type 2 diabetes. *Patient Prefer. Adherence* **2015**, *9*, 1243–1253. [PubMed]
49. Griffin, S.J.; Kinmonth, A.L.; Veltman, M.W.; Gillard, S.; Grant, J.; Stewart, M. Effect on health-related outcomes of interventions to alter the interaction between patients and practitioners: A systematic review of trials. *Ann. Fam. Med.* **2004**, *2*, 595–608. [CrossRef] [PubMed]
50. Satia, J.A. Diet-related disparities: Understanding the problem and accelerating solutions. *J. Am. Diet. Assoc.* **2009**, *109*, 610–615. [CrossRef] [PubMed]
51. Attridge, M.; Creamer, J.; Ramsden, M.; Cannings-John, R.; Hawthorne, K. Culturally appropriate health education for people in ethnic minority groups with type 2 diabetes mellitus. *Cochrane Database Syst. Rev.* **2014**, *9*. [CrossRef] [PubMed]
52. Krueger, R.A.; Casey, M.A. *Focus Groups: A Practical Guide for Applied Research*, 4th ed.; SAGE Publications Inc.: Thousand Oaks, CA, USA, 2009.
53. Lawrence, H.; Nathan Reynolds, A.; Joseph Venn, B. Perceptions of the healthfulness of foods of New Zealand adults living with prediabetes and type 2 diabetes: A pilot study. *J. Nutr. Educ. Behav.* **2017**, *49*, 339–345.e1. [CrossRef] [PubMed]
54. Forouhi, N.G.; Misra, A.; Mohan, V.; Taylor, R.; Yancy, W. Dietary and nutritional approaches for prevention and management of type 2 diabetes. *BMJ* **2018**, *361*. [CrossRef] [PubMed]
55. Gray, A. Nutritional Recommendations for Individuals with Diabetes. Available online: https://www.ncbi.nlm.nih.gov/pubmed/25905243 (accessed on 23 August 2018).
56. Unwin, D.; Unwin, J. Low carbohydrate diet to achieve weight loss and improve HbA1c in type 2 diabetes and pre-diabetes: Experience from one general practice. *Pract. Diabetes* **2014**, *31*, 76–79. [CrossRef]
57. Wens, J.; Vermeire, E.; Royen, P.V.; Sabbe, B.; Denekens, J. GPs' perspectives of type 2 diabetes patients' adherence to treatment: A qualitative analysis of barriers and solutions. *BMC Fam. Pract.* **2005**, *6*. [CrossRef] [PubMed]
58. Franz, M.J.; Monk, A.; Barry, B.; McClain, K.; Weaver, T.; Cooper, N.; Upham, P.; Bergenstal, R.; Mazze, R.S. Effectiveness of medical nutrition therapy provided by dietitians in the management of non-insulin-dependent diabetes mellitus: A randomized, controlled clinical trial. *J. Am. Diet. Assoc.* **1995**, *95*, 1009–1017. [CrossRef]
59. Coppell, K.J.; Kataoka, M.; Williams, S.M.; Chisholm, A.W.; Vorgers, S.M.; Mann, J.I. Nutritional intervention in patients with type 2 diabetes who are hyperglycaemic despite optimised drug treatment—Lifestyle Over and Above Drugs in Diabetes (LOADD) study: Randomised controlled trial. *BMJ* **2010**, *341*. [CrossRef] [PubMed]

12

Metabolic Responses to Carbohydrate Ingestion during Exercise: Associations between Carbohydrate Dose and Endurance Performance

Michael L. Newell [1,*], Gareth A. Wallis [2], Angus M. Hunter [3], Kevin D. Tipton [3] and Stuart D. R. Galloway [3]

1 Department of Life Sciences, Faculty of Science and Technology University of Westminster, London W1W 6UW, UK
2 School of Sport, Exercise and Rehabilitation Sciences, University of Birmingham, Birmingham B15 2TT, UK; g.a.wallis@bham.ac.uk
3 Physiology, Exercise and Nutrition Research Group, Faculty of Health Sciences and Sport, University of Stirling, Stirling FK9 4LA, UK; a.m.hunter1@stir.ac.uk (A.M.H.); k.d.tipton@stir.ac.uk (K.D.T.); s.d.r.galloway@stir.ac.uk (S.D.R.G.)
* Correspondence: m.newell@westminster.ac.uk

Abstract: Carbohydrate (CHO) ingestion during exercise lasting less than three hours improves endurance exercise performance but there is still debate about the optimal dose. We utilised stable isotopes and blood metabolite profiles to further examine metabolic responses to CHO (glucose only) ingestion in the 20–64 $g{\cdot}h^{-1}$ range, and to determine the association with performance outcome. In a double-blind, randomized cross-over design, male cyclists (n = 20, mean ± SD, age 34 ± 10 years, mass 75.8 ± 9 kg, peak power output 394 ± 36 W, VO_{2max} 62 ± 9 $mL{\cdot}kg^{-1}{\cdot}min^{-1}$) completed four main experimental trials. Each trial involved a two-hour constant load ride (185 ± 25 W) followed by a time trial, where one of three CHO beverages, or a control (water), were administered every 15 min, providing 0, 20, 39 or 64 g $CHO{\cdot}h^{-1}$. Dual glucose tracer techniques, indirect calorimetry and blood analyses were used to determine glucose kinetics, exogenous CHO oxidation (EXO), endogenous CHO and fat oxidation; and metabolite responses. Regression analysis revealed that total exogenous CHO oxidised in the second hour of exercise, and suppression of serum NEFA concentration provided the best prediction model of performance outcome. However, the model could only explain ~19% of the variance in performance outcome. The present data demonstrate that consuming ~40 $g{\cdot}h^{-1}$ of CHO appears to be the minimum ingestion rate required to induce metabolic effects that are sufficient to impact upon performance outcome. These data highlight a lack of performance benefit and few changes in metabolic outcomes beyond an ingestion rate of 39 $g{\cdot}h^{-1}$. Further work is required to explore dose-response effects of CHO feeding and associations between multiple metabolic parameters and subsequent performance outcome.

Keywords: glucose; fat oxidation; exogenous; fatty acids; hepatic glucose output

---

1. Introduction

During prolonged steady state exercise, endogenous glycogen stores and circulating plasma glucose are key substrates for energy provision. Fatigue is often reported to coincide with the depletion of endogenous carbohydrate (CHO) stores and the dysregulation of circulating plasma glucose concentration [1–3]. Ingesting CHO improves performance and extends exercise duration via a range of proposed mechanisms including: better maintenance of circulating plasma glucose [1], higher rates of exogenous [4] and total CHO oxidation, and endogenous glycogen sparing [5]. These proposed mechanisms do not occur in isolation but occur together facilitating force production and improving performance and exercise capacity.

Early research by Coyle et al. [1] reported that feeding CHO maintained blood glucose concentration and CHO oxidation rates, and in turn, exercise capacity increased 33% (3.02 versus 4.02 h) significantly in comparison to a water control. In a follow-up study [2] participants exercised to exhaustion and were then provided with either no CHO, ingested CHO, or infused CHO. Both CHO provision conditions increased exercise duration on commencement of exercise in comparison to no CHO. However, only the infusion condition maintained blood glucose concentration sufficiently to subsequently extend exercise duration above that of the CHO ingestion trial. The authors concluded that the maintenance of blood glucose concentration was the critical factor for maintaining sufficient CHO oxidation rates to extend exercise capacity.

Further research has indicated that the maintenance of higher CHO oxidation can be primarily explained by an increase in exogenous CHO oxidation rates [4]. An elevation in exogenous CHO oxidation rate and enhanced endurance exercise performance are now believed to be directly associated, despite little systematic evaluation to date. As a result, increasing exogenous CHO oxidation rate is thought to be essential for the enhancement of endurance performance when ingesting CHO throughout a range of 20–100 $g \cdot h^{-1}$. This relationship has led some researchers to hypothesise that maximising exogenous CHO oxidation rate, through use of glucose: fructose combinations at high feeding rates will result in further performance gains [6]. However, most studies examining performance benefits of multiple transportable CHO ingestion have been conducted in comparison to isocaloric single source CHO. The findings using this model are likely to be confounded by gastrointestinal issues when ingesting single source CHO at high feeding rates. At lower feeding rates, Smith et al. [4] demonstrated that the largest improvement in performance occurred when ingesting 60 $g \cdot h^{-1}$ in comparison to 15 or 30 $g \cdot h^{-1}$. The 60 $g \cdot h^{-1}$ ingestion rate also resulted in the highest exogenous CHO oxidation rate. These authors reported a non-significant but 'likely' 2.3% improvement in performance when comparing 60 vs. 30 $g \cdot h^{-1}$ suggesting a dose-response effect of CHO feeding rate. We recently reported that a 2.3% performance gain would not necessarily be 'likely' due to typical variance observed in performance outcome measures [7] when using a more suitably powered design. In addition, there has yet to be an extensive exploration of the association between multiple metabolic variables and subsequent exercise performance outcomes using a dose-response investigation. Thus, more work remains to be done to determine the key factors driving performance improvement in exercise lasting <3 h. In our previous work [7] a lack of any further improvement in performance when feeding 64 $g \cdot h^{-1}$ in comparison to 39 $g \cdot h^{-1}$ suggests that the metabolic alterations with feeding rates as low as 39 $g \cdot h^{-1}$ could be sufficient to maximise performance gains within this feeding rate range. As such, peak exogenous carbohydrate oxidation rate may not be the sole, or key, determining factor for performance enhancement during exercise lasting less than 3 h with the single source CHO doses studied.

Feeding CHO during exercise influences the usage of endogenous glycogen stores. Several studies have assessed endogenous glycogen utilisation using stable isotopes during 1–2 h of moderate intensity exercise. McConnell et al. [8] provided participants with 100 $g \cdot h^{-1}$ of CHO during 2 h of exercise at 69 ± 1% VO_{2peak}. Hepatic glucose output was suppressed in comparison to a control trial and remained close to baseline rates throughout the exercise bout. The authors calculated that a 51% reduction in hepatic glucose production occurred as a result of consuming 100 $g \cdot h^{-1}$ CHO in comparison to the control. Furthermore, Jeukendrup et al. [5] provided 30 and 180 $g \cdot h^{-1}$ of a glucose based CHO beverage during a 2 h moderate intensity exercise bout. They reported reduced fat oxidation rates, increased rate of appearance (Ra) and rate of disappearance (Rd) of glucose, and an increase in the oxidation of exogenous CHO particularly with the higher glucose dose. Endogenous muscle glycogen oxidation rates were not altered with either 30 or 180 $g \cdot h^{-1}$ of CHO in their study. However, liver glycogen breakdown was reduced when consuming 30 $g \cdot h^{-1}$, and completely inhibited when consuming 180 $g \cdot h^{-1}$ of CHO. These observations suggest that only when very high doses of glucose are ingested can hepatic glucose production be completely inhibited. Smith et al. [4] estimated a stepped reduction in the contribution of liver glycogen to total CHO oxidation during the second hour of their submaximal exercise bout whilst consuming 15, 30 and 60 g·h^{-1} of CHO. Interestingly, all three studies indicate that muscle glycogen was not spared with any ingestion rate provided. These data suggest that a focus on hepatic glycogen sparing is required when considering factors likely to influence subsequent performance outcomes.

The amount of CHO to ingest for optimal endurance performance has been widely debated. A consensus has been reached that the maximal exogenous CHO oxidation rate that can be achieved with glucose (single source CHO) ingestion is around ~1 g·min^{-1}. As previously mentioned, Smith et al. [4] suggested the existence of a dose response relationship between CHO ingestion rate and endurance exercise performance enhancement when feeding 0, 15, 30 and 60 g·h^{-1} of glucose. However, their initial study was underpowered. Their study was followed up with a multicentre investigation which presented evidence for a curvilinear dose response relationship with ingestion rates of a multi-source CHO beverage spanning 0 to 120 g·h^{-1} with a statistically optimal ingestion rate reported as 78 g·h^{-1}. However, whether maximal exogenous oxidation rates driven by higher CHO ingestion rates result in optimal performances during endurance tasks requires further metabolic analysis. Until now our previously published work is the most suitably powered and most statistically robust study design to indicate the lack of a clear dose response relationship with ingestion rates between 20 and 64 g·h^{-1} [7]. However, from these data alone we are unable to determine what the underlying physiological explanations were for the plateau in performance. We now present the metabolic data to explore these performance changes more comprehensively.

As such, in the present manuscript we aimed to explore the metabolic responses to submaximal endurance exercise with CHO ingestion rates between 0 and 64 g·h^{-1}. We specifically aimed to: examine glucose kinetics and quantify or estimate the total substrate usage from exogenous and endogenous glycogen stores by utilising stable isotopic tracers; measure key circulating metabolites; quantify the percentage contribution of key substrates throughout the exercise bout. We hypothesised that during exercise lasting <3 h there would be a minimum effective dose of CHO required to result in optimal metabolic responses, and endogenous CHO sparing, linked to improved performance outcome. We also hypothesized that both exogenous CHO oxidation rate and reduction in hepatic glucose production would be the key parameters most closely associated with performance outcomes.

2. Materials and Methods

2.1. Participants

Twenty trained male cyclists were recruited from regional cycling and triathlon clubs. The mean (±SD) characteristics of the participants were: age 34.0 (±10.2) years, body mass 74.6 (±7.9) kg, stature 178.3 (±8.0) cm, peak power output (PPO) 393 (±36) W, power output (PO) at lactate threshold 206 (±30) W and VO_{2max} 62 (±9) mL·kg^{-1}·min^{-1}. Participants were required to have been training for >6 h/week for >3 years. Each individual had the procedures and associated risks explained prior to providing written informed consent to participate in the study. The study was approved by the University of Stirling, Research Ethics Committee (SSREC number 604) in accordance with the Declaration of Helsinki. In some circumstances, not all participants were included in all datasets. Unfortunately, 2 participants had to be removed from all stable isotope and substrate use data due to measurement errors. Hence, the characteristics of participants included in the stable isotope analyses were: body mass 76.9 (±8.4) kg, stature 178.7 (±8.1) cm, PPO 392 (±34) W, VO_{2max} 61.2 (±8.2) mL·kg^{-1}·min^{-1} and PO at lactate threshold 206 (±30) W.

2.2. Pretesting

Following pre-screening, on week one of six, after a ten hour overnight fast, participants performed a two-part incremental cycle test (Lode Excalibur Sport, The Netherlands) to determine lactate threshold (LT), maximal oxygen uptake (VO_{2max}), and peak power output as described previously [7]. The mean ± SD lactate concentration at LT was 2.1 ± 0.4 mmol·L^{-1} corresponding to an intensity of 52 ± 6% of PPO for LT which is typical of other studies utilising a similar protocol [9]. The test end time and power output of the final stage was used to calculate peak power output (PPO) using the following Equation (1) [10]:

$$PPO = W_{final} + ([t/60] \times PI) \quad (1)$$

where, W_{final} = the power output of the final completed stage in (watts), t = the time spent in the final uncompleted stage (seconds), 60 = the duration of each stage (seconds) and PI = the increase in power output between each stage (W). Maximal oxygen uptake (VO_{2max}) was assessed via an automated online gas analyser (Oxycon Pro, Jaeger, Wuerzerberg, Germany). VO_{2max} was determined as the highest average VO_2 captured over a 30 s period.

2.3. Design

In a double blind, placebo controlled, randomised cross-over study design participants visited the laboratory for 5 experimental trials (1 preliminary and 4 intervention) over a five-week period. They completed one visit per week commencing each trial on the same day of the week and at the same time of day. On the first of these trial visits participants completed a full familiarisation. The familiarisation trial and the four subsequent intervention trials consisted of a 120 min steady state submaximal cycle ergometer ride at 95% lactate threshold (185 ± 25 W). Participants were asked to record their habitual dietary intake for 48 h prior to visit one and replicate this dietary intake for the two days prior to each subsequent visit. Additionally, participants were asked to arrive at the laboratory following a ~10 h overnight fast. Water was ingested before and during the familiarisation trial and was consumed at a rate of 1 L·h^{-1}. Thereafter, participants consumed in a counterbalanced randomized cross-over design either: 0%, 2%, 3.9% or 6.4% CHO solutions before and during exercise at a fluid ingestion rate of 1 L·h^{-1}. The 0% trial was a water control trial. Blood samples, expired gas collection and subjective measures were obtained every 15 min throughout the submaximal ride.

2.4. Experimental Trials

On arrival at the laboratory, participants emptied their bladder and bowel prior to nude body mass measurement. Participants then changed into cycling clothing. Teflon catheters were placed into an antecubital vein in each arm. One catheter was attached to a three way stop cock to enable stable isotopic tracer infusion. The second was attached to a 10-cm extension line for multiple venous blood sampling. The sampling line was kept patent with a sterile saline solution flush (2 mL) following each sample collection. A baseline blood sample was drawn (10 mL) prior to commencing the primed (18.54 μmol·kg^{-1}) continuous (0.32 μmol·kg^{-1}·min^{-1}) infusion of 6,6,$^2H_2$ glucose via a calibrated syringe pump (Asena GS Syringe Pump; Alaris Medical Systems, Basingstoke, UK) over 60 min at rest. Further blood samples were drawn at 30 min prior to and at the start of exercise for later determination of isotopic enrichments. The concentration of isotopic tracer in the infusate and the pre and post syringe weights were both determined to confirm the actual infusion rate achieved.

2.5. Immediately Pre Exercise

Five minutes prior to the start of exercise, a resting breath sample was collected into an expired gas-sampling bag (Quintron QT00892 GaSampler, Milwaukee, WI 53215, USA). 10 mL gas samples were immediately drawn into a 10 mL syringe from the bag and secured with a three way stop cock. Samples were then extracted with a 21G needle directly, and in duplicate, into evacuated exetainer tubes (Labco, High Wycombe, UK) for the determination of the CO_2 isotopic ratio of $^{13}C/^{12}C$. Two minutes prior to the start of exercise, a further blood sample was collected and the first bolus of CHO test solution was provided (240 mL). The infusion rate of the deuterated glucose tracer was then doubled at the start of exercise (to 0.64 μmol·kg^{-1}·min^{-1}) to accommodate for the increased turnover of glucose during exercise and to maintain plasma enrichment.

2.6. The 2 h Preload Ride and Performance Task

Participants then completed a 2 h submaximal ride at 95% LT (185 ± 25 W, 59 ± 7% of VO_{2max}). In the last 3 min of each 15 min time segment a breath by breath gas capture was obtained for the determination of VO_2 and VCO_2 (Oxycon Pro, Mannheim, Germany). Immediately following the expired gas collection participants removed the mouth piece and provided a single end-tidal breath sample into a breath sample bag (Quintron QT00892 GasSampler, Milwaukee, WI 53215, USA) for the determination of $^{13}C/^{12}C$ ratio as per the baseline sample. Following the breath sampling a 10 mL blood sample (10 mL) was drawn and stored on ice prior to centrifugation. Finally, participants were asked to rate their perceived exertion [11] before ingesting a volume of test drink (220 mL). This was repeated every 15 min throughout the 2 h ride. Following this a performance task lasting approximately 30 min was conducted and is reported elsewhere [7].

2.7. Carbohydrate Solutions

During the 2 h preload ride, each of four solutions were consumed in randomized double-blind fashion: 0% water (control); 2.0%; 3.9%; or 6.4% glucose (single source CHO) based commercially available solutions. All test solutions were maintained at 10 °C and were consumed at a rate of 1 L·h^{-1} providing 0, 20, 39 and 64 g·h^{-1} of CHO respectively. The 20 g·h^{-1} solution contained 37 mg of sodium per 100 mL with the 39 and 64 g·h^{-1} solutions both containing 50 mg per 100 mL. Each solution was initially provided two minutes prior to the start of exercise (240 mL) with subsequent volumes (220 mL) consumed every 15 min. The final drink was provided at 120 min of exercise. All solutions except for the 0% were enriched by adding 50 mg L^{-1} of U-$^{13}C_6$ glucose (Cambridge Isotopes, Cambridge, UK) during preparation by the laboratory technician. The trial day experimental protocol is shown in Figure 1.

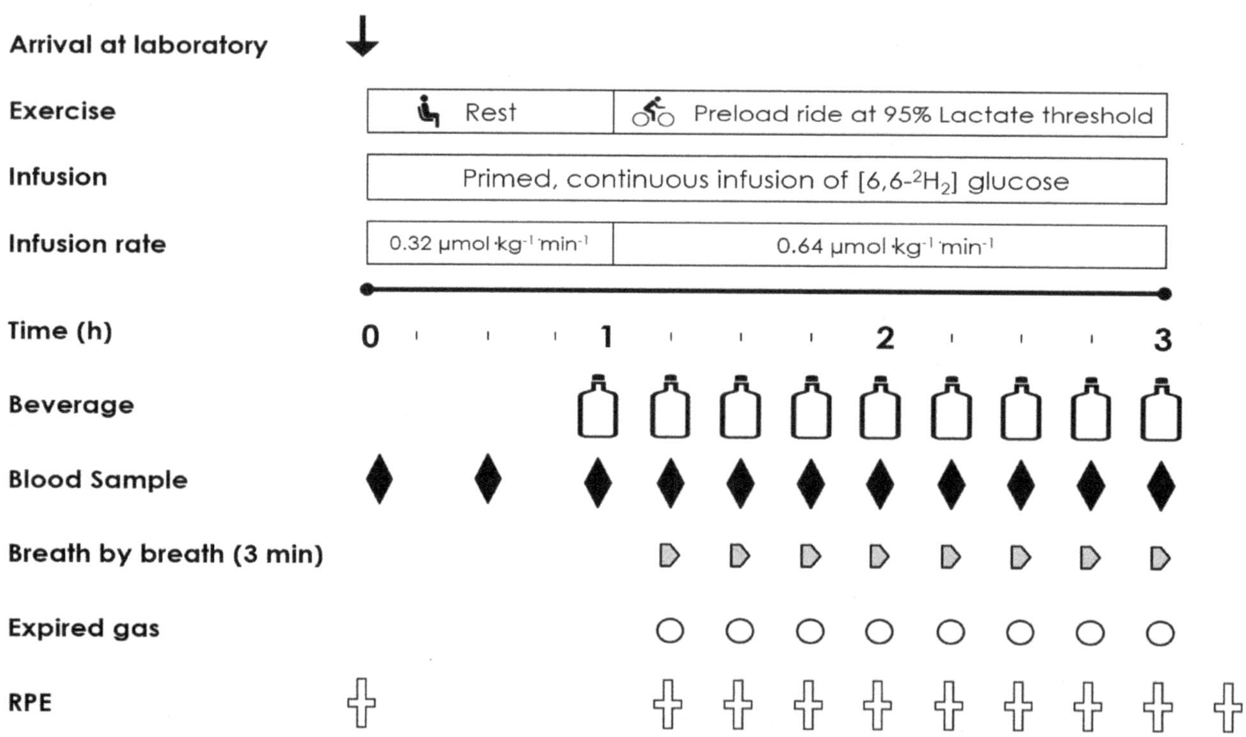

Figure 1. Trial visit time line indicating the infusion rate and time course and the frequency of measures taken throughout each experimental trial visit.

2.8. Analyses and Calculations

2.8.1. Blood

Blood samples were collected in EDTA-containing vacutainers and spun in a centrifuge at 3500 rpm for 10 min at 4 °C. Aliquots of plasma were then frozen and stored at −80 °C until further analysis. Plasma glucose, non-esterified fatty acids (NEFA), and lactate were analysed using enzymatic methods on an automated analyser (Ilab Aries, Instrumentation Laboratory, Warrington, UK). Plasma insulin and adrenaline concentrations were analysed using commercially available ELISA kits (Dimedic International, Hamburg, Germany and IBL International, Hamburg, Germany respectively). Both ELISAs were carried out following the manufacturer's instructions.

Plasma samples were derivatised for the analysis of [$^2H_2$] glucose and [^{13}C] glucose content. Briefly, 150 µL of plasma and 150 µL of distilled water with added hydrochloric acid (pH 2) was added to a glass vial and mixed vigorously for 10 s. 3 mL of methanol: chloroform (2.3:1) (500 mL = 348:152) was then added and mixed on a plate shaker (300 rpm) for 3 min. Samples were then centrifuged at 4 °C at 3500 rpm for 15 min. The supernatant was then pipetted into a new glass vial. Here 2 mL of chloroform and 1 mL of distilled water (pH 2) were added and mixed for 15 min on a plate shaker at 300 rpm. Samples were then centrifuged at 4 °C for 15 min at 3500 rpm. The supernatant was then pipetted into a new glass tube. The glass tubes were then transferred to a nitrogen drying rack and incubated at 40 °C for ~2 h until the vials were dry. Once dried 150 µL of butaneboronic acid (10 mg/1 mL pyridine) was added and mixed on a plate shaker for 15 min. Once mixed samples were then incubated at 95 °C for 30 min before 150 µL of acetic anhydride was added and mixed at 300 rpm for 90 min. Samples were then dried under nitrogen gas and incubated at 40 °C until dry. Samples were prepared for the GC-MS and GC-C-IRMS by adding 150 µL of ethylacetate and mixing for 10 min. [6,6,$^2H_2$] enrichment was determined by gas chromatography mass spectroscopy (GCMS) using selected ion monitoring at molecular weights of 297 and 299 ([^{12}C] and [$^2H_2$] respectively). Plasma [^{13}C] content was assessed using gas chromatography combustion isotope ratio mass spectroscopy (GC-C-IRMS). Plasma ^{13}C glucose enrichment was determined using the method of Pickert et al. [12], modified for use with gas chromatography-combustion-IRMS (GC-C-IRMS). The glucose derivative (1 µL) was injected into the GC (split ratio 1:15) and analysed by GC-C-IRMS (GC, Trace GC Ultra; C, GC Combustion III; IRMS, Delta Plus XP; all Thermo Finnigan, Herts, UK).

2.8.2. ^{13}C Breath Samples

Breath samples were analysed in duplicate for $^{13}C/^{12}C$ ratio by continuous-flow IRMS (GC, Trace GC Ultra; IRMS, Delta Plus XP; both Thermo Finnigan, Herts, UK).

2.8.3. Substrate Oxidation

Expired gas analysis was used to estimate rates of substrate oxidation from VO_2 and VCO_2 every 15 min. These breath measures were averaged every 4 breaths and the mean of these were taken from the last 60 s of a 3-min sampling period. Whole body substrate oxidation calculations were based on those proposed by Jeukendrup and Wallis [13]:

$$\text{CHO oxidation rate } (\text{g}\cdot\text{min}^{-1}) = 4.210\ VCO_2 - 2.962\ VO_2 \tag{2}$$

$$\text{Fat oxidation rate } (\text{g}\cdot\text{min}^{-1}) = 1.695\ VO_2 - 1.701\ VCO_2 \tag{3}$$

where VCO_2 and VO_2 are measured in litres per minute. Once the rate of substrate usage was determined during each 15-min breath by breath capture, the rates calculated in grams per minute were multiplied by 15 and summed from each time point to provide an estimate of the total substrate use during the whole exercise bout. Protein oxidation was considered as negligible.

2.8.4. Tracer Calculations

The isotopic enrichment in the expired breath samples was expressed as mean difference between the $^{13}C/^{12}C$ ratio of the sample and a known laboratory reference standard using the following formula to enable calculation of exogenous carbohydrate oxidation:

$$\text{Exogenous CHO oxidation } (g \cdot min^{-1}) = VCO_2\ [(R_{exp} - R_{ref})/(R_{exo} - R_{ref})]/k \quad (4)$$

where VCO_2 is in litres per minute, R_{exp} is the observed isotopic composition of expired CO_2, R_{ref} is the isotopic composition of expired CO_2 with the ingestion of the placebo, R_{exo} is the isotopic composition of exogenous glucose ingested in the drink and k (0.747 $L \cdot g^{-1}$) is the volume of CO_2 produced by the complete oxidation of glucose.

2.8.5. Percentage Contribution of Substrates (Second Hour of Exercise)

Once the total amount of exogenous carbohydrate oxidation had been determined, this rate was extrapolated over the previous 15 min period to determine total grams of exogenous carbohydrate oxidised in each time period from 60 min of exercise onwards. Only the second hour of exercise was considered as exogenous carbohydrate oxidation rates are stable. The total exogenous carbohydrate oxidised was subtracted from the total carbohydrate oxidised over the same time period to give an estimate of endogenous carbohydrate oxidation. The endogenous and exogenous carbohydrate oxidised totals were then multiplied by 4.07 to provide total carbohydrate energy expenditure in kcal for each carbohydrate source. The total fat oxidised was multiplied by 9.75 to give total energy expenditure (kcal) for fat oxidation [13]. The total energy expenditure from all three substrates was then summed and each component was expressed as a percentage of the total energy expenditure over the second hour of exercise.

2.8.6. Glucose Kinetics

From the $6,6,^2H_2$ tracer infusion the Ra and Rd of glucose were calculated with the single pool non-steady state equations of Steele, as modified for use with stable isotopes [14]. Total Ra represents the total splanchnic glucose from ingested CHO and liver derived glucose:

$$R_a \text{ total} = F - (pV \times (C_1 + C_2)/2 \times (E_2 - E_1)/(t_2 - t_1))/(E_2 + E_1)/2) \quad (5)$$

$$R_d \text{ total} = R_a \text{ total} - V \times (C_1 + C_2/t_2 - t_1) \quad (6)$$

where F is the infusion rate ($mg \cdot kg^{-1} \cdot min^{-1}$); E_1 and E_2 are the [$^2H_2$] glucose enrichments (MPE) in plasma at time points t_1 and t_2 (min), respectively; C_1 and C_2 are glucose concentrations ($mg \cdot mL^{-1}$) at t_1 and t_2, respectively; and pV is volume of distribution which was set at 40 $mL \cdot kg^{-1}$ to coincide with the findings of Wolfe et al. [15].

2.8.7. Estimation of Liver Glucose Contribution

Liver glucose contribution has been estimated from the following calculation:

$$\text{Whole body glucose Ra } (Ra_{body})\ g \cdot min^{-1} = Ra \times \text{body mass} \times 1000 \quad (7)$$

$$\text{Estimation of liver glucose contribution to glucose Ra } (\%) = 100 - ((EXO/Ra_{body}) \times 100) \quad (8)$$

where Ra is the total Ra previously calculated ($mg \cdot kg^{-1} \cdot min^{-1}$), and the body mass is the pre-trial body mass measure taken before each trial (kg). The factor of 1000 is to convert from mg to grams. EXO is the exogenous CHO oxidation rate ($g \cdot min^{-1}$) calculated previously. These calculations serve as an estimation of hepatic glucose contribution during the second hour of exercise [5].

2.9. Data Presentation and Statistical Analysis

All data are presented as mean (±SD) unless otherwise stated. Unfortunately, two participants had to be removed from all stable isotope and substrate use data due to measurement errors making these data $n = 18$. Specific reference to how many participants are included in each dataset is made for each variable considered. Three factor repeated measures analysis of variance was used to determine treatment, time, period (order) main effects and treatment x time interaction effects. Where a significant period effect was observed then period was used as a covariate and the analysis re-run. Significant main and interaction effects were explored using post hoc Tukey's comparisons to indicate where these differences occurred. Pearson correlation analysis was performed to examine associations between individual metabolic parameters and the performance outcome differences on 20, 39 and 64 $g{\cdot}h^{-1}$ trials compared to 0 $g{\cdot}h^{-1}$. Stepwise linear regression analysis was used to find the best prediction model for performance outcome using multiple metabolic parameters. An alpha value of 0.15 was used for inclusion and exclusion of variables from the model at any given step. An alpha value of 0.15 was chosen to ensure variables were not included or excluded too easily from the model. In addition, a best subsets regression analysis was performed on all metabolic variables. In all cases statistical significance was accepted at $p < 0.05$.

3. Results

3.1. Participants

Twenty male competitive cyclists completed all trials in this study. All treatments were tolerated well by participants. Tremendous effort was made to ensure all data points were collected, though some data sets had to be removed due to technical problems. As such, all data for substrate oxidation are for $n = 18$ due to the absence of ^{13}C tracer on one CHO trial for one participant, and expired gas analysis analytical problems during exercise with one other participant. All other data are for $n = 20$.

3.2. Performance Task Outcomes

Performance task data ($n = 20$) has been reported elsewhere [7]. Briefly, endurance cycling performance was equally improved with carbohydrate provision when ingested at a rate of 39 or 64 $g{\cdot}h^{-1}$ in comparison to water placebo (0 $g{\cdot}h^{-1}$). No significant difference in performance task time was noted between 20 $g{\cdot}h^{-1}$ and 0 $g\ h^{-1}$ treatments, or between 39 and 64 $g{\cdot}h^{-1}$ treatments (Table 1).

Table 1. Performance task outcome data on trials where 0, 20, 39 and 64 $g{\cdot}h^{-1}$ of carbohydrate was ingested.

Variable	Performance Time (min)	Percentage Change from 0 $g{\cdot}h^{-1}$ (%)	Cohen's Size Effect from 0 $g{\cdot}h^{-1}$
0 $g{\cdot}h^{-1}$	37:01.9 ± 05:35.0	-	-
20 $g{\cdot}h^{-1}$	35:17.6 ± 04:16.3	3.7 (95% CI −1.5–8.8; $p = 0.13$)	0.6 (95% CI −0.1–1.4)
39 $g{\cdot}h^{-1}$	34:19.5 ± 03:07.1	6.1 (95% CI 1–11.3; $p = 0.02$)	1.0 (95% CI 0.2–1.7)
64 $g{\cdot}h^{-1}$	34:11.3 ± 03:08.5	7.0 (95% CI 1–12, $p = 0.01$)	1.0 (95% CI 0.3–1.8)

3.3. Substrate Oxidation

3.3.1. Respiratory Exchange Ratio

RER data analysis ($n = 18$) revealed a significant main effect of time ($p < 0.01$), treatment ($p < 0.01$), and period ($p < 0.01$) but no interaction ($p = 0.39$). Period was subsequently treated as a covariate for all further analyses. Pairwise comparisons of time indicated that RER values declined with exercise duration. Comparisons of treatment indicated the 0 $g{\cdot}h^{-1}$ treatment RER was significantly ($p < 0.01$) lower in comparison to 20, 39 and 64 $g{\cdot}h^{-1}$ (Figure 2A). Mean (SD) RER on the trials was 0.90 (0.03), 0.91 (0.03), 0.92 (0.03) and 0.92 (0.03) for 0, 20, 39 and 64 $g{\cdot}h^{-1}$ respectively.

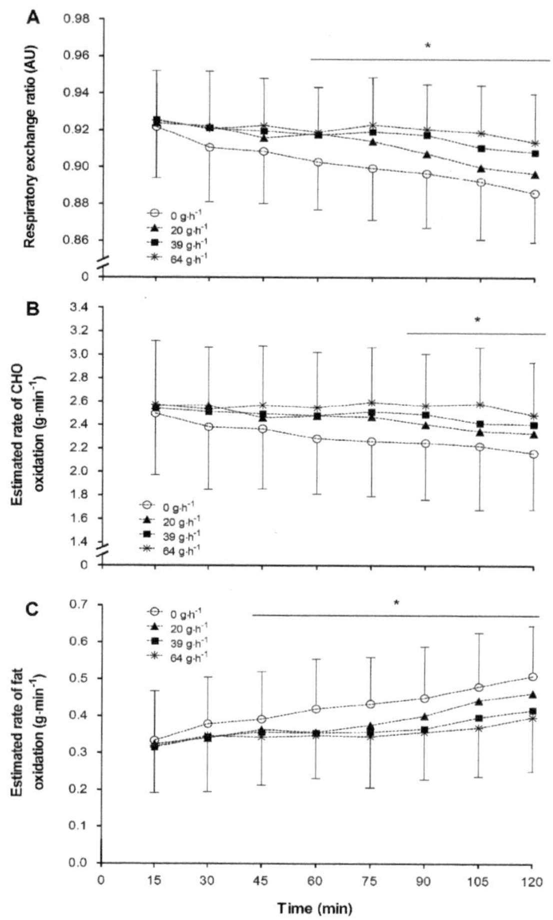

Figure 2. Mean (SD) (**A**) respiratory exchange ratio; (**B**) estimated rate of carbohydrate oxidation and (**C**) estimated rate of fat oxidation during submaximal exercise when consuming 0, 20, 39 and 64 $g{\cdot}h^{-1}$ of CHO. RER values are significantly (* $p < 0.01$) lower from time point 60 min onwards in comparison to 15 min values, with the 0 $g{\cdot}h^{-1}$ treatment eliciting a significantly ($p < 0.01$) lower mean RER over the two hours in comparison to 20, 39 and 64 $g{\cdot}h^{-1}$. A comparison of time indicated CHO oxidation rates at 90 min onwards were significantly lower than 15 min with the 0 $g{\cdot}h^{-1}$ treatment being significantly lower than 20, 39 and 64 $g{\cdot}h^{-1}$. Post hoc comparisons indicated the mean rate of fat oxidation was significantly lower when consuming 39 and 64 $g{\cdot}h^{-1}$ of CHO compared to 0 $g{\cdot}h^{-1}$. Additionally, time comparisons indicated an increase in fat oxidation from 45 min onwards in comparison to rates at 15 min.

3.3.2. Whole Body Substrate Oxidation

Analysis of the carbohydrate oxidation data ($n = 18$) indicated a significant effect of time ($p < 0.01$), treatment ($p < 0.01$), and period ($p < 0.01$) but no interaction effect ($p < 0.58$). Period was treated as a covariate for all subsequent analysis. Pairwise comparisons over time indicated that estimated rate of CHO oxidation was declining over time with measures from 90 min onwards being significantly lower than 15 min values. Treatment pairwise comparisons revealed that the lowest CHO oxidation rate occurred when consuming the 0 $g{\cdot}h^{-1}$ treatment with significant increases in oxidation when consuming 20 and further increases when consuming 39 and 64 $g{\cdot}h^{-1}$ in comparison to 20 $g{\cdot}h^{-1}$ (Figure 2B). Total CHO oxidation on the trials was 279 (58), 298 (52), 302 (47) and 312 (56) g for 0, 20, 39 and 64 $g{\cdot}h^{-1}$ respectively of which 0 was significantly different ($p < 0.01$) from 64 $g{\cdot}h^{-1}$.

Results for estimated rate of fat oxidation ($n = 18$) indicated a significant effect of time, treatment and period (all $p < 0.01$) but no interaction effect ($p = 0.82$). Period was treated as a covariate with all further comparisons. Pairwise comparisons of time indicated an increase in fat oxidation rates with increase in exercise duration. Fat oxidation was higher from 45 min onwards compared with 15 min values. Additional pairwise comparisons revealed that consuming the 0 g·h^{-1} treatment resulted in the significantly higher mean fat oxidation rates in comparison to 39 and 64 g·h^{-1} (Figure 2C). Estimated total fat oxidation was 51 (15), 45 (15), 43 (15) and 42 (15) g for 0, 20, 39 and 64 g·h^{-1} respectively of which no total oxidation was significantly different from another.

3.3.3. Exogenous Carbohydrate Oxidation and Whole-Body Substrate Contribution to Total Energy Expenditure

Data for exogenous carbohydrate oxidation (n = 18) indicated significant main effects of treatment ($p < 0.01$), time ($p < 0.01$), period ($p < 0.01$) and an interaction effect between treatment and time ($p < 0.01$). Period was included as a covariate for all further comparisons. Pairwise comparisons indicated that exogenous CHO oxidation rates were significantly different between all treatments from the 60-min time point until the end of exercise. Specifically, exogenous CHO oxidation rates were higher in comparison to the 20 g·h^{-1} treatment by 0.13 (95% CI: 0.10 to 0.15) and 0.29 (95% CI: 0.27–0.31) g·min^{-1} on the 39 and 64 g·h^{-1} treatments. Additionally, the 64 g·h^{-1} treatment increased exogenous oxidation rates at 75, 90, 105 and 120 min above the 60 min rates highlighting that exogenous CHO oxidation was still rising from 60 min onwards on this trial. Similarly, when consuming 39 g·h^{-1} the values at 90, 105 and 120 min also were significantly increased above the 60 min values, and at 105 and 120 min in comparison to 60 min for the 20 g·h^{-1} treatment (Figure 3A).

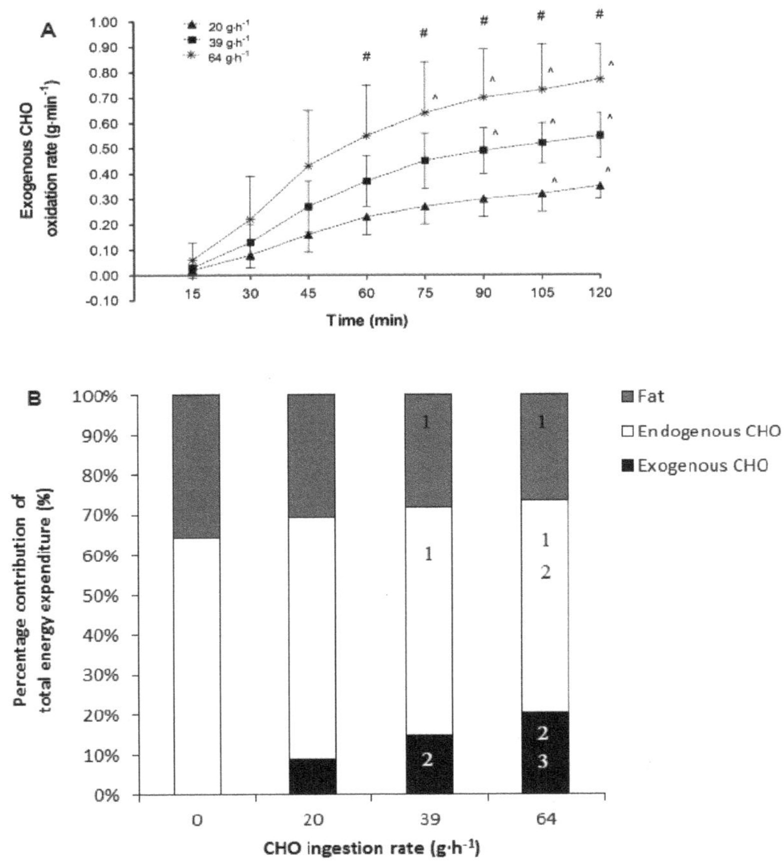

Figure 3. Mean (SD) exogenous carbohydrate (CHO) oxidation rates during submaximal exercise (**A**) while consuming 0, 20, 39 and 64 g·h^{-1} of CHO. ^ indicates time point values significantly ($p < 0.01$) different in comparison to 60 min values; # indicates that all trials are significantly ($p < 0.01$) different from each other at the indicated time point; (**B**) Percentage contribution of total carbohydrate oxidation rates from endogenous and exogenous sources during the second hour of exercise; 1 Indicates significantly different from 0 g·h^{-1}; 2 indicates significantly different from 20 g·h^{-1}; and 3 indicates significantly different from 39 g·h^{-1}.

Percentage contribution of fat oxidised in the second hour of exercise ($n = 18$) revealed significant effects of treatment ($p < 0.01$) and period ($p < 0.01$). Following inclusion of period as a covariate, pairwise comparisons of treatment indicated the percentage contribution of fat oxidation was significantly lower when consuming 39 (−7.5, 95% CI: −1.6 to −13.4%) and 64 (−8.9, 95% CI: −3.1 to −14.8%) $g \cdot h^{-1}$ in comparisons to consuming 0 $g \cdot h^{-1}$. Endogenous carbohydrate percentage contribution highlighted significant effects of treatment ($p < 0.01$) but not period ($p = 0.39$). Pairwise comparisons of treatment indicated that endogenous carbohydrate percentage contribution was significantly suppressed in the 39 and 64 $g \cdot h^{-1}$ trials (−7.3, 95% CI: −1.6 to −13.1 and −11.2, 95% CI: −5.5 to −16.9 respectively) compared to the 0 $g \cdot h^{-1}$ treatment, respectively. Additionally, consuming carbohydrate at 64 $g \cdot h^{-1}$ suppressed endogenous carbohydrate percentage contribution by −7.2% (95% CI: −1.5–13.0%) in comparison to the 20 $g \cdot h^{-1}$ treatment. Exogenous carbohydrate oxidation percentage contribution demonstrated a significant effect of treatment ($p < 0.01$). Pairwise comparisons indicated that for exogenous carbohydrate oxidation all treatments were significantly different from one another (Figure 3B).

Glucose Ra values ($n = 18$) were mirrored by that of the Rd values, and as such statistical analysis outcomes for both data sets were almost identical. Analysis of the glucose Ra and Rd indicated significant effects of treatment ($p < 0.01$), time ($p < 0.01$), period ($p < 0.01$) and an interaction of treatment by time ($p < 0.01$). Period was treated as a covariate for all subsequent analysis. Post hoc comparisons revealed that consuming CHO resulted in a significantly higher glucose Ra of 1.98 (95% CI: 1.37–2.58), 2.12 (95% CI: 1.52–2.72), and 3.65 (95% CI: 3.05–4.25) $mg \cdot kg^{-1} \cdot min^{-1}$ for the 20, 39 and 64 $g \cdot h^{-1}$ treatments respectively, when compared to the 0 $g \cdot h^{-1}$ condition. Post hoc interaction comparisons indicated a significant increase in glucose Ra when consuming 39 and 64 $g \cdot h^{-1}$ compared to 0 $g \cdot h^{-1}$ at time points from 75 min onwards. Additionally, during the 20 $g \cdot h^{-1}$ trial glucose Ra was significantly increased over the control condition at time points from 90 min onwards. Glucose Ra values were significantly increased over the 60 min time point value from 75 to 120 min in the 64 $g \cdot h^{-1}$, 105 to 120 min with 39 $g \cdot h^{-1}$, and only at 120 min in the 20 $g \cdot h^{-1}$ Trial (Figure 4A,B).

In the analysis of the contribution of liver glucose to total Ra ($n = 18$), significant effects of treatment ($p < 0.01$) but not time ($p = 0.13$) or interaction ($p = 0.89$) were observed. Pairwise comparisons of treatment indicated that the percentage contribution of liver glucose to total Ra was significantly reduced between 20 and 39 $g \cdot h^{-1}$ feeding rates (−17.8%, 95% CI: −22.8 to −12.8%), and further significantly reduced when comparing 39 to 64 $g \cdot h^{-1}$ (−11.6%, 95% CI: −16.6 to −6.6%). These reductions represent a mean percentage suppression of liver glucose output of 43 (14%), 61 (14%) and 72 (23%) for the 20, 39 and 64 $g \cdot h^{-1}$ treatments, respectively, in comparison to the 0 $g \cdot h^{-1}$ (Figure 4C).

3.4. Blood Plasma Measures

3.4.1. Glucose

There were main effects of time ($p < 0.01$), treatment ($p < 0.01$), period ($p < 0.01$) and an interaction effect ($p < 0.01$) of treatment by time observed for plasma glucose response ($n = 20$). Period was then used as a covariate for all further analyses. Mean glucose concentration was higher when consuming 39 $g \cdot h^{-1}$ and 64 $g \cdot h^{-1}$ (0.41 $mmol \cdot L^{-1}$ (95% CI: 0.31–0.51) and 0.46 $mmol \cdot L^{-1}$ (95% CI 0.36–0.56), respectively) when pairwise comparisons to the 0 $g \cdot h^{-1}$ treatment were made. Consuming 39 and 64 $g \cdot h^{-1}$ also resulted in increased mean plasma glucose concentration by 0.23 (95% CI: 0.13–0.33) and 0.28 (95% CI: 0.18–0.38) $mmol \cdot L^{-1}$, respectively, in comparison to consuming 20 $g \cdot h^{-1}$. There was no evidence of a difference between 39 and 64 $g \cdot h^{-1}$ treatments. Treatment by time interaction analysis revealed that plasma glucose concentration was significantly increased above 0 min in the 64 $g \cdot h^{-1}$ treatment from 15 min until the end of the exercise period. Additionally, the 39 $g \cdot h^{-1}$ treatment significantly increased plasma glucose concentration from the 0 min value at 15, 30, 45 and 60 min, as did the 20 $g \cdot h^{-1}$ treatment at 30 and 45 min (Figure 5).

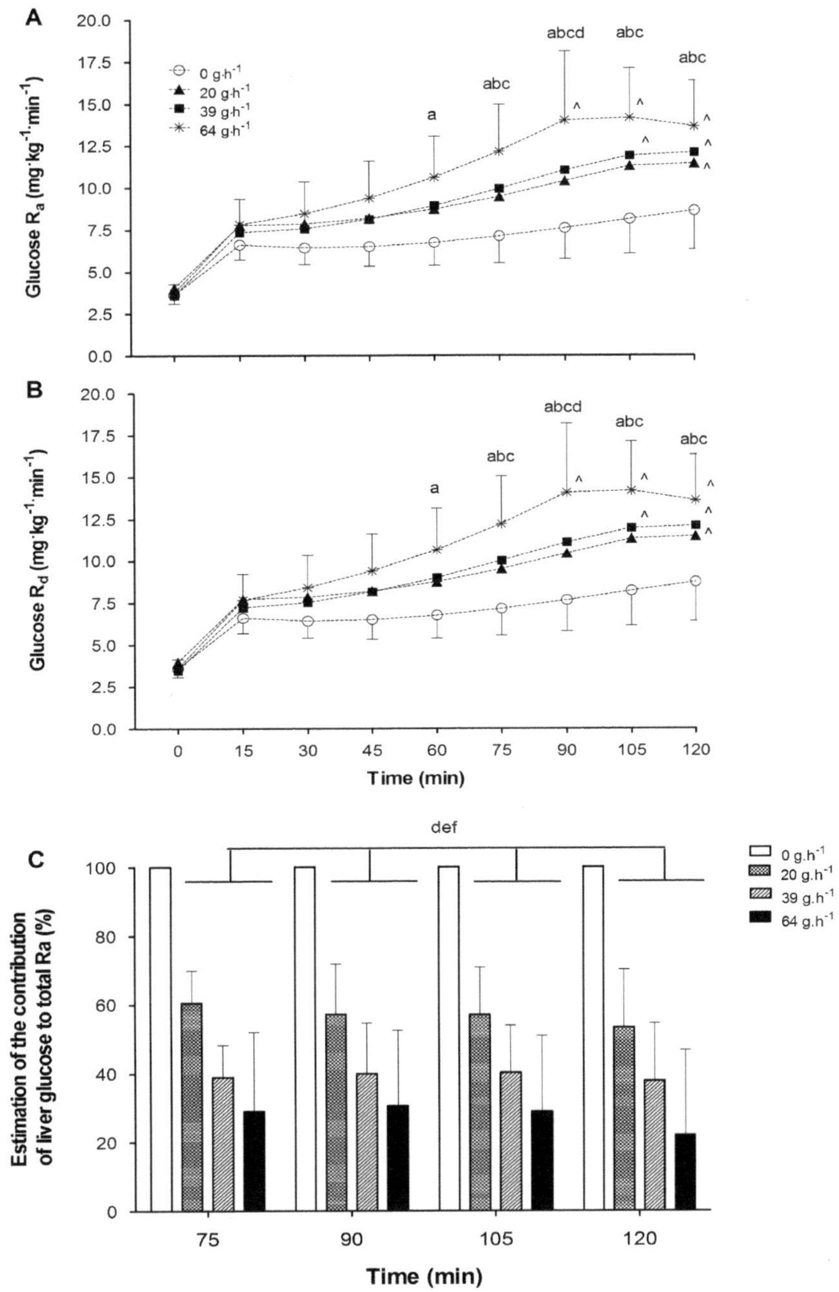

Figure 4. Mean (SD) glucose rate of appearance (**A**) and rate of disappearance (**B**) during submaximal exercise while consuming 0, 20, 39 and 64 g·h^{-1} of CHO. a, b and c indicates 64, 39 and 20 g·h^{-1} value is significantly different from 0 g·h^{-1} at the marked time point; d indicates 64 g·h^{-1} is significantly different from 20 g·h^{-1} at marked time point. ^ indicates time point values significantly ($p < 0.01$) different in comparison to 60 min values. Mean (SD) estimation of the contribution of liver glucose to total glucose Ra during submaximal exercise (**C**) while consuming 20, 39 and 64 g·h^{-1} of CHO. There was a significant treatment effect whereby 64 g·h^{-1} was significantly different from 20 g·h^{-1} (d) and 39 g·h^{-1} (e); and 39 g·h^{-1} was significantly ($p < 0.01$) different from 20 g·h^{-1} (f).

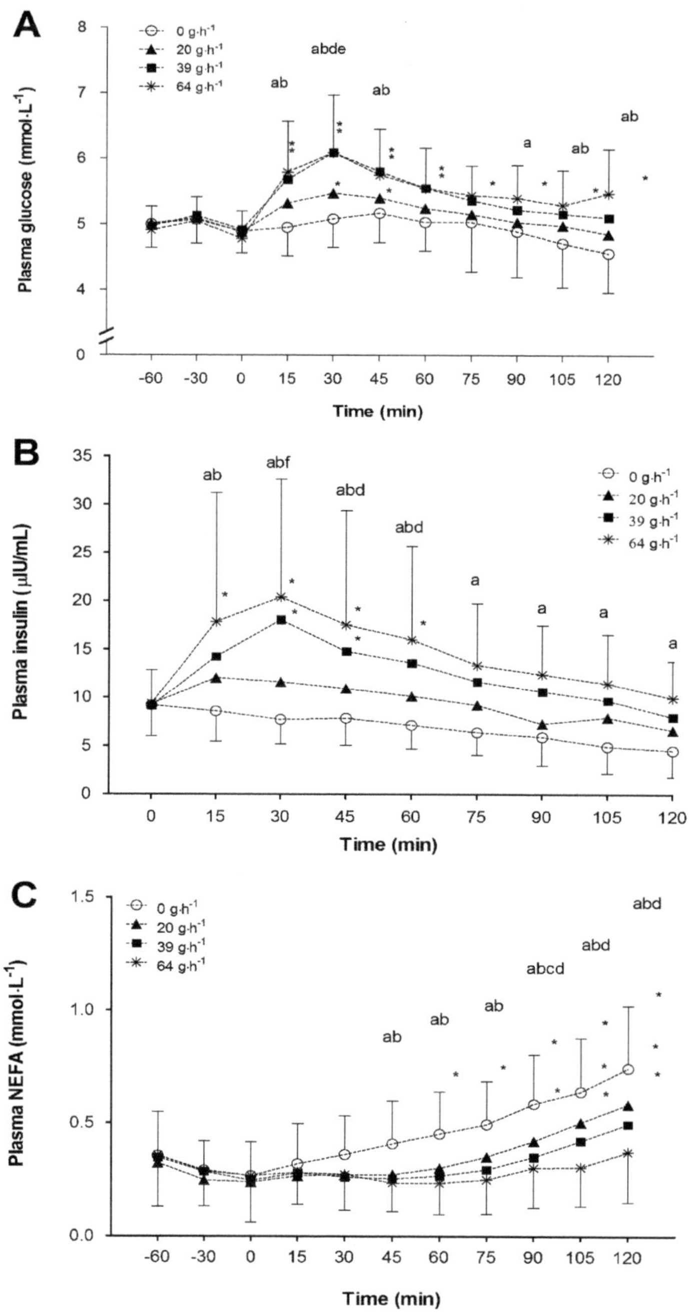

Figure 5. Mean (SD) plasma glucose (**A**); insulin (**B**); and non-esterified fatty acids (**C**) concentration during rest (−60, −30 and 0 min), and during submaximal exercise, (15–120 min), while consuming 0, 20, 39 and 64 g·h^{-1} of CHO. * Values significantly different from 0 min time point. a, b and c indicates 64, 39 and 20 g·h^{-1} value is significantly different from 0 g·h^{-1} at the marked time point; d indicates 64 g·h^{-1} is significantly different from 20 g·h^{-1} at marked time point; e indicates 39 g·h^{-1} is significantly different from 20 g·h^{-1} at marked time point; f indicates 39 and 64 g·h^{-1} are both different from the 20 g·h^{-1} at the marked time point.

3.4.2. Insulin

There were main effects of time ($p < 0.01$), treatment ($p < 0.01$), and an interaction effect between treatment and time ($p < 0.01$) on plasma insulin response ($n = 20$). There was no effect of period ($p = 0.14$). On average insulin concentration increased by 2.5 (95% CI: 1.3–3.7), 5.2 (95% CI: 4.0–6.4) and 7.3 (95% CI: 6.1–8.5) μIU·mL when consuming 20, 39 and 64 g·h^{-1} CHO, respectively, compared to the 0 $g{\cdot}h^{-1}$ trial. Insulin concentration significantly increased from pre ingestion (0 min) values at 15–60 min time points for 64 $g{\cdot}h^{-1}$, and at 30 and 45 min for 39 $g{\cdot}h^{-1}$. Further pairwise comparisons revealed that insulin concentration was significantly elevated in the 39 and 64 $g{\cdot}h^{-1}$ treatments when compared to the 0 $g{\cdot}h^{-1}$ at time points between 15 and 45 min. At 30 min, consuming 39 and 64 $g{\cdot}h^{-1}$ also significantly elevated insulin concentration over that of consuming 20 $g{\cdot}h^{-1}$. The 64 $g{\cdot}h^{-1}$ treatment also significantly increased insulin concentration at time points 45 and 60 min when compared to the 20 $g{\cdot}h^{-1}$ treatment (Figure 5).

3.4.3. Non-Esterified Fatty Acids

There were main effects of time ($p < 0.01$), treatment ($p < 0.01$), period ($p < 0.01$) and an interaction of treatment by time ($p < 0.01$) on plasma NEFA ($n = 20$). Period was included as a covariate for all further analyses. Pairwise comparisons between treatments revealed that on the 0 $g{\cdot}h^{-1}$ treatment mean NEFA concentration was 0.10 (95% CI: 0.07–0.13), 0.12 (95% CI: 0.10–0.16) and 0.16 (95% CI: 0.13–0.19) $mmol{\cdot}L^{-1}$ higher than when consuming the 20, 39 and 64 $g{\cdot}h^{-1}$ treatments, respectively. Additionally, the NEFA concentration throughout exercise on 20 $g{\cdot}h^{-1}$ was significantly higher (0.06 $mmol{\cdot}L^{-1}$, 95% CI: 0.03–0.09) than when consuming 64 $g{\cdot}h^{-1}$. When consuming 0 $g{\cdot}h^{-1}$ all NEFA concentrations were significantly increased above the 0 min time point from 60 min onwards. On the 20 $g{\cdot}h^{-1}$ treatment plasma NEFA concentration was elevated compared to the 0 min time point at 90, 105 and 120 min. Additionally, on the 39 $g{\cdot}h^{-1}$ treatment NEFA concentration increased at time points 105 and 120 min compared to 0 min. No increase was observed on 64 $g{\cdot}h^{-1}$ treatment. Post hoc interaction comparisons revealed that mean NEFA concentration in the 0 $g{\cdot}h^{-1}$ treatment was significantly elevated compared to the 39 and 64 $g{\cdot}h^{-1}$ treatments from the 45 min time point until the end of exercise. Additionally, the 20 $g{\cdot}h^{-1}$ treatment was significantly different from 64 $g{\cdot}h^{-1}$ at 90, 105 and 120 min. Finally, the 20 $g{\cdot}h^{-1}$ treatment significantly elevated plasma NEFA concentration in comparison to the 0 $g{\cdot}h^{-1}$ at time point 90 min (Figure 5).

3.4.4. Lactate

Plasma lactate concentration ($n = 20$) revealed a significant effect of time ($p < 0.01$) and an effect of treatment ($p = 0.02$) but no interaction ($p = 0.84$), and no period effect ($p = 0.57$). Post hoc comparisons of time indicated that all exercising lactate concentrations were elevated above resting values, though there was no significant difference between trials. Mean plasma lactate concentration was 1.06 (0.38), 1.09 (0.35), 1.04 (0.29) and 1.10 (0.36) $mmol{\cdot}L^{-1}$ for 0, 20, 39 and 64 $g{\cdot}h^{-1}$ trials, respectively.

3.4.5. Adrenaline

Analysis of adrenaline concentration ($n = 20$) revealed there was a main effect of period ($p < 0.01$) time ($p < 0.01$), treatment ($p < 0.01$), but no interaction ($p = 0.10$). Period was treated as a covariate for all subsequent analysis. Pairwise comparisons of time indicated adrenaline concentrations were increasing over the duration of the exercise bout. Additionally, comparisons between treatments indicated that adrenaline concentration was highest on the 0 $g{\cdot}h^{-1}$ trial (0.99 ± 0.69 ng mL^{-1}) in comparison to the 39 $g{\cdot}h^{-1}$ (0.78 ± 0.38 ng mL^{-1}) and 64 $g{\cdot}h^{-1}$ (0.78 ± 0.41 ng mL^{-1}) trials. Mean adrenaline concentration on the 20 $g{\cdot}h^{-1}$ trial was 0.87 (0.48) ng mL^{-1}.

3.5. *Associations between Metabolic Responses and Prediction of Subsequent Performance Outcomes*

Association analysis between a number of key metabolic parameters during 2 h of exercise and subsequent change in performance task outcome are shown in Table 2. This analysis revealed a moderate positive association between increases in total exogenous CHO oxidized in the second hour of exercise, and total glucose rate of disappearance in the second hour of exercise, with an improvement in performance outcome. In addition, there was a tendency towards a moderate negative association between change in circulating NEFA concentration and subsequent performance outcome.

Factors such as liver glucose output suppression, mean plasma glucose, and mean plasma insulin concentrations were not associated with the changes in performance task outcome.

Table 2. Association analysis for selected metabolic parameters, obtained on the 20, 39 and 64 $g{\cdot}h^{-1}$ ingestion trials, with change in performance outcome compared to 0 $g{\cdot}h^{-1}$.

Variable	Pearson's Correlation	p-Value
Liver glucose suppression (%)	−0.055	0.691
Total exogenous CHO oxidation in 2nd hour (g)	0.269	0.049 *
Total glucose Rd in 2nd hour (g)	0.291	0.033 *
Mean glucose concentration	−0.045	0.747
Mean insulin concentration	0.158	0.253
Δ NEFA concentration from 0 $g{\cdot}h^{-1}$	−0.262	0.056 †

* Significant association between parameter and change in performance outcome from 0 $g{\cdot}h^{-1}$ trial; † tendency towards significant association.

Using these metabolic parameters in a stepwise linear regression analysis revealed that the combination of exogenous CHO oxidation in the second hour of exercise ($p = 0.011$) and the suppression of circulating NEFA ($p = 0.010$) provided the best model to predict subsequent performance outcomes as shown in Table 3. However, this model only explained ~19% of the variance in performance outcome observed. The regression equation that resulted was:

$$\text{Performance change from 0 (\%)} = 1.13 + 0.405\ (\text{Exo CHO}) - 34.6\ (\Delta\ \text{NEFA}) \tag{9}$$

where Exo CHO is the total exogenous CHO oxidation in 2nd hour in grams and Δ NEFA is the difference in NEFA concentration ($mmol{\cdot}L^{-1}$) in comparison to consuming the 0 $g{\cdot}h^{-1}$. Finally, a best subsets analysis was conducted on all variables included in the regression. Including all variables reported in Table 2, except for mean glucose concentration, explained 23% of the variance in performance.

Table 3. Stepwise regression analysis of metabolic variables, obtained on the 20, 39 and 64 $g{\cdot}h^{-1}$ ingestion trials, with change in performance outcome compared to 0 $g{\cdot}h^{-1}$.

Model	Variable (ID)	R^2	p (Variable ID)
1	(1) Total glucose Rd in 2nd hour (g)	0.087	0.033 (1) *
2	(2) +Δ NEFA concentration from 0 $g{\cdot}h^{-1}$	0.126	0.129 (2), 0.074 (1) *
3	(3) +Total exogenous CHO oxidation in 2nd hour (g)	0.192	0.048 (3) *, 0.032 (2) *, 0.48 (1)
4	(4) −Total glucose Rd in 2nd hour (g)	0.184	0.011 (2) *, 0.010 (3) *

Alpha-to-enter = 0.15; Alpha-to-remove = 0.15; * indicates a significant ($p < 0.05$) component in the model.

3.6. Heart Rate and RPE

There were significant effects of time, treatment and period ($p < 0.01$) but no interaction effect ($p > 0.99$) for heart rate. Period was treated as a covariate for all subsequent analysis. Pairwise comparisons indicated that heart rate tended to increase with increasing exercise duration. In addition, post hoc comparisons of treatment indicated a significant difference between 0 and 64 $g{\cdot}h^{-1}$ with a mean difference of 4 (95% CI: 2, 6) beats per minute between the two trials. The mean heart rates for each treatment were 135, 137, 136 and 139 for 0, 20, 39 and 64 $g{\cdot}h^{-1}$ respectively.

There was a significant effect of time ($p < 0.01$) and period ($p = 0.02$), but not treatment ($p = 0.83$) or interaction ($p = 0.94$) effects on RPE responses to exercise. Period was treated as a covariate for all further comparisons. Post hoc comparisons indicated that mean RPE scores increased from 13 to 14 from minute 60 to minute 120.

4. Discussion

During this investigation, we aimed primarily to characterize the metabolic response of trained cyclists to the ingestion of graded amounts of CHO during a two-hour submaximal ride to explore the dose-response. Our secondary aim was to determine the strength of association between selected metabolic parameters and prediction of the performance task outcomes, previously reported elsewhere [7]. We observed that increasing rates of CHO ingestion (particularly at 39 and 64 $g{\cdot}h^{-1}$) during non-exhaustive submaximal exercise resulted in: (1) a reduction in the contribution of endogenous carbohydrate and fat stores to total energy provision; (2) a decrease in hepatic glucose output in a dose response manner; (3) an increase in the contribution of exogenous CHO oxidation to total energy contribution in a dose response manner; (4) an increase in rate of total carbohydrate oxidation and plasma glucose turnover; (5) increased circulating blood glucose and insulin concentration; and (6) a blunting of the circulating NEFA response to exercise. While individually these responses to increasing doses of CHO feeding are not unforeseen the novel aspect of the present study is the examination of dose-response effects in all of these responses. Moreover, the correlation and regression analyses indicate that the rate of exogenous CHO oxidation and suppression of NEFA are the two most closely linked to a significant prediction of subsequent performance task outcome.

The significant alterations in fuel selection observed with the ingestion of 39 and 64 $g{\cdot}h^{-1}$ of CHO in comparison to 0 or 20 $g{\cdot}h^{-1}$ closely compliment the performance task outcome data previously reported [7]. In addition, the ingestion of 64 $g{\cdot}h^{-1}$ had no added effect, over 39 $g{\cdot}h^{-1}$, on many of the key metabolic responses to exercise, but it did result in an increased rate of exogenous substrate oxidation, and a further blunting of hepatic glucose output, when compared with the 39 $g{\cdot}h^{-1}$ trial. A difference in exogenous CHO oxidation rate and hepatic glucose output, two key metabolic parameters, between the 39 and 64 $g{\cdot}h^{-1}$ trials might be expected to impact subsequent performance, but no impact was observed. Interestingly, the best subsets regression analysis indicated that some other metabolic parameters were also associated with change in performance in relation to graded doses of CHO ingestion. These other predictors were mean insulin concentration, and suppression in circulating plasma NEFA. The lack of difference in insulin or NEFA response between the 39 and 64 $g{\cdot}h^{-1}$ trials suggests that, with ingestion of a dose of single source CHO up to 64 $g{\cdot}h^{-1}$ over a two-hour exercise bout, there seems little metabolic advantage of going beyond ~40 $g{\cdot}h^{-1}$.

Many investigators have observed a significant difference in plasma insulin and NEFA concentration with the ingestion of CHO during submaximal exercise, and a subsequent alteration of fuel utilization [5,16]. However, the only previous dose-response study [4] did not observe differences in insulin or NEFA response between the two highest CHO doses ingested (30 and 60 $g{\cdot}h^{-1}$). The present study data corroborate these observations and, with a more suitably powered design, suggest that moderate amounts of CHO in the region of only 40 $g{\cdot}h^{-1}$ are sufficient to modulate metabolic responses enough to impact upon subsequent performance task outcome. By utilizing stable isotopes researchers have been able to quantify the movement of glucose into and out of the plasma pool during exercise when carbohydrate is consumed [15]. During exercise, blood glucose can be maintained or increased by the augmented release of glucose from the liver. In the present study, the 20 $g{\cdot}h^{-1}$ treatment reduced hepatic glucose output by 43% but the performance outcome (3.7% improvement) previously reported [7] was too variable for it to be considered a significant performance enhancement. Hepatic glucose output calculations in the current investigation reveal that all CHO ingestion rates resulted in a reduction in hepatic glucose output, and that the magnitude of reduction essentially followed a dose-response pattern. Higher CHO ingestion rates of 39 and 64 $g{\cdot}h^{-1}$ both suppressed hepatic glucose output to a greater extent than the 20 $g{\cdot}h^{-1}$ treatment. Interestingly, the magnitude of suppression in the 39 and 64 $g{\cdot}h^{-1}$ trials was similar or greater than that observed by McConnell et al. [8] when they fed CHO at 100 $g{\cdot}h^{-1}$. This observation could suggest that even low doses of CHO at 39 and 64 $g{\cdot}h^{-1}$ are resulting in a near maximal suppression of hepatic glucose output, which is not exceeded unless very high doses of CHO are ingested (i.e., 180 $g{\cdot}h^{-1}$; Jeukendrup [5]). The lack of any association between hepatic glucose output suppression and performance outcome suggests that even modest reductions in liver glucose output, induced by feeding only 39 $g \cdot h^{-1}$ of CHO during two hours of exercise, are sufficient to impact upon subsequent endurance task performance.

Exogenous CHO oxidation rates increase when CHO is ingested, but when a single source of CHO is ingested these typically only reach rates of ~1 $g \cdot min^{-1}$ [5,17,18]. In the present study, rates of exogenous CHO oxidation followed a dose-response pattern with the highest rates of around 0.75 $g \cdot min^{-1}$ achieved on the 64 $g \cdot h^{-1}$ trial. On the 39 $g \cdot h^{-1}$ trial exogenous CHO oxidation rates reached 0.55 $g \cdot min^{-1}$. These data are slightly higher than those obtained by Smith et al. [4] in their dose-response study. Smith et al. [4] noted rates of ~0.3 and ~0.5 $g \cdot min^{-1}$ for their 30 and 60 $g \cdot h^{-1}$ CHO ingestion trials, respectively. The lack of performance task improvement with increasing rate of oxidation of exogenous CHO in the present study, and in the Smith et al. [4] study, suggests that capacity to oxidize exogenous CHO at a high rate is not for the key factor driving performance improvement. In addition, there was only a weak, albeit significant, association observed between exogenous CHO oxidation rate and subsequent performance outcome, as well as a modest contribution from exogenous CHO oxidation rate to prediction of performance outcome in the regression analyses. Overall, these data suggest that higher exogenous CHO delivery and higher subsequent oxidation likely contribute to endogenous (hepatic) glycogen sparing during two hours of endurance cycling, and can have some impact upon subsequent performance task outcome. However, as a note of caution, these observations may be particular to the exercise model investigated. For example, in longer exercise task durations exceeding three hours of total activity it may well is that higher feeding rates and higher exogenous CHO oxidation would translate to improved performance.

The blunting of fat oxidation observed only on the two highest CHO doses (39 and 64 $g \cdot h^{-1}$) subsequently would drive fuel utilization towards a CHO dependent state. The suppression of fat oxidation and circulating NEFA concentration was similar on both 39 and 64 $g \cdot h^{-1}$ feeding rates. Thus, it seems that feeding of only 39 $g \cdot h^{-1}$ is sufficient to sustain exercise. Van Loon et al. [19] reported that a suppression in adipose tissue lipolysis increases glycogen utilization in exercising humans. While a greater dependence upon CHO oxidation was observed between 39 and 64 $g \cdot h^{-1}$ feeding rates compared with 0 $g \cdot h^{-1}$, there was no difference in CHO usage between the two highest feeding rates in the present study. These observations suggest that near optimal substrate metabolism changes occurred with a feeding rate of close to 40 $g \cdot h^{-1}$.

Our results highlight that CHO provision leading to an increased oxidation of exogenous CHO, increased total glucose disposal, and reduction in circulating NEFA, have the closest associations with subsequent performance task outcome. Higher CHO feeding rates that reach a threshold level to blunt circulating NEFA concentration, increase reliance on CHO oxidation, and enhance exogenous CHO oxidation, will have the biggest impact upon subsequent performance task outcome. The threshold required for these outcomes appears to be around 40 $g \cdot h^{-1}$ in the present study. However, these associations are low to moderate and the threshold of CHO ingestion rate could well be influenced by the total task duration and/or training status of participants. With longer task durations (>3 h) an increased reliance on exogenous CHO oxidation later in exercise could enhance liver glycogen sparing and could improve subsequent performance outcomes. Furthermore, with improved training status comes improved capacity to oxidize substrates [20,21] which might drive the CHO provision threshold beyond 40–60 $g \cdot h^{-1}$.

Prediction of performance task outcome from metabolic parameters was not particularly strong, with only 19–23% of the variance in subsequent performance task outcome explained by the key metabolic parameters in the model. Interestingly, the prediction model containing only the two variables of exogenous CHO oxidation rate and suppression of plasma NEFA response provided almost all of the predictive power of the model. Given that these two parameters are most closely aligned to the actual CHO dose administered, it would seem plausible to suggest that higher doses of CHO should result in better performance outcomes. However, further investigation into higher rates of CHO provision and performance outcome are required before this can be categorically stated. Of particular interest would be studies in which comparisons are made between ingestion rates within the 40–60 $g \cdot h^{-1}$ range using single source CHO, with those in the 90–120 $g \cdot h^{-1}$ range using multiple transportable CHO. To date, only one study, by Baur et al. [22], has compared a single source trial with a practically relevant feeding rate of glucose, against a multiple transportable CHO trial designed to maximize rate of exogenous CHO oxidation. Their study compared feeding rates of glucose at 62 and 93 $g \cdot h^{-1}$ with a 2:1 glucose: fructose beverage ingested at 93 $g \cdot h^{-1}$, during three hours of endurance cycling. Their data revealed that when compared to the 62 $g \cdot h^{-1}$ glucose trial, there was no clear evidence of a benefit to performance compared with ingestion of 93 $g \cdot h^{-1}$ of the glucose: fructose beverage. These data indicate that aiming to increase exogenous CHO oxidation through consumption of composite CHO drinks at high feeding rates will not necessarily lead to meaningful performance gains. Thus, it seems that there is a need for further investigation of CHO dose and performance outcome. So, at high ingestion rates the use of multiple transportable CHO will likely reduce gastrointestinal symptoms, but this does not necessarily translate into enhanced endurance exercise performance. These previous findings may explain the lack of a strong association between exogenous CHO oxidation rate and subsequent performance outcome in the present dataset. Thus, it seems that in endurance tasks lasting <3 h, a feeding rate of 40 $g \cdot h^{-1}$ of single source CHO could be considered near optimal to provide sufficient metabolic advantages to maximize performance gains.

5. Conclusions

Researchers have been aiming to identify the optimal ingestion rate of CHO to elicit the greatest improvements in endurance performance for many years. We have reported that the ingestion of 39 and 64 $g \cdot h^{-1}$ of single source CHO were equally effective at improving endurance exercise performance in comparison to a control condition (0 $g \cdot h^{-1}$). The data presented in the current manuscript further demonstrate that the ingestion of 39 $g \cdot h^{-1}$ of CHO appears sufficient to alter substrate utilization during a two-hour submaximal exercise bout, and lead to performance gains. These performance gains partly come from preservation of endogenous glycogen stores, most likely hepatic stores, and maintaining high rates of CHO oxidation through suppression of circulating NEFA concentration. Ingestion of CHO at a lower rate (20 $g \cdot h^{-1}$) is insufficient for these particular metabolic changes to occur, while increasing the rate of ingestion to 64 $g \cdot h^{-1}$ does not appear to have any additional benefit. The lack of any additional change in many metabolic parameters when consuming 64 $g \cdot h^{-1}$ could be partly responsible for a lack of any additional improvement in subsequent performance task outcome. From these present observations, we conclude that an ingestion rate of 39 $g \cdot h^{-1}$ is a dose beyond which there a no further performance or metabolic benefits, suggesting that it could be an optimal ingestion rate, to elicit a sufficient alteration in fuel provision during submaximal exercise. While a 39 $g \cdot h^{-1}$ dose appears effective in this investigation, the observations should be confined to the particular task duration and participant group studied. Further work is required to explore the metabolic advantages and potential performance enhancement from higher feeding rates in more well-trained/elite competitors, in female participants, and in tasks lasting longer than three hours.

Acknowledgments: Funding for the present work was provided by Lucozade Ribena Suntory Ltd., Uxbridge, U.K. to University of Stirling. We would like to thank Gillian Dreczkowski for her assistance with the analytical components of the trials.

Author Contributions: S.D.R.G., K.D.T. and A.M.H. conceived and designed the experiments; M.L.N., A.M.H. and S.D.R.G. performed the experiments; M.L.N., S.D.R.G. and G.A.W. analysed the data; G.A.W. contributed reagents/materials/analysis tools; M.L.N. and S.D.R.G. wrote the paper. All other authors contributed to editing of the final manuscript.

References

1. Coyle, E.F.; Coggan, A.R.; Hemmert, M.K.; Ivy, J.L. Muscle glycogen utilization during prolonged strenuous exercise when fed carbohydrate. *J. Appl. Physiol. (1985)* **1986**, *61*, 165–172. [CrossRef] [PubMed]
2. Coggan, A.R.; Coyle, E.F. Reversal of fatigue during prolonged exercise by carbohydrate infusion or ingestion. *J. Appl. Physiol. (1985)* **1987**, *63*, 2388–2395. [CrossRef] [PubMed]
3. Nybo, L. CNS Fatigue and prolonged exercise: Effect of glucose supplementation. *Med. Sci. Sports Exerc.* **2003**, *35*, 589–594. [CrossRef] [PubMed]
4. Smith, J.W.; Zachwieja, J.J.; Peronnet, F.; Passe, D.H.; Massicotte, D.; Lavoie, C.; Pascoe, D.D. Fuel selection and cycling endurance performance with ingestion of [^{13}C] glucose: Evidence for a carbohydrate dose response. *J. Appl. Physiol. (1985)* **2010**, *108*, 1520–1529. [CrossRef] [PubMed]
5. Jeukendrup, A.E.; Wagenmakers, A.J.; Stegen, J.H.; Gijsen, A.P.; Brouns, F.; Saris, W.H. Carbohydrate ingestion can completely suppress endogenous glucose production during exercise. *Am. J. Physiol.* **1999**, *276*, E672–E683. [CrossRef] [PubMed]
6. Rowlands, D.S.; Houltham, S.; Musa-Veloso, K.; Brown, F.; Paulionis, L.; Bailey, D. Fructose–glucose composite carbohydrates and endurance performance: Critical review and future perspectives. *Sports Med.* **2015**, *45*, 1561–1576. [CrossRef] [PubMed]
7. Newell, M.L.; Hunter, A.M.; Lawrence, C.; Tipton, K.D.; Galloway, S.D. The ingestion of 39 or 64 $g \cdot h^{-1}$ of carbohydrate is equally effective at improving endurance exercise performance in cyclists. *Int. J. Sport Nutr. Exerc. Metab.* **2015**, *25*, 285–292. [CrossRef] [PubMed]
8. McConell, G.; Fabris, S.; Proietto, J.; Hargreaves, M. Effect of carbohydrate ingestion on glucose kinetics during exercise. *J. Appl. Physiol. (1985)* **1994**, *77*, 1537–1541. [CrossRef] [PubMed]
9. Neal, C.M.; Hunter, A.M.; Brennan, L.; O'Sullivan, A.; Hamilton, D.L.; De Vito, G.; Galloway, S.D. Six weeks of a polarized training-intensity distribution leads to greater physiological and performance adaptations than a threshold model in trained cyclists. *J. Appl. Physiol. (1985)* **2013**, *114*, 461–471. [CrossRef] [PubMed]
10. Kuipers, H.; Verstappen, F.; Keizer, H.; Geurten, P.; Van Kranenburg, G. Variability of aerobic performance in the laboratory and its physiologic correlates. *Int. J. Sports Med.* **1985**, *6*, 197–201. [CrossRef] [PubMed]
11. Borg, G.A. Psychophysical bases of perceived exertion. *Med. Sci. Sports Exerc.* **1982**, *14*, 377–381. [CrossRef] [PubMed]
12. Pickert, A.; Overkamp, D.; Renn, W.; Liebich, H.; Eggstein, M. Selected ion monitoring Gas Chromatography/Mass Spectrometry using uniformly labelled (^{13}C) glucose for determination of glucose turnover in man. *Biol. Mass Spectrom.* **1991**, *20*, 203–209. [CrossRef] [PubMed]
13. Jeukendrup, A.; Wallis, G. Measurement of substrate oxidation during exercise by means of gas exchange measurements. *Int. J. SPORTS Med.* **2005**, *26*, S28–S37. [CrossRef] [PubMed]
14. Proietto, J. Estimation of glucose kinetics following an oral glucose load. Methods and applications. *Horm. Metab. Res. Suppl.* **1990**, *24*, 25–30. [PubMed]
15. Wolfe, R.R.; Chinkes, D.L. *Isotope Tracers in Metabolic Research: Principles and Practice of Kinetic Analysis*; John Wiley & Sons: Hoboken, NJ, USA, 2005.
16. Wallis, G.A.; Yeo, S.E.; Blannin, A.K.; Jeukendrup, A.E. Dose-response effects of ingested carbohydrate on exercise metabolism in women. *Med. Sci. Sports Exerc.* **2007**, *39*, 131–138. [CrossRef] [PubMed]
17. Jentjens, R.L.; Shaw, C.; Birtles, T.; Waring, R.H.; Harding, L.K.; Jeukendrup, A.E. Oxidation of combined ingestion of glucose and sucrose during exercise. *Metab. Clin. Exp.* **2005**, *54*, 610–618. [CrossRef] [PubMed]
18. Harvey, C.R.; Frew, R.; Massicotte, D.; Peronnet, F.; Rehrer, N.J. Muscle glycogen oxidation during prolonged exercise measured with oral [^{13}C] glucose: Comparison with changes in muscle glycogen content. *J. Appl. Physiol. (1985)* **2007**, *102*, 1773–1779. [CrossRef] [PubMed]
19. Van Loon, L.J.; Thomason-Hughes, M.; Constantin-Teodosiu, D.; Koopman, R.; Greenhaff, P.L.; Hardie, D.G.; Keizer, H.A.; Saris, W.H.; Wagenmakers, A.J. Inhibition of adipose tissue lipolysis increases intramuscular lipid and glycogen use in vivo in humans. *Am. J. Physiol. Endocrinol. Metab.* **2005**, *289*, E482–E493. [CrossRef] [PubMed]
20. Lund, J.; Tangen, D.S.; Wiig, H.; Stadheim, H.K.; Helle, S.A.; Birk, J.B.; Ingemann-Hansen, T.; Rustan, A.C.; Thoresen, G.H.; Wojtaszewski, J.F. Glucose metabolism and metabolic flexibility in cultured skeletal muscle

cells is related to exercise status in young male subjects. *Arch. Physiol. Biochem.* **2017**, 1–12. [CrossRef] [PubMed]

21. Hargreaves, M.; Spriet, L.L. Exercise metabolism: Fuels for the fire. *Cold Spring Harb Perspect. Med.* **2017**. [CrossRef] [PubMed]
22. Baur, D.A.; Schroer, A.B.; Luden, N.D.; Womack, C.J.; Smyth, S.A.; Saunders, M.J. Glucose-fructose enhances performance versus isocaloric, but not moderate, glucose. *Med. Sci. Sports Exerc.* **2014**, *46*, 1778–1786. [CrossRef] [PubMed]

13

Kiwifruit Exchanges for Increased Nutrient Richness with Little Effect on Carbohydrate Intake, Glycaemic Impact or Insulin Response

John Monro [1,2,*], Kerry Bentley-Hewitt [1] and Suman Mishra [1]

1 New Zealand Institute for Plant & Food Research, Private Bag 11600, Palmerston North 4442, New Zealand; kerry.bentley-hewitt@plantandfood.co.nz (K.B.-H.); suman.mishra@plantandfood.co.nz (S.M.)
2 Riddet Institute, Massey University, Palmerston North 4442, New Zealand
* Correspondence: john.monro@plantandfood.co.nz

Abstract: Background: Kiwifruit are nutrient-rich and have properties which indicate a low glycaemic impact compared with many cooked cereal foods, suggesting that they may be used for dietary enrichment of vitamin C without glycaemic cost. Aim: To develop tables for equi-carbohydrate and equi-glycaemic partial exchange of kiwifruit for glycaemic carbohydrate foods. Method: The available carbohydrate content of Zespri® Green and Zespri® SunGold kiwifruit was determined as sugars released during in vitro digestive analysis. Glycaemic potency was determined as grams of glucose equivalents (GGEs) in a clinical trial using 200 g (a two-kiwifruit edible portion) of each cultivar, non-diabetic subjects (n = 20), and a glucose reference. GGE values were also estimated for a range of carbohydrate foods in the New Zealand Food Composition Database for which available carbohydrate and glycaemic index values were available. The values allowed exchange tables to be constructed for either equi-carbohydrate or equi-glycaemic partial exchange of kiwifruit for the foods. Results: GGE values of both kiwifruit cultivars were low ("Hayward", 6.6 glucose equivalents/100 g; "Zesy002", 6.7 glucose equivalents/100 g). Partial equi-carbohydrate substitution of foods in most carbohydrate food categories substantially increased vitamin C with little change in glycaemic impact, while equi-glycaemic partial substitution by kiwifruit could be achieved with little change in carbohydrate intake. Conclusion: Equi-carbohydrate partial exchange of kiwifruit for starchy staple foods is a means of greatly increasing nutrient richness in a diet without the physiological costs of increased glycaemia and insulin responses or carbohydrate intake.

Keywords: kiwifruit; carbohydrate exchanges; glycaemic response; glycaemic glucose equivalents; vitamin C

---

1. Introduction

Kiwifruit is one of the most nutrient-rich of readily available fruits, and can make a valuable contribution to dietary intakes of micronutrients and phytochemicals that foster good health through a variety of protective mechanisms. So much so that it has recently been recommended that kiwifruit should be considered as part of a natural and effective dietary strategy to address some of the major global health and wellness concerns [1]. One kiwifruit per day has been shown to be sufficient to achieve "healthy" plasma levels of vitamin C [2] and to saturate muscle tissue vitamin C concentrations [3].

Fruits are also generally rich in available carbohydrate in the form of approximately equal proportions of glucose and fructose. In kiwifruit, for instance, sugars make up about 12% of the edible portion of the fresh fruit, consisting of glucose, fructose, and sucrose (about 2:2:1), and represent a major proportion of the skin-free dry matter (New Zealand Food Composition Database, 2015). Consequently, with an increasing global incidence of diabetes and obesity, the high content of sugars is often seen as reason to avoid fruit, ignoring the fact that fruit phytochemicals, including vitamin C, may have a valuable role in counteracting body states and processes such as glycaemia-induced oxidative stress and inflammation [4], which are implicated in the development of diabetic complications [5]. It is therefore important that the need to control intakes of glycaemic carbohydrate should not be misconstrued as a need to decrease intakes of fruits, particularly as fruit structure, fruit sugar (fructose), and other fruit constituents that retard glycaemic response, such as cell wall debris (dietary fibre), organic acids, and phenolics acting in the gut, may lead to a relatively low glycaemic response to sugars in fruit. We have shown that in kiwifruit, both the available carbohydrates and other components, contribute to an improved glycaemic response upon equal-carbohydrate partial substitution of kiwifruit for starchy breakfast cereal [6].

One of the strategies for glycaemia management that has been used in dietetic practice is to substitute highly glycaemic carbohydrates in the diet with less glycaemic carbohydrates using the "carbohydrate exchange" system [7]. Carbohydrate exchanges are generally carried out by substituting low glycaemic impact carbohydrate for higher glycaemic impact carbohydrate sources, while maintaining a more or less constant nutrient composition. However, rather than simply substituting one carbohydrate source for another, carbohydrate exchanges provide an opportunity to improve the nutrient richness of the diet by partially substituting nutrient-rich carbohydrate products, such as fresh kiwifruit, for less nutrient-rich foods such as starch-based staples and refined cereal products.

To facilitate the more general use of kiwifruit in food exchange for nutrient enrichment or glycaemic control we determined the available carbohydrate content of two cultivars of kiwifruit (*Actinidia chinensis* var. *deliciosa* "Hayward" marketed as Zespri® Green kiwifruit, and *Actinidia chinensis* var. *chinensis* "Zesy002", marketed as Zespri® SunGold kiwifruit) by in vitro digestive analysis, and their glycaemic potencies relative to a glucose reference in a human intervention study. The results allowed quantities to be calculated for either equi-carbohydrate or equi-glycaemic substitution of a range of foods, and construction of tables of kiwifruit exchanges to show:

(1) How much of a range of carbohydrate foods could be substituted by one kiwifruit while keeping available carbohydrate content constant.
(2) Approximately how much glycaemic impact would be altered by equal carbohydrate partial substitution of one kiwifruit for a food.
(3) Approximately how much of a number of foods could be substituted by one kiwifruit while keeping glycaemic impact constant.

The aim of the study was to demonstrate the feasibility and glycaemic safety of using kiwifruit exchanges to increase intake of nutrients such as vitamin C within the diet with little effect on its glycaemic impact or carbohydrate load.

2. Methods

2.1. Test Components

"Hayward" (GR) and "Zesy002" (SG) kiwifruit were provided by Zespri Group Ltd., Tauranga, New Zealand, in a ready-to-eat state of ripeness, and processed within a few days of receipt. They were peeled and the hard apical core removed from the green kiwifruit, then halved and frozen (−20 °C). The frozen fruit were allowed to thaw partially and were then crushed to a coarse pulp by briefly (10 s) chopping in a Halde food processor. The pulp was then divided accurately into individual 200-g portions, each stored frozen within a plastic, capped, freezer-proof sundae container until required.

The glucose used was dextrose monohydrate (Davis Food Ingredients, Palmerston North, New Zealand), which contains 91% glucose. It is henceforth referred to as glucose, and an allowance was made for its water content in all calculations and weight measurements.

2.2. Carbohydrate Analysis of Kiwifruit

The available carbohydrate contents of the fruit (GR and SG) were determined by a standard digestive analysis, involving simulated gastric (pepsin pH 2.5, 30 min) and small intestinal digestion (pancreatin/amyloglucosidase, pH 6.2, 120 min), with the available carbohydrate content of the digested pulp measured after invertase digestion using a reduced scale modification of the dinitrosalicylic acid method [8]. The fructose content was measured by the thiobarbituric acid procedure [9].

2.3. Formulation of Meals

The subjects consumed three materials:

(1) 40 g of glucose (reference).
(2) 200 g of "Hayward" kiwifruit alone
(3) 200 g of "Zesy002" kiwifruit alone.

2.4. Human Intervention Study

This study was conducted according to the guidelines laid down in the Declaration of Helsinki and all procedures involving human subjects were approved by the Human and Disabilities Ethics Committee of the New Zealand Ministry of Health (ethics approval number 14/CEN/207). Written informed consent was obtained from all subjects. The trial was registered with the Australia New Zealand Clinical Trials Registry (Trial ID: ACTRN12615000222549) (URL: http://www.anzctr.org.au). The participant flow chart shows ethical approval, recruitment, and intervention processes for the trial (Figure 1).

The trial was run as a non-blinded randomised repeated measures study. It was not possible to blind the subjects to the meals they were consuming. However, the data and statistical analysis were performed by an analyst who was blinded to the treatments. Meal order was randomised for each subject using a computerised random number generator.

Participants: Twenty participants, eight male and 12 female, were recruited by flyer and email. Respondents were interviewed and given an information pack including a description of the study and a consent form. Prospective participants were asked to complete a health questionnaire and provide a capillary blood glucose sample for glucose and glycated haemoglobin analysis. Exclusion criteria included known intolerance of kiwifruit, glucose intolerance as indicated by the fasting blood glucose and HbA1c, and recent ill health. The characteristics (mean $\pm$ SD) of the study group were as follows: age 36.7 $\pm$ 8.1 years, BMI 24.5 $\pm$ 5.2 kg.m^{-2}, fasting glucose 4.6 $\pm$ 0.4 mmol.L^{-1}, HbA1c 33.9 $\pm$ 4 mmol.mol^{-1}).

Ingestion: The kiwifruit were thawed in a microwave with care to avoid heating, immediately before being consumed. The glucose and kiwifruit were consumed with enough water to give an equal intake volume (300 mL) in all meals.

Glycaemic response: Subjects were asked to eat moderately the evening before and to fast overnight and present themselves at 0830 h for the dietary intervention. They were asked to consume the meals within a 10-min period and avoid physical exertion for three hours afterward, during which time blood glucose determinations were made. Blood glucose concentrations were measured by finger-prick analysis of capillary blood using a HemoCue (Ängelholm, Sweden) blood glucose analyser. Blood samplings were made immediately before consuming the diets (duplicate, baseline), and at 15, 30, 45, 60, 90, 120, and 180 min after the start of food consumption.

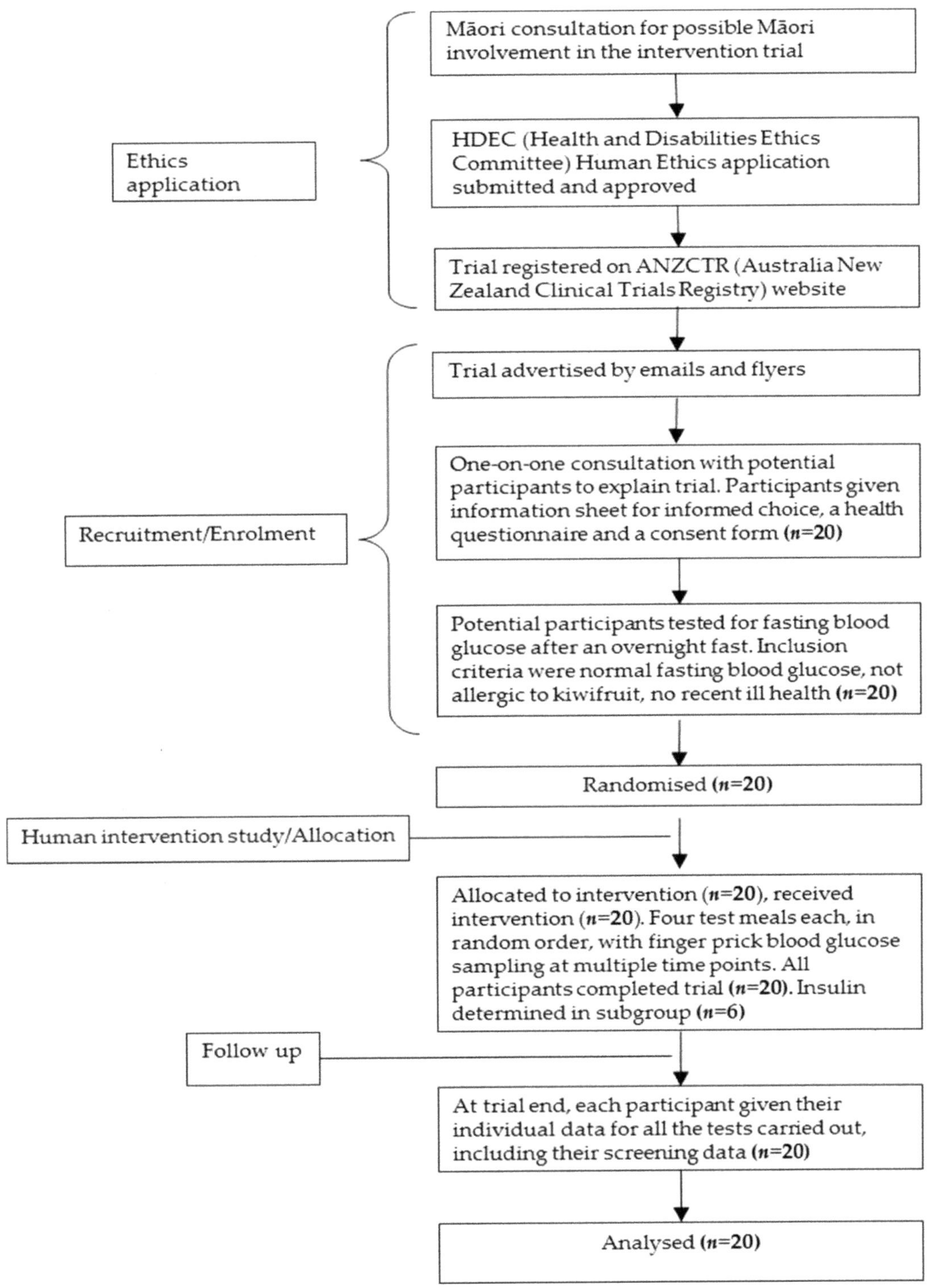

Figure 1. Participant flow chart for clinical determination of the relative glycaemic potency of kiwifruit.

Plasma insulin: Plasma insulin was determined with a Human Insulin Elisa kit (Millipore Hertfordshire, UK) using 0.8-mL capillary blood glucose samples collected at the same time as capillary blood glucose measurements of the glucose reference and SG kiwifruit. A subset of six subjects was used for insulin determination, with their response to SG compared with response to the glucose reference. The aim was to show that kiwifruit exchange did not induce a disproportionately high insulin response. An obvious outlier was removed from the glucose and kiwifruit groups because of technical problems with the glucose analysis, so the analysis involved five subjects. Removal of the outlier did not affect conclusions drawn from the results.

2.5. Data Analysis

Glycaemic potency of kiwifruit carbohydrate: Incremental blood glucose responses were calculated by subtracting each individual's average baseline value from their subsequent measurements and were then used to determine the incremental area under the curve (IAUC) for each individual by trapezoid summation of positive increments [10]. Data were entered into a Microsoft® Excel spreadsheet for preliminary analysis. For statistical comparison of means (ANOVA), GenStat software was used (version 11.1, VSNi Ltd., Hemel Hempstead, UK). Data were analysed using unbalanced analysis of variance (ANOVA), testing differences between meals after adjusting for participant and order effects.

Relative glycaemic potency of the carbohydrate (CHO) in kiwifruit (grams of glucose equivalents (GGEs)/100 g CHO) was used as an estimate of glycaemic index and calculated from the areas under the blood glucose response curves for the kiwifruit ($IAUC_{200\ g\ KF}$) relative to the glucose reference ($IAUC_{40\ g\ Glucose}$), with adjustment for weights of carbohydrate involved (Table 1):

$$\text{Relative glycaemic potency (RGP)} = (IAUC_{KF}/IAUC_{glucose}) \times (\text{Wt. glucose/Wt. KF}) \times 100 \quad \text{GGE/100 g CHO} \tag{1}$$

$$RGP = (IAUC_{200\ g\ KF}/IAUC_{40\ g\ Glucose}) \times (40/200) \times 100 \quad \text{GGE/100 g CHO} \tag{2}$$

GGE expresses the effects of foods on blood glucose on a whole-food basis relative to glucose, as grams of glucose equivalents (GGEs) [11]. The GGE has weight (g) units, so it can be expressed per serving or per reference amount customarily consumed, or per 100 g of food. Thus, it behaves like a nutrient value, and has been termed a virtual food component [12]. It allows direct comparison of foods, and indicates how much glucose a food quantity would be equivalent to in its glycaemic effect. A food composition table containing GGE values allows one to see not only what a food is, but also what it does in terms of its relative glycaemic effect.

Kiwifruit equivalents and kiwifruit exchanges: From a knowledge of the available carbohydrate and GGE content of various foods, including kiwifruit, it was possible to construct tables as guides to incorporating kiwifruit into diets while managing postprandial glycaemia as follows. Because the glycaemic potencies of the two kiwifruit cultivars were similar, the exchange tables have been based on the SunGold values for carbohydrate (12.3 g/100 g) and GGE (6.7 g/100 g) content.

(1) Equi-carbohydrate exchanges (Table 2)

The amount of a food that could be exchanged for (substituted by) one kiwifruit without altering carbohydrate intake was calculated from the available carbohydrate content (%) of kiwifruit and the substituted food.

Where $\%CHO_f$ is the percentage of available carbohydrate in the food (New Zealand Food Composition Database), and $\%CHO_k$ is the percentage of carbohydrate in the kiwifruit, 100 g kiwifruit (one kiwifruit) would exchange: $(\%CHO_k/\%CHO_f) \times 100$ g of the food, or $((\%CHO_k/\%CHO_f) \times 100)/Sf$ servings of the food, where Sf is the serving size (g) of the food.

(2) Glycaemic impact of carbohydrate-based kiwifruit exchange

From the glycaemic potencies (GGE contents) of kiwifruit and foods, and their carbohydrate contents, one may estimate the reduction in relative glycaemic impact that could be expected by equi-carbohydrate partial substitution of kiwifruit for a food. This would allow estimation of possible changes in glycaemic response, for the purposes of blood glucose management.

The proportional reduction in glycaemic impact as a result of substitution by kiwifruit is the relative glycaemic potency of the food (GGE/serving) after substituting plus the GGE added in the substituting kiwifruit, as a proportion of the relative glycaemic potency of the unsubstituted food. The relative glycaemic potency of the food (RGP_f) may be estimated as glycaemic load from its carbohydrate content and glycaemic index (Table 1).

The glycaemic potency of the food before substituting (GGE_B) is:

$$(GGE_B) = \text{Wt food} \times RGP_f/100 \quad (3)$$

After substituting (GGE_A), it is:

$$GGE_A = ((\text{Wt food} \times \%\ CHO) - CHO_{KF}) \times RGP_f/\%\ CHO \quad (4)$$

where CHO_{KF} is the carbohydrate in the substituting kiwifruit. Including the GGE contribution from the substituting kiwifruit (6.7 GGE), the proportional (%) decrease as a result of substitution would be:

$$\%\ \text{decrease in GGE} = (GGE_A + 6.7) \times 100/GGE_B \quad (5)$$

(3) Equi-glycaemic partial substitution (Table 3)

From the relative glycaemic potencies of kiwifruit and a food (GGE/100 g = RGP) one can estimate the amount of the food that should be removed from a meal to include a kiwifruit without increasing postprandial glycaemia. This approach may be useful where the aim is to include fruits in the diet while maintaining a constant blood glucose response.

If the RGP of a food is RGP_f, and the RGP of kiwifruit is RGP_{KF}, the weight of food (W_f) equivalent to 100 g of kiwifruit is given by:

$$W_f = RGP_f/RGP_{KF} \times 100 \quad (6)$$

Similarly, the weight of kiwifruit (W_{KF}) that is the glycaemic equivalent of any given food quantity (W_f), such as a serving, is easily calculated from the relationship between the relative glycaemic potencies of the kiwifruit (RGP_{KF}) and the food (RGP_f):

$$W_{KF} = W_f \times RGP_{KF}/RGP_f \quad (7)$$

This information may be useful where it is desired to replace a complete item with kiwifruit without altering glycaemic response.

Table 1. Estimation of relative glycaemic potency (RGP) of foods as glycaemic load for a selection of foods with available glycaemic index (GI) and available carbohydrate (% CHO avail.) values.

Description	Portion Size [1] (CSM)	Weight [2] (g)	GI [3] (%)	CHO Avail. (%)	RGP [4] (GGE/100 g)	GGEs/CSM [5]
Bakery Products						
Bread, white	1 medium slice	26	70	43.4	30.4	7.9
Crispbread	1 biscuit	6	65	64.4	41.9	2.5
Mixed grain bread "heavy"	1 medium slice	28	45	36.7	16.5	4.6
Bread, wholemeal	1 medium slice	28	69	37.1	25.6	7.2
Muffin, bran	1 muffin	80	60	32.5	19.5	15.6
Breakfast Cereal						
Bran cereal	1 cup	45	42	37.4	15.7	7.1
Corn flakes	1 cup	31	80	84.8	67.8	21.0
Porridge, prepared	1 cup	260	61	10.5	6.4	16.7
Cereal Grain						
Rice, brown, boiled	1 cup	206	55	29.2	16.1	33.1
Rice, white, boiled	1 cup	144	56	17.5	9.8	14.1
Dairy						
Yoghurt, fat red, unsweetened	1 pottle	150	20	14.8	3.0	4.4
Fruit						
Apple, dessert, flesh, raw	1 apple	130	36	10.7	3.9	5.0
Apricot, dried	10 halves	35	31	48.8	15.1	5.3
Banana, raw	1 banana	128	53	24.1	12.8	16.3
Cherries	10 cherries	67	22	14.0	3.1	2.1
Grapefruit	1 grapefruit	236	25	10.1	2.5	6.0
Grapes, black and white	10 grapes	54	43	15.8	6.8	3.7
Kiwifruit	1 kiwi fruit	100	52	10.0	5.2	5.2
Mango	1 cup slices	176	55	14.6	8.0	14.1

Table 1. *Cont.*

Description	Portion Size [1] (CSM)	Weight [2] (g)	GI [3] (%)	CHO Avail. (%)	RGP [4] (GGE/100 g)	GGEs/CSM [5]
Orange, raw	1 orange	128	43	7.7	3.3	4.2
Pawpaw	1 slice	140	58	6.9	4.0	5.6
Pineapple, raw	1 cup chopped	164	66	11.4	7.5	12.3
Peaches, canned in juice	1 cup slices	264	30	22.2	6.7	17.6
Pear, raw	1 pear	148	33	12.8	4.2	6.3
Plum, raw	1 plum	49	24	13.9	3.3	1.6
Rock melon	1 cup sliced	168	65	6.4	4.1	7.0
Raisins	1 cup	154	64	71.3	45.6	70.3
Watermelon	1 cup flesh	169	72	5.1	3.7	6.2
Legumes						
Chickpeas, cooked	1 cup	173	33	8.6	2.8	4.9
Haricot beans, boiled	1 cup	180	31	15.2	4.7	8.5
Kidney beans, red, boiled	1 cup	187	27	15.9	4.3	8.0
Lentils, red, cooked	1 cup	209	26	10.4	2.7	5.7
Pasta						
Spaghetti, boiled	1 cup	148	40	23.9	9.6	14.1
Macaroni, boiled	1 cup	149	45	16.8	7.6	11.3
Noodles, instant, chicken	1 packet	200	47	5.8	2.7	6.0
Treats						
Jelly beans	10 jelly beans	20	80	91.8	73.4	14.7
Potato crisps	1 small packet	50	54	47.6	25.7	12.9
Honey	1 tablespoon	21	73	79.6	58.1	12.2
Vegetables						
Beetroot, boiled	1 cup slices	180	64	9.8	6.3	11.3
Broad beans, boiled	1 cup	170	79	8.6	6.8	11.5
Carrot, boiled	1 carrot	49	71	5.5	3.9	1.9
Corn-sweet, boiled	1 cob	128	55	20.9	11.5	14.7
Kumara, baked	1 kumara	114	44	23.3	10.3	11.7
Parsnip, boiled	1 parsnip	160	97	12.3	11.9	19.1
Peas, green	1 cup	164	48	7.1	3.4	5.6
Potato, rua, boiled	1 potato	114	56	18.2	10.2	11.6
Potato, mashed	1 cup	209	70	14.5	10.2	21.2
Pumpkin, boiled	1 cup	220	75	4.0	3.0	6.6
Swede	1 cup chopped	150	72	3.7	2.7	4.0
Taro corms, cooked	1 cup sliced	142	54	27.4	14.8	21.0
Yams, boiled	1 cup cubes	144	51	27.1	13.8	19.9

[1] Portion size used was a "Common Standard Measure" (CSM); [2] Weight of a portion (g); [3] From the international tables of glycaemic index and glycaemic load a [13]; [4] GI·% available carbohydrate (CHO avail (%)); [5] Relative glycaemic impact per portion expressed as glucose equivalents.

Table 2. Kiwifruit exchanges that would maintain a constant carbohydrate intake, based on the available carbohydrate content of selected carbohydrate foods.

Description	Portion Size	Weight	SG Equivalents		1 Zespri® SunGold Kiwifruit (SG) Replaces		GGE
		(g)	per 100 g [1]	per Portion [2]	(g) [3]	Portions [4]	(g) [5]
Bakery Products							
Bread, white	1 medium slice	26	3.53	0.9	28	1.09	−1.9
Crispbread	1 biscuit	6	5.24	0.3	19	3.18	−1.3
Mixed grain bread	1 medium slice	28	2.98	0.8	34	1.20	1.2
Bread, wholemeal	1 medium slice	28	3.02	0.8	33	1.18	−1.8
Muffin, bran	1 muffin	80	2.64	2.1	38	0.47	−0.7
Breakfast Cereal							
Bran cereal	1 cup	45	3.04	1.4	33	0.73	1.5
Corn flakes	1 cup	31	6.89	2.1	15	0.47	−3.1
Porridge, prepared	1 cup	260	0.85	2.2	117	0.45	−0.8
Cereal Grain							
Rice, brown, boiled	1 cup	206	2.37	4.9	42	0.20	−0.1
Rice, white, boiled	1 cup	144	1.42	2.0	70	0.49	−0.2
Dairy							
Yoghurt, fat red, unsweetened	1 pottle	150	1.20	1.8	83	0.55	4.2
Fruit							
Apple, dessert, raw	1 apple	130	0.87	1.1	115	0.88	2.3
Apricot, dried	10 halves	35	3.97	1.4	25	0.72	2.9
Banana, raw	1 banana	128	1.96	2.5	51	0.40	0.2

Table 2. *Cont.*

Description	Portion Size	Weight (g)	SG Equivalents per 100 g [1]	SG Equivalents per Portion [2]	1 Zespri® SunGold Kiwifruit (SG) Replaces (g) [3]	1 Zespri® SunGold Kiwifruit (SG) Replaces Portions [4]	GGE (g) [5]
Cherries	10 cherries	67	1.14	0.8	88	1.31	4.0
Grapefruit	1 grapefruit	236	0.82	1.9	122	0.52	3.6
Grapes	10 grapes	54	1.28	0.7	78	1.44	1.4
Kiwifruit	1 kiwi fruit	100	1.00	1.0	100	1.00	0
Mango	1 cup slices	176	1.19	2.1	84	0.48	−0.1
Orange, raw	1 orange	128	0.63	0.8	160	1.25	1.4
Pawpaw	1 slice	140	0.56	0.8	178	1.27	−0.4
Pineapple, raw	1 cup	164	0.93	1.5	108	0.66	−1.4
Peaches, canned	1 cup slices	264	1.80	4.8	55	0.21	3.0
Pear, raw	1 pear	148	1.04	1.5	96	0.65	2.6
Plum, raw	1 plum	49	1.13	0.6	88	1.81	3.7
Rock Melon	1 cup sliced	168	0.52	0.9	193	1.15	−1.3
Raisins	1 cup	154	5.80	8.9	17	0.11	−1.2
Watermelon	1 cup flesh	169	0.41	0.7	241	1.43	−2.2
Legumes							
Chickpeas, cooked	1 cup	173	0.70	1.2	143	0.83	2.6
Haricot beans, boiled	1 cup	180	1.24	2.2	81	0.45	2.9
Kidney beans, boiled	1 cup	187	1.29	2.4	77	0.41	3.4
Lentils, red, cooked	1 cup	209	0.85	1.8	118	0.57	3.5
Pasta							
Spaghetti, boiled	1 cup	148	1.94	2.9	51	0.35	1.8
Macaroni, boiled	1 cup	149	1.37	2.0	73	0.49	1.2
Noodles, instant	1 packet	200	0.47	0.9	212	1.06	0.9
Treats							
Jelly beans	10 jelly beans	20	7.46	1.5	13	0.67	−3.1
Potato crisps	1 small packet	50	3.87	1.9	26	0.52	0.1
Honey	1 tablespoon	21	6.47	1.4	15	0.74	−2.3
Vegetables							
Beetroot, boiled	1 cup slices	180	0.80	1.4	126	0.70	−1.2
Broad beans, boiled	1 cup	170	0.70	1.2	143	0.84	−3.0
Carrot, boiled	1 carrot	49	0.45	0.2	224	4.56	−2.0
Corn, sweet, boiled	1 cob	128	1.70	2.2	59	0.46	−0.1
Kumara, baked	1 kumara	114	1.89	2.2	53	0.46	1.3
Parsnip, boiled	1 parsnip	160	1.00	1.6	100	0.63	−5.2
Peas, green	1 cup	164	0.58	0.9	173	1.06	0.8
Potato, rua, boiled	1 potato	114	1.48	1.7	68	0.59	−0.2
Potato, mashed	1 cup	209	1.18	2.5	85	0.41	−1.9
Pumpkin, boiled	1 cup	220	0.33	0.7	308	1.40	−2.5
Swede	1 cup	150	0.30	0.5	332	2.22	−2.2
Taro corms, cooked	1 cup sliced	142	2.23	3.2	45	0.32	0.1
Yams, boiled	1 cup cubes	144	2.20	3.2	45	0.32	0.4

[1] % carbohydrate in food/12.3 (12.3 = % available carbohydrate in kiwifruit); [2] (Portion weight × % carbohydrate in food/100)/12.3; [3] (12.3 × 100)/% available carbohydrate in food; [4] ((12.3 × 100)/% available carbohydrate in food)/portion weight; [5] 6.7—(12.3 × GI of food/100). GGEs = grams of glucose equivalents.

Table 3. Equi-glycemic kiwifruit exchanges based on the relative glycaemic potency of Zespri® SunGold Kiwifruit (SG) and a selection of carbohydrate foods for which relative glycaemic potency (RGP) could be estimated from GI and available carbohydrate as grams of glucose equivalents (GGEs)/100 g, to maintain a constant glycaemic response.

Description	Portion Size	Weight (g)	SG Equivalents (per 100 g) [1]	SG Equivalents (per Portion) [2]	1 SG Replaces (g) [3]	1 SG Replaces (Portions) [4]
Bakery Products						
Bread, white	1 medium slice	26	4.5	1.2	22	0.8
Crispbread	1 biscuit	6	6.2	0.4	16	2.7
Mixed grain bread "heavy"	1 medium slice	28	2.5	0.7	41	1.4
Bread, wholemeal	1 medium slice	28	3.8	1.1	26	0.9
Muffin, bran	1 muffin	80	2.9	2.3	34	0.4
Breakfast Cereal						
Bran cereal	1 cup	45	2.3	1.1	43	0.9
Corn flakes	1 cup	31	10.1	3.1	10	0.3
Porridge, prepared	1 cup	260	1.0	2.5	105	0.4
Cereal Grain						
Rice, brown, boiled	1 cup	206	2.4	4.9	42	0.2
Rice, white, boiled	1 cup	144	1.5	2.1	68	0.5

Table 3. *Cont.*

Description	Portion Size	Weight (g)	SG Equivalents (per 100 g) [1]	(per Portion) [2]	1 SG Replaces (g) [3]	(Portions) [4]
Dairy						
Yoghurt, fat red, unsweetened	1 pottle	150	0.4	0.7	226	1.5
Fruit						
Apple, dessert, flesh, raw	1 apple	130	0.6	0.7	174	1.3
Apricot, dried	10 halves	35	2.3	0.8	44	1.3
Banana, raw	1 banana	128	1.9	2.4	52	0.4
Cherries	10 cherries	67	0.5	0.3	218	3.2
Grapefruit	1 grapefruit	236	0.4	0.9	265	1.1
Grapes, black and white	10 grapes	54	1.0	0.5	99	1.8
Kiwifruit	1 kiwifruit	100	1.0	1.0	97	1.0
Mango	1 cup slices	176	1.2	2.1	83	0.5
Orange, raw	1 orange	128	0.5	0.6	202	1.6
Pawpaw	1 slice	140	0.6	0.8	167	1.2
Pineapple, raw	1 cup chopped	164	1.1	1.8	89	0.5
Peaches, canned in juice	1 cup slices	264	1.0	2.6	101	0.4
Pear, raw	1 pear	148	0.6	0.9	159	1.1
Plum, raw	1 plum	49	0.5	0.2	201	4.1
Rock melon	1 cup sliced	168	0.6	1.0	162	1.0
Raisins	1 cup	154	6.8	10.5	15	0.1
Watermelon	1 cup flesh	169	0.5	0.9	182	1.1
Legumes						
Chickpeas, cooked	1 cup	173	0.4	0.7	236	1.4
Haricot beans, boiled	1 cup	180	0.7	1.3	142	0.8
Kidney beans, red, boiled	1 cup	187	0.6	1.2	156	0.8
Lentils, red, cooked	1 cup	209	0.4	0.8	248	1.2
Pasta						
Spaghetti, boiled	1 cup	148	1.4	2.1	70	0.5
Macaroni, boiled	1 cup	149	1.1	1.7	89	0.6
Noodles, instant, chicken	1 packet	200	0.4	0.9	246	1.1
Treats						
Jelly beans	10 jelly beans	20	11.0	2.2	9	0.5
Potato crisps	1 small packet	50	3.8	1.9	26	0.5
Honey	1 tablespoon	21	8.7	1.8	12	0.5
Vegetables						
Beetroot, boiled	1 cup slices	180	0.9	1.7	107	0.6
Broad beans, boiled	1 cup	170	1.0	1.7	99	0.6
Carrot, boiled	1 carrot	49	0.6	0.3	172	3.5
Corn, sweet, boiled	1 cob	128	1.7	2.2	58	0.5
Kumara, baked	1 kumara	114	1.5	1.7	65	0.6
Parsnip, boiled	1 parsnip	160	1.8	2.8	56	0.4
Peas, green	1 cup	164	0.5	0.8	197	1.2
Potato, rua, boiled	1 potato	114	1.5	1.7	66	0.6
Potato, mashed	1 cup	209	1.5	3.2	66	0.3
Pumpkin, boiled	1 cup	220	0.4	1.0	223	1.0
Swede	1 cup chopped	150	0.4	0.6	252	1.7
Taro corms, cooked	1 cup sliced	142	2.2	3.1	45	0.3
Yams, boiled	1 cup cubes	144	2.1	3.0	48	0.3

[1] RGP (Table 1)/6.7; [2] GGE per CSM (Table 1)/6.7; [3] 6.7 × 100/RGP; [4] 6.7/(GGE per CSM (Table 1)).

3. Results

Analysis of kiwifruit: Digestive analysis showed the available carbohydrate contents of the kiwifruit to be as follows: "Hayward" green kiwifruit, 11.2% *w*/*w*; "Zesy002" gold kiwifruit, 12.3% *w*/*w*.

The figures were close to values from previous analyses of six cultivars of kiwifruit (New Zealand Food Composition Database). The sugars consisted of approximately equal proportions of glucose and fructose, with a lesser sucrose component, in the approximate ratio 2:2:1.

Blood glucose responses: All 20 subjects completed the trial and the results from all of them were used in the data analysis. The between-subject variations were large, as is typical of such studies, but no outliers were removed. The different diets induced blood glucose responses that were clearly distinctive (Figure 2). The responses to the two kiwifruit cultivars were very similar and less than for the glucose reference.

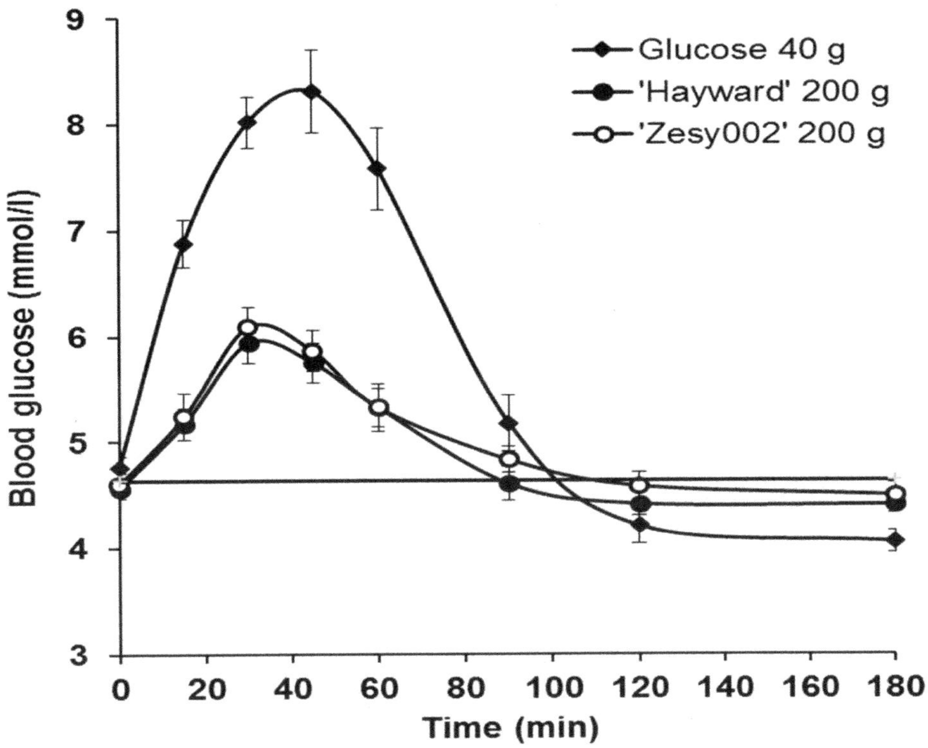

Figure 2. Mean (± SEM) blood glucose responses used to determine the relative glycaemic potency of "Hayward" (GR) and "Zesy002" (SunGold, SG) kiwifruit.

Relative glycaemic potency: The relative glycaemic potency (RGP; grams of glucose equivalents (GGE)) of the whole fruit, calculated from the glycaemic response to 200 g kiwifruit compared with the response to 40 g of glucose reference (Figure 2), and based on the area under the blood glucose response curve, showed that in terms of blood glucose-raising potential, one 100-g piece of "Hayward" kiwifruit would have a blood glucose-raising (glycaemic) potency equivalent to that of 6.6 g of glucose, and one 100-g piece of "Zesy002" kiwifruit would have a glycaemic potency equivalent to 6.7 g glucose (Table 4).

Table 4. Relative glycaemic potency (RGP) expressed as grams of glucose equivalents (GGEs) per 100 g of kiwifruit, determined from the relative areas under the blood glucose response curves (incremental area under the curve, IAUC) shown in Figure 2.

	IAUC		GGE/200 g		RRGP (GGEs/100 g) (GGEs/100 g)	
	Mean	SEM	Mean	SEM	Mean	SEM
Glucose (40 g)	234.7	18.8				-
"Hayward" kiwifruit (200 g)	75.1	7.3	13.2	1.25	6.6	0.8
"Zesy002" kiwifruit (200 g)	76.2	8.5	13.4	1.44	6.7	0.4

The RGP of the available carbohydrate alone in "Hayward", its approximate glycaemic index, was 59 ± 7.03 GGE/100 g carbohydrate (mean ± SEM) and that of "Zesy002" was 54 ± 3.05 GGE/100 g carbohydrate (mean ± SEM), with the difference between the values non-significant.

Insulin responses: On an equal carbohydrate basis, insulin response was lower for kiwifruit carbohydrate than for than for glucose (Table 5), consistent with the lower insulinaemic potential of fructose compared with glucose [14]. A lower insulin response to kiwifruit than to rice in equal carbohydrate meals has similarly been measured recently [15]. When expressed per GGE the insulin responses were very similar (Table 5), indicating that it is physiologically valid to express glycaemic potency of mixed sugars in fruit as glucose equivalents, as indicated in previous studies of the relative effects of glucose and fructose on the insulin response [14].

With the one removed outlier subject included in the analysis the median insulin response (μU mL^{-1}.min^{-1}) per gram of carbohydrate was: glucose 39.7, SunGold 24.1; and the insulin response per GGE was: glucose 39.7, SunGold 42.1.

Table 5. Insulin response to glucose and to glycaemic glucose equivalents (GGEs) in kiwifruit.

	Insulin Response (μU mL^{-1}.min^{-1}) per g Carbohydrate		**Insulin Response (μU mL^{-1}.min^{-1}) per GGE**	
	Mean	**SEM**	**Mean**	**SEM**
Glucose	40.9	2.2	40.9	2.2
Kiwifruit	28.8	5.3	39.6	4.5

4. Discussion

The tables of equi-carbohydrate (Table 2) and equi-glycaemic (Table 3) exchanges of kiwifruit show that kiwifruit exchanges over a range of food categories will result in very small changes in glycaemic impact, based purely on the glycaemic potency of the sugars involved. The change in GGE intake using one kiwifruit exchange is within the range $\pm$ 5 GGE for most of the foods considered (Figure 3). Because the exchange is on a carbohydrate basis, whether kiwifruit exchange increases or decreases glycaemic impact will depend on the glycaemic index (GI) of the food being substituted relative to the GI of kiwifruit. Substitution of any foods with a GI less than that of kiwifruit (GI = 54) will increase glycaemic impact, and substitution of foods with a GI greater than 54 will reduce glycaemic impact. However, because the substitution involves quite small amounts of carbohydrate, due to the high water content of kiwifruit and the fact that kiwifruit has a low GI, the change in GGE intake will be small. Food groups in which kiwifruit substitution would slightly increase glycaemic impact include pasta, pulses, and some fruits. Kiwifruit substitution of cereal-based starchy foods such as bakery products and breakfast cereals would reduce glycaemic impact most.

The exchange tables indicate the change in relative glycaemic impact that may be attributed to carbohydrate exchange (Table 2, Figure 3). However, kiwifruit substitution is likely to cause a greater reduction in glycaemic impact than would be predicted from carbohydrate substitution alone because of the presence of organic acids, dietary fibre, and other fruit components such as phenolics. Thus, where kiwifruit exchange indicates an increase in relative glycaemic impact, as in the case of pulses and pasta, the increase is likely to be smaller than indicated in Figure 3. Furthermore, the pattern of food intake can have a sizeable effect on glycaemic response: if the kiwifruit portion of the substituted meal is consumed 30 min before the rest of the meal, the overall glycaemic response can be substantially suppressed [15], by as much as 30%.

The results of insulin analysis in a subset of participants (Table 5) showed that the insulin response per kiwifruit GGE was almost identical to the response per gram of glucose. Therefore, substitution of kiwifruit carbohydrate for food carbohydrate would not lead to a disproportionately large increase in insulin response compared with glucose. Because the exchange involves no more than 6–7 GGEs per kiwifruit, any disproportionate increase in insulin per GGE from kiwifruit would in any case give a small net change in insulin for the meal. Kiwifruit exchanges will not, therefore, appreciably increase insulin demand.

The vitamin C content of the kiwifruit was not determined for the present study because it has been previously well established as consistently higher than in most other fruits [1], with a concentration of about 150 mg per 100 g SunGold fruit—enough for a single fruit to raise vitamin C intake to the recommended daily allowance. The present analysis of the effects of kiwifruit exchanges has shown that using kiwifruit to improve intakes of vitamin C or other fruit components would have very little effect on glycaemic impact over a range of food categories, and is therefore glycaemically safe.

With the aid of exchange tables, kiwifruit may be used to improve vitamin C intakes while maintaining either a constant carbohydrate intake, or a more or less constant glycaemic impact and insulin demand.

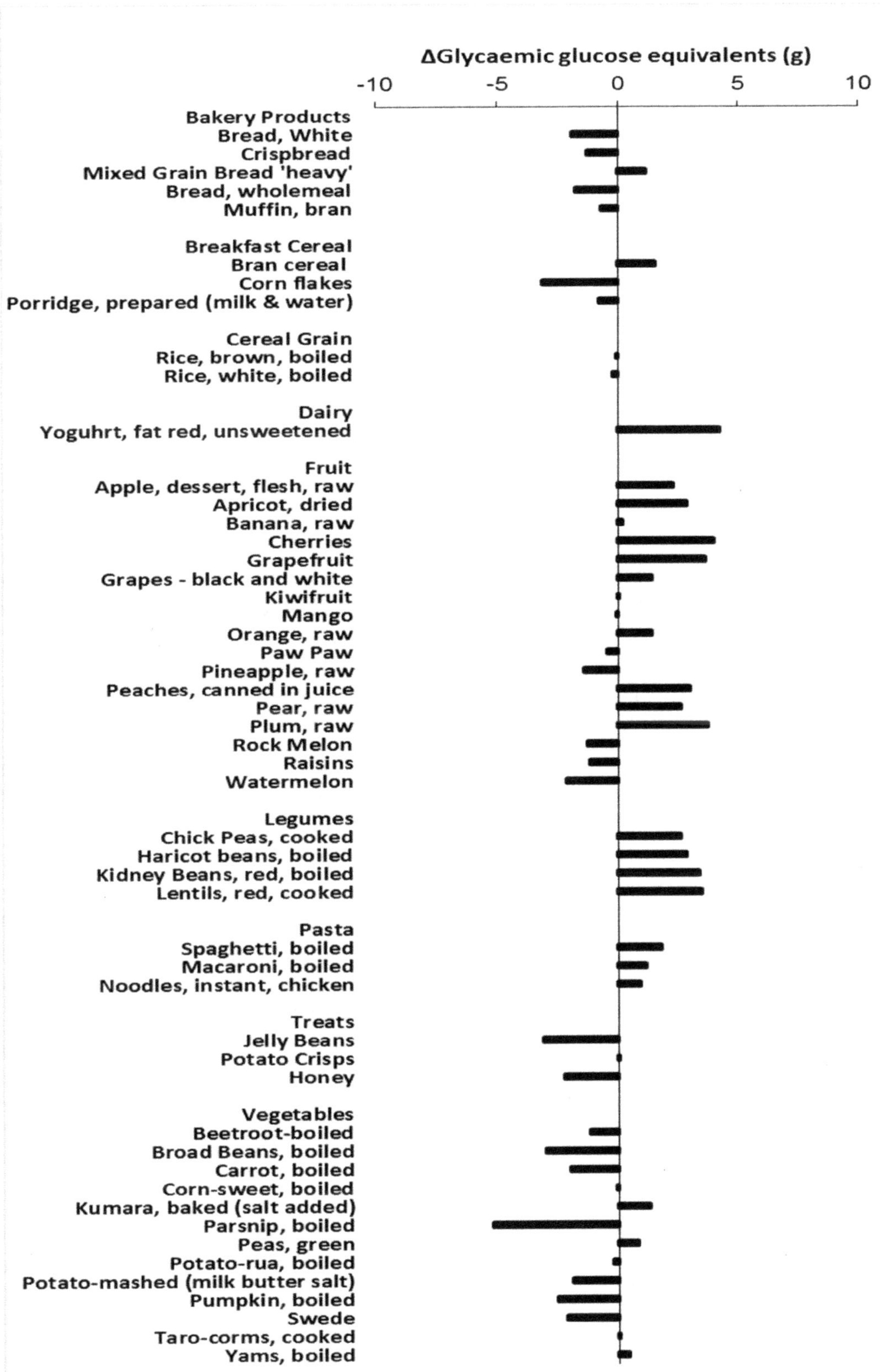

Figure 3. Change in glycaemic potential (GGE (g)) upon equi-carbohydrate substitution of one SunGold kiwifruit for various foods.

Although the focus has been on vitamin C in this paper, it is noteworthy that kiwifruit have a high content of potassium, 315 mg per 100 g (about one fruit) [1]. When kiwifruit exchange involves substitution of refined cereal products, including many breakfast cereals, a substantial increase in potassium may result. For instance, one cup of cornflakes containing 24.4 g of available carbohydrate provides 27 mg of potassium. Exchange for two SunGold kiwifruit providing 24.6 g of available carbohydrate, according to the analysis in this paper, would provide 630 mg of potassium, a 24-fold increase. Similarly, substitution of highly refined cereal products by kiwifruit on an equal carbohydrate basis may help to address the shortfall in dietary fibre in many modern diets.

The utility of the exchange tables in dietary management of glycaemia, and how accurately they achieve this purpose, requires further validation, particularly for the equi-glycaemic exchanges which are based on glycaemic response. The equal carbohydrate exchanges can be conducted accurately, because the measurements on which they are based are purely chemical analyses of available carbohydrate content of foods. If measured directly, available carbohydrate is accurate, although it is often measured indirectly "by difference", which is not as accurate. However, measures involving glycaemic responses such as GGEs, RGP, and GI involve intrinsically larger errors [16], arising from individual differences and variations in physiological response to foods.

Calculating the glucose equivalence of 200 g kiwifruit with a 40-g glucose reference involves a small error because of the non-linearity of the glucose dose–blood glucose response curve [11]. The present study was about the glycaemic impact of foods, not about GI per se, so there was no need to use a 50-g glucose reference as specified for GI determination. Instead, the reference glucose dose of 40 g was closer to the carbohydrate dose of 23 g ingested in the realistic 200 g intake of kiwifruit, which is the edible portion of two fresh kiwifruit, used in the clinical trial of the present study. Therefore, no adjustment for non-linearity was required when calculating the glucose equivalence (GGE content) of the kiwifruit [17]. We have also shown that the difference between GGE estimated as glycaemic load from GI and carbohydrate content, and GGE measured directly, is small [18]. Thus, glycaemic load values may be used as estimates of RGP with little loss of accuracy in guiding food choices for glycaemia management [19].

The present study has shown the glycaemic potencies of "Hayward" and "Zesy002" in comparison to a glucose reference (their relative glycaemic potencies) to be very low. Both kiwifruit cultivars had an RGP of 6–7 GGEs per 100 g. That is, 100 g (one kiwifruit edible portion) would have the same glycaemic effect as 6–7 g of glucose. Converting the GGE content to a per 100-g carbohydrate basis gave estimates of GI for "Hayward" and "Zesy002" of 59 and 54, respectively. The values were slightly higher than previously published [20] perhaps because the fruit were consumed after disintegration and freezing. However, with the very low relative glycaemic potency and low available carbohydrate content of kiwifruit, a difference of 10 GI units would translate to a difference of about 1 g of glucose equivalents per kiwifruit. With a carbohydrate content of about 10%, a difference of 10 GI units would make a difference of only about 1 GGEs (the effect equivalent to 1 g glucose) in a 100 g edible portion of kiwifruit. This underlines the irrelevance of GI to management of intakes of kiwifruit and other fresh fruits for postprandial glycaemic control, and the need to use more realistic means of expressing glycaemic potency, such as RGP. So even if consumed on an equal carbohydrate basis as a partial replacement of low GI foods there would be little glycaemic cost compared with the benefit of a greatly increased intake of vitamin C.

Similarly, when kiwifruit is used in an exchange format to partially substitute other carbohydrate foods, the net effect on GGE intake of removing carbohydrate in the substituted food and adding it in the substituting kiwifruit is only a few GGE units (Figure 3). Furthermore, partially substituting fresh kiwifruit, with a vitamin C content of about 100 mg per fruit, for starch-based foods such as breakfast cereals and cereal-based cooked staples, has the potential to enormously improve vitamin C status. As vitamin C is heat-labile and most cereal products and other starchy staples are cooked and therefore contain very low amounts of vitamin C, partial substitution by one or two kiwifruit would be a useful strategy for naturally improving vitamin C intakes.

Substituting kiwifruit for unsweetened starchy products would increase fructose intakes slightly, but by an amount that would not produce the metabolic changes that are associated with high fructose intakes in sweetened processed foods [21]. In fact, a modest intake of fructose has the benefit of enhancing glucose metabolism and facilitating glucose disposal [22]. We have found that consuming two kiwifruit per day for 12 weeks did not cause any of the metabolic changes that have been reported for high intakes of fructose (paper in preparation).

The present paper has illustrated the concept of kiwifruit exchange tables, but the practicality of using the exchange tables, and the range of foods they contain also needs further development. While the tables in their present form would be easily understood by nutritionists and dieticians, how the information could be best used in a user-friendly format for public use, could be the subject of consumer research. Further research in long-term trials should also be conducted to determine whether or not sustained use of kiwifruit exchanges leads to improvements, or delays decline, in key biomarkers of health outcomes.

The exchange tables are based on a value for ready-to-eat ripe fruit, but such a value is likely to depend on the stage of ripeness of the fruit when consumed, so it is also important to determine the stability of the GGE values determined in the present study. In that respect, the values are likely to be similar to any other values in a food composition database that are guides, but do not pretend to be exact predictors of effects of any given food ingestion event.

Overall, the results indicate that including kiwifruit or other fruits in diets by equi-carbohydrate substitution of highly digestible and therefore high GI starch components will generally lead to glycaemic benefits, while also enriching the diets functionally and nutritionally. At the very least, despite the perception of fruits as sweet-flavoured and therefore high in glycaemic sugars, the glycaemic change associated with consuming fresh fruits in a carbohydrate exchange format is small. Including fresh fruit in the diet need not have a negative glycaemic impact when its introduction is guided by tables of exchanges based on carbohydrate or glycaemic equivalents, as presented here for kiwifruit.

Author Contributions: Conceptualisation: J.M. Funding acquisition: J.M. Ethics application: S.M., J.M. Clinical trial management and sampling: S.M. In vitro digestive analysis: S.M. Insulin analysis: K.B.-H. Data curation and analysis: S.M., J.M. Preparation of manuscript: J.M.

Acknowledgments: The research was funded as part of the "Kiwi, fruity and friendly" research programme in the High Value Nutrition theme of the New Zealand National Science Challenge (subcontract UOAX1421), and by the New Zealand Institute for Plant & Food Research (Contract no. 33115). Technical help from Sue Middlemiss-Kraak is gratefully acknowledged.

References

1. Richardson, D.P.; Ansell, J.; Drummond, L.N. The nutritional and health attributes of kiwifruit: A review. *Eur. J. Nutr.* **2018**. [CrossRef] [PubMed]
2. Carr, A.C.; Pullar, J.M.; Moran, S.; Vissers, M.C.M. Bioavailability of vitamin C from kiwifruit in non-smoking males: Determination of 'healthy' and 'optimal' intakes. *J. Nutr. Sci.* **2012**, *1*, e14. [CrossRef] [PubMed]
3. Carr, A.C.; Bozonet, S.M.; Pullar, J.M.; Simcock, J.M.; Vissers, M.C.M. Human skeletal muscle ascorbate is highly responsive to changes in vitamin C intake and plasma concentrations. *Am. J. Clin. Nutr.* **2013**, *97*, 800–807. [CrossRef] [PubMed]
4. Frei, B.; England, L.; Ames, B.N. Ascorbate is an outstanding antioxidant in human-blood plasma. *Proc. Natl. Acad. Sci. USA* **1989**, *86*, 6377–6381. [CrossRef] [PubMed]
5. Brownlee, M. Biochemistry and molecular cell biology of diabetic complications. *Nature* **2001**, *414*, 813–820. [CrossRef] [PubMed]
6. Mishra, S.; Edwards, H.; Hedderley, D.; Podd, J.; Monro, J. Kiwifruit Non-Sugar Components Reduce Glycaemic Response to Co-Ingested Cereal in Humans. *Nutrients* **2017**, *9*, 1195. [CrossRef] [PubMed]

7. Wheeler, M.L.; Franz, M.; Barrier, P.; Holler, H.; Cronmiller, N.; Delahanty, L.M. Macronutrient and energy database for the 1995 Exchange Lists for Meal Planning: A rationale for clinical practice decisions. *J. Am. Diet. Assoc.* **1996**, *96*, 1167–1171. [CrossRef]
8. Monro, J.A.; Mishra, S.; Venn, B. Baselines representing blood glucose clearance improve in vitro prediction of the glycemic impact of customarily consumed food quantities. *Br. J. Nutr.* **2010**, *103*, 295–305. [CrossRef] [PubMed]
9. Blakeney, A.; Mutton, L. A simple colourimetric method for determination of sugars in fruit and vegetables. *J. Sci. Food Agric.* **1980**, *31*, 889–897. [CrossRef]
10. Brouns, F.; Bjorck, I.; Frayn, K.; Gibbs, A.; Lang, V.; Slama, G.; Wolever, T. Glycaemic index methodology. *Nutr. Res. Rev.* **2005**, *18*, 1–28. [CrossRef] [PubMed]
11. Monro, J.A.; Shaw, M. Glycemic impact, glycemic glucose equivalents, glycemic index, and glycemic load: Definitions, distinctions and implications. *Am. J. Clin. Nutr.* **2008**, *87*, S237–S243. [CrossRef] [PubMed]
12. Monro, J.A. Virtual food components: Functional food effects expressed as food components. *Eur. J. Clin. Nutr.* **2004**, *58*, 219–230. [CrossRef] [PubMed]
13. Foster-Powell, K.; Holt, S.H.A.; Brand-Miller, J.C. International table of glycemic index and glycemic load values: 2002. *Am. J. Clin. Nutr.* **2002**, *76*, 5–56. [CrossRef] [PubMed]
14. Lee, B.M.; Wolever, T.M.S. Effect of glucose, sucrose and fructose on plasma glucose and insulin responses in normal humans: Comparison with white bread. *Eur. J. Clin. Nutr.* **1998**, *52*, 924–928. [CrossRef] [PubMed]
15. Lubransky, A.; Monro, J.; Mishra, S.; Yu, H.; Haszard, J.J.; Venn, B.J. Postprandial Glycaemic, Hormonal and Satiety Responses to Rice and Kiwifruit Preloads in Chinese Adults: A Randomised Controlled Crossover Trial. *Nutrients* **2018**, *10*, 1110. [CrossRef] [PubMed]
16. Venn, B.J.; Green, T.J. Glycemic index and glycemic load: Measurement issues and their effect on diet-disease relationships. *Eur. J. Clin. Nutr.* **2007**, *61*, S1221–S1231. [CrossRef] [PubMed]
17. Wallace, A.; Monro, J.; Brown, R.; Frampton, C. A glucose reference curve is the optimum method to determine the Glycemic Glucose Equivalent values of foods in humans. *Nutr. Res.* **2008**, *28*, 753–759. [CrossRef] [PubMed]
18. Venn, B.J.; Wallace, A.J.; Monro, J.A.; Perry, T.; Brown, R.; Frampton, C.; Green, T.J. The glycemic load estimated from the glycemic index does not differ greatly from that measured using a standard curve in healthy volunteers. *J. Nutr.* **2006**, *136*, 1377–1381. [CrossRef] [PubMed]
19. Monro, J.A.; Mishra, S. Database values for food-based dietary control of glycaemia. *J. Food Compos. Anal.* **2010**, *23*, 406–410. [CrossRef]
20. Monro, J.A. Kiwifruit, carbohydrate availability, and the glycemic response. *Adv. Food Nutr. Res.* **2013**, *68*, 257–271. [PubMed]
21. Stanhope, K.L. Role of Fructose-Containing Sugars in the Epidemics of Obesity and Metabolic Syndrome. *Ann. Rev. Med.* **2012**, *63*, 329–343. [CrossRef] [PubMed]
22. Laughlin, M.R. Normal Roles for Dietary Fructose in Carbohydrate Metabolism. *Nutrients* **2014**, *6*, 3117–3129. [CrossRef] [PubMed]

14

Carbohydrate Counting in Children and Adolescents with Type 1 Diabetes

Giorgia Tascini, Maria Giulia Berioli, Laura Cerquiglini, Elisa Santi, Giulia Mancini, Francesco Rogari, Giada Toni and Susanna Esposito *

Pediatric Clinic, Department of Surgical and Biomedical Sciences, Università degli Studi di Perugia, 06132 Perugia, Italy; giorgia.tascini@gmail.com (G.T.); mgiuliaberioli@gmail.com (M.G.B.); laura.cerquiglini@ospedale.perugia.it (L.C.); elisa.santi1988@gmail.com (E.S.); giu87manci@gmail.com (G.M.); rogari.francesco@virgilio.it (F.R.); toni.giada@gmail.com (G.T.)

* Correspondence: susanna.esposito@unimi.it

Abstract: Carbohydrate counting (CC) is a meal-planning tool for patients with type 1 diabetes (T1D) treated with a basal bolus insulin regimen by means of multiple daily injections or continuous subcutaneous insulin infusion. It is based on an awareness of foods that contain carbohydrates and their effect on blood glucose. The bolus insulin dose needed is obtained from the total amount of carbohydrates consumed at each meal and the insulin-to-carbohydrate ratio. Evidence suggests that CC may have positive effects on metabolic control and on reducing glycosylated haemoglobin concentration (HbA_{1c}). Moreover, CC might reduce the frequency of hypoglycaemia. In addition, with CC the flexibility of meals and snacks allows children and teenagers to manage their T1D more effectively within their own lifestyles. CC and the bolus calculator can have possible beneficial effects in improving post-meal glucose, with a higher percentage of values within the target. Moreover, CC might be integrated with the counting of fat and protein to more accurately calculate the insulin bolus. In conclusion, in children and adolescents with T1D, CC may have a positive effect on metabolic control, might reduce hypoglycaemia events, improves quality of life, and seems to do so without influencing body mass index; however, more high-quality clinical trials are needed to confirm this positive impact.

Keywords: carbohydrate counting; glycosylated haemoglobin; hypoglycaemia; insulin; type 1 diabetes

1. Introduction

Type 1 diabetes (T1D), formerly called insulin-dependent diabetes or juvenile diabetes, is an autoimmune disorder characterised by a severe deficiency or absence of endogenous insulin, which results in chronic hyperglycaemia. The achievement of optimal glucose control is facilitated by intensive insulin treatment in patients with T1D [1,2]. The current recommendations are based on the basal bolus paradigm, with subcutaneous long-acting insulin or continuous subcutaneous infusion of rapid-acting insulin to cover basal requirements and with rapid-acting insulin to prevent or correct glucose excursions. Frequent self-measurements of capillary blood glucose allow for insulin dose adjustments, with the aim of achieving good metabolic control [3]. Furthermore, continuous glucose monitoring (CGM) provides information about the glucose level every 5 min and allows patients to view their glycaemic data either on their insulin pump or on a separate receiver [4].

Despite advances in medical treatment and technology, nutritional therapy continues to be a cornerstone of diabetes care [5]. Nutritional recommendations for a healthy lifestyle for the general population are also appropriate for children and adolescents with T1D, with the only difference compared to healthy peers being the need for insulin therapy. The International Society for Paediatric and Adolescent Diabetes (ISPAD) Consensus Guidelines of 2014 stressed the importance of and special issues applying to nutritional management for children with diabetes [6]. The Guidelines recommended that a proper diet should allow for optimal growth, maintain an ideal weight, and prevent acute and chronic complications. The approximate energy intake and essential nutrients should be distributed as follows: carbohydrates 50–55%; fat 30–35%; and protein 10–15%.

Carbohydrates are the primary macronutrient that has an effect on the postprandial glycaemic response; their dietary intake should not be limited to ensure proper growth in children and adolescents with T1D. Adjusting the insulin dose to carbohydrate intake could produce potential improvements in glycaemic control and quality of life. Carbohydrate counting (CC) is a meal-planning tool for patients with T1D, based on an awareness of foods that contain carbohydrates and their effect on blood glucose. The bolus insulin dose needed is obtained from the total amount of carbohydrates consumed at each meal and the insulin-to-carbohydrate ratio (ICR) [7]. The current guidelines recommend the algorithms for prandial insulin be based on the carbohydrate amount taken in during a meal. They recognise the additional benefits to glycaemic control due to the use of the glycaemic index (GI) and that fats and proteins in the diet may influence postprandial glycaemia [6,8,9]. The aim of this review is to analyse the impact of CC in children and adolescents with T1D.

2. Educational Program on Carbohydrate Counting (CC)

With the discovery of insulin, researchers recognised that the total amount of dietary carbohydrates should be used to determine the need for insulin at meals. In the 1980s, the conventional insulin therapy imposed very rigid eating patterns with restricted and controlled carbohydrates portions. Subsequently, in the 1990s, the Diabetes Control and Complication Trial (DCTT) was a turning point for the treatment of diabetes. From this study, it was found that intensive insulin therapy, using multiple daily injection (MDI) or insulin pumps (CSII), improved glycaemic control and reduced complications related to the disease. In the DCTT, CC, one of the methods of meal planning, was considered effective in achieving good glycaemic control and allowing more flexibility in food choices [10,11].

An experienced team, including the role of the dietitian, is essential for the patient with T1D and his or her family so that they can then partake in the educational program and learn the method of CC as well as healthy-eating principles [11]. Children and those who care for them can learn to estimate the amount of carbohydrates with reasonable accuracy; however, continuing education therapy is needed. Carbohydrates have the most significant impact on raising postprandial blood glucose. A careful counting of carbohydrates will lead to the correct calculation of the required insulin dose, which in turn will lead to normalising postprandial glycaemia [12]. The American Academy of Nutrition and Dietetics have identified three levels of CC [8]:

- Level 1, Patients should understand that carbohydrates raise blood glucose, and they must be encouraged to consume a consistent amount of carbohydrates per meal. Simple methods to quantify the carbohydrates must be provided: gram increments of carbohydrates, 10–12 g carbohydrate portions, and 15 g carbohydrate exchanges. In particular, this level is helpful for patients in therapy with twice-daily insulin doses and who need consistent carbohydrate intake [13];
- Level 2, Pattern management. This represents an intermediate step, in which patients learn to evaluate changes in blood glucose compared to carbohydrates consumed, which are modified by insulin and physical activity. Therefore, patients supported by paediatric teams can make changes to their insulin. However, ever more frequently, paediatric teams use other methods, such as carbohydrate intake or the insulin-to-carb ratio (ICR);
- Level 3, Advanced CC. Patients in MDI or CSII learn ICR and how to use it.

3. Insulin-to-Carb Ratio (ICR), Insulin Sensitivity Factor (ISF), and Glycaemic Index (GI)

The insulin-to-carb ratio (ICR) is individualised and depends on one's sensitivity to insulin, which is how many grams of carbohydrates 1 unit of insulin covers. ICR allows children to obtain their insulin needs at mealtimes on the basis of the carbohydrates that will be consumed at that time, their blood glucose level, and their anticipated physical activity [6,9]. For the identification of the carbohydrates-to-insulin ratio, the empirical method of the 500 rule or 300–450 rule, for very young children who need less than 10 units of insulin a day, is often used [14–17]. It consists of dividing 500, 300, or 450 by the total daily insulin dose (TDD). ICR is not constant during the day; it tends to be higher in the morning, lower for lunch, and higher in the evening [18]. ICR varies more in children than in adults, which is linked to the more frequent changes occurring in the daily activity of the child [9].

The insulin sensitivity factor (ISF) is a correction algorithm of pre-prandial glycaemia. In particular, ISF indicates how many mmol/L (or mg/dL) 1 unit of insulin lowers blood glucose by; it is obtained by dividing 1800 (rapid analogue) or 1500 (regular insulin) by the TDD [19]. ISF also needs to be individualised for each patient. Regarding infants and toddlers, ISF is generally higher, approximately 100–150 mg/dL [19]. A recent study showed that the bolus insulin for meals was more than the one calculated by the 500 rule, in particular at breakfast and in pre-pubescent children. Moreover, for corrections, insulin need was slightly less than that calculated by the 100 rule (100 divided by total daily insulin dose) [19].

The GI expresses the glycaemic response after eating a known amount of carbohydrates contained in food, but in relation to the same amount of carbohydrates contained in white bread. The glycaemic area measured 120 min after food intake is expressed as a percentage of the standard. Using the GI and eating low-GI food may produce modest benefits in the control of postprandial hyperglycaemia. Moreover, to consider both the quality and the amount of carbohydrates, the concept of glycaemic load was introduced [20]. In patients with T1D, GI should be used with a method of carbohydrate quantification [21].

3.1. Glycaemic Control

In previous studies conducted in adult subjects, glycaemic variations were assessed after the ingestion of different amounts and qualities of carbohydrates: complex carbohydrates in a mixed meal and simple sugar dextrose [22]. Blood sugar was higher, but for a shorter time, after the dextrose load than after the mixed meals. The total amount released by the artificial pancreas to return glycaemia to basal levels did not differ when exposed to different types of carbohydrates, but a difference did occur in the release kinetics. Furthermore, there was a linear relation between carbohydrate intake and insulin need.

A systematic review and meta-analysis was recently performed to evaluate the effectiveness of CC on glycaemic control in people with T1D [22]. It included 10 studies, published from 2000 to 2014, involving 773 participants. Four studies enrolled children and adolescents [23–26], and six studies included adults [27–32]. Overall, CC, compared with other diabetes diet methods or usual diabetes diets, improved HbA_{1c} values, in line with a previous systematic review and a meta-analysis [28,33,34]. A non-significant improvement of HbA_{1c} was found in the subgroup analysis restricted to trials that compared CC with other T1D diet methods [14].

One systematic review and meta-analysis aimed to summarise all available evidence from both observational and randomised controlled studies on the effects of advanced CC on glycaemic control, psychosocial measures, body weight, and severe hypoglycaemic events in patients of all age groups with T1D [26]. Six randomised controlled trials and 21 before/after studies were included; four uncontrolled trials (Table 1) [35–38] and one randomised controlled trial (Table 2) [39] were conducted in children and adolescents with a mean age $\pm$ standard deviation of 12 $\pm$ 4 years. In only one study, in which 28 adolescents were included, the improvement in HbA_{1c} was not demonstrated after advanced CC. These 28 patients switched from a prescriptive to a flexible meal plan and insulin. According to the authors, this result could be related to inaccurate CC, incorrect calculation of insulin dose, or inappropriate insulin injection technique.

Table 1. Characteristics of uncontrolled studies with carbohydrate counting (CC) used in children and adolescents with type 1 diabetes (T1D).

Authors and Year	Design	Follow-Up (Months)	Sample Size	Insulin Regimen	Insulin Type (Short-Acting/Long-Acting)	Age (Years)	T1D Duration (Years)	HbA_{1c} at Baseline (mmol/mol)	HbA_{1c} at Baseline (%)	Psychosocial Measures	Weight (kg)/BMI (kg/m^2)/BMI SDS at Baseline	Hypoglycaemia Reporting
Uncontrolled Trials												
Abaci et al., 2009 [35]	Before/after	12	9	MDI	Analogue/NPH	15	4	78	9.3	Not reported	—/—/1.1	Yes
Alemzadeh et al., 2003 [36]	Before/after	12	44	MDI	Analogue/NPH or analogue	11	5	78	9.3	Not reported	—/19.3/—	Yes
Alemzadeh et al., 2005 [37]	Before/after	12	35	MDI	Analogue/analogue	5	3	73	8.8	Not reported	—/17.1/—	Yes
Hayes et al., 2012 [38]	Before/after	9	28	MDI	Human or analogue/analogue	14 (median)	4 (median)	61 (median)	7.7 (median)	DQOL-Y	—/—/0.99	Not reported

BMI: body mass index; BMI SDS: body mass index standard deviation score; DQOL-Y: Diabetes Quality of Life for Youth scale; HbA1c: glycosylated haemoglobin concentration; MDI: multiple dose injections; NPH: neutral protamine Hagedorn.

Table 2. Characteristics of controlled, randomised study with carbohydrate counting (CC) used in children and adolescents with type 1 diabetes (T1D).

Author and Year	Country	Population	No. of Patients	Intervention	Control	HbA_{1c} (%) (M ± SD) Intervention/Control	Hypoglycaemia (M ± SD)	Insulin Dose (U/kg) (M ± SD)	BMI (M ± SD)	Follow Up
Enander et al. [39]	Sweden	Children and young people	45; 26/30; 14/15	Dietary education in carbohydrate counting	Dietary education in the traditional methodology (the plate exchange method)	7.43 ± 0.83 to 7.69 ± 1.00 7.70 ± 1.00 to 8.00 ± 1.00	-	0.78 ± 0.24 to 0.80 ± 0.19 0.81 ± 0.22 to 0.83 ± 0.22	-	12 months

BMI: body mass index; HbA1c: glycosylated haemoglobin concentration.

Bell et al. only included one study of children in their systematic review [28]. The results favoured the alternative approach, i.e., a low glycaemic index over CC. However, the improvement of the glycaemic control found in adults needed to be interpreted with care, as more studies had a concurrent intensification of insulin therapy in the intervention group.

Compliance and the ability to accurately estimate the amount of carbohydrates consumed by children and adolescents with T1D is another aspect that should be considered. The greater ability of parents to count carbohydrates led to lower values of HbA_{1c} in their children and adolescents [40–44]. At the same time, there are wide variations in this ability, with studies where participants may estimate carbohydrates to within 10–15 g or within 15–20% of the actual amount, while in others, only half could accurately evaluate the carbohydrate amount or had large differences in calculations [28,40–45].

An important aspect that should not be overlooked is the effect of time on changes in HbA_{1c}. The effects of diabetes self-management training programmes were short-lived. Thus, as recommended in many countries, regular reinforcement of advanced CC is critical in patient management [41,46,47]. In the review by Schmidt et al., the study with the longest period of evaluation was also the study with the smallest improvement in HbA_{1c} [34]. The accuracy of counting carbohydrates is associated with an improvement in glycaemic control; at the same time, intense glucose monitoring is an independent variable related to the reduction in HbA_{1c} [43,48].

Considering the available data, in several studies the CC method has been compared to a control arm consisting of usual or standard care rather than alternative methods for calculating bolus insulin. In addition, observational studies generally conclude showing no improvement in glycaemic control. Furthermore, results in the paediatric and adolescent population seem better than those observed in adults, probably also for the psychological aspects associated with CC. All these considerations highlight the need of further well-designed, double-blind large studies that confirm the role of CC in patients with T1D of different age groups.

3.2. Hypoglycaemia

The calculation of carbohydrate amount for the adjustment of insulin dose is useful for better glycaemic control, and, for the practical CC, the small quantification errors are permissive. A 10 g variation in the carbohydrate quantity did not induce differences in blood glucose. Furthermore, patients may have episodes of hypo- and hyperglycaemia for an overestimation or underestimation of 20 g in a meal of 60 g carbohydrates [35,37,49]. Adolescents may be less accurate in the calculation and have a decay of glycaemic control. Hypoglycaemia is not reported or defined uniformly [40]. Uncontrolled studies showed a significant reduction in severe hypoglycaemia in children with T1D using CC [29,30]. Other data suggested that CC did not significantly decrease hypoglycaemia events [14]. In a before/after study in nine children, an insignificant increase in non-severe hypoglycaemia was observed [28]. CC might reduce the frequency of hypoglycaemia; probably, the reduction in HbA_{1c} concentration is a result of stabilised glycaemic control rather than just an overall lowering of blood glucose [15].

3.3. Growth, Weight, and Psychological Effects

Intensive and appropriate insulin therapy and, consequently, better metabolic control have enabled an improvement in the growth prognosis of paediatric patients with T1D [30,50]. Modern T1D care prevents abnormalities of the GH-IGF-I axis, which means that children with T1D can achieve a final height similar to their healthy peers [51].

Some clinicians believe that flexibility in the diet, which can be permitted by CC, may lead to the development of obesity [8,9]. The DAFNE study demonstrated that a freedom diet did not increase cardiovascular risk factors, including obesity [26]. Paediatric studies have shown that therapy MDI associated with the calculation of carbohydrates does not cause obesity in children with T1D. Some studies documented a decrease in body mass index (BMI), and some studies reported an increase; nevertheless, only minor variations in weight after the use of CC were found [30,52–54]. The increased weight documented in children and adolescents with T1D was attributed to changes in growth occurring during puberty progression [29]. In another study, Marigliano et al. evaluated the impact of CC and nutritional education on changes in dietary habits, body fat composition, and fat body distribution in diabetic children in therapy with CSII [55]. The results revealed that CC and a proper nutrition education did not have a negative effect on dietary habits, body composition, or body fat distribution. Moreover, a reduction of intake of fat and protein, with an increase in carbohydrates intake, was observed in a subgroup of subjects showing a significant improvement in metabolic control.

Females at a young age with T1D face a higher risk of eating behaviour disorders and, consequently, are more likely to have impaired metabolic control and diabetic complications [56]. Furthermore, a cross-sectional case-controlled study has shown that there was an increased frequency of food disturbances in pre-teen and early-teenage girls with T1D [57]. Rigid dietary patterns that do not conform to the habits and needs of patients might have an effect on the psychological development of children with T1D. An Australian 9-month before/after study that evaluated diabetes-related quality of life reported significant improvements in patient-rated life satisfaction after the introduction of CC. Often, the lack of flexibility in the management of meals and snacks is one of the worst aspects of living with diabetes, and adolescents especially ignore dietary advice. Thus, CC is an important tool allowing children and teenagers to manage their T1D more effectively within their own lifestyles [1,31]. This psychological effect of CC could also be useful during the honeymoon period and the transition from adolescence to adulthood.

In addition, it is extremely important to highlight that for the children and adolescents with T1D, the psychological aspects, such as the quality of life, adherence, and motivation, are key points of good glycaemic control. The reports of the Dose Adjustment for Normal Eating (DAFNE) study emphasised the positive effect of CC on the quality of life [58]. So far, many kinds of structural education programs for T1D have been reported [59,60]. Most of these programs included CC and showed the improvement of patients' adherence, as well as motivation. Therefore, CC has a positive effect on patients' adherence and motivation too. In addition, it has been observed that CC also has a positive effect on the parents and caregivers, who are the key persons for the treatment of infants and young children with T1D [59,60].

3.4. Bolus Calculator

The bolus calculator is a useful tool both for patients with T1D who require MDI and patients with an insulin pump, which allows the calculation of the prandial insulin dose based on the amount of carbohydrates, the pre-prandial blood glucose value, and active insulin [61]. Its use is associated with improved metabolic control and greater satisfaction in treating adults, children, and adolescents [62]. Few studies found the bolus calculator to be effective in children using CSII. The bolus calculator and CC may have beneficial effects in reducing HbA_{1c} by improving post-meal glucose, with a higher percentage of values within the target range [63–65]. Moreover, an insulin pump offers the possibility to tailor insulin delivery to the meal composition through the use of different bolus options: normal, dual wave, or square wave. Evidence suggests that children who apply at least one D-W/S-W bolus a day are better at achieving the recommended HbA_{1c} level [66]. In an 18-month observational study, Rabbone et al. investigated the effect of CC, with or without an automated bolus calculator, in children treated with MDI. This study showed that bolus calculator use led to greater improvements in HbA_{1c} [67].

3.5. Fat and Protein Counting

Learning about CC is important because it also increases knowledge about other macronutrients [57]. Low carbohydrate diets have been popularised by social media for those who wish to lose weight [68]. However, the promotion of a low carbohydrate diet in lay media is in contrast to published paediatric diabetes guidelines that endorse a balanced diet from a variety of foods for optimal growth and development in children with T1D [69]. De Bock et al. described a series of six cases where the adoption of a low carbohydrate diet in children impacted growth and cardiovascular risk factors with potential long-term sequelae [69]. Meals enriched in fat and protein result in a prolonged blood glucose rise by 3–4 h after food ingestion, and frequently, a relative insulin resistance is observed [70]. The American Diabetes Association recommends an appropriate glycaemic impact education regarding protein and fat. Recent studies and the use of continuous glucose monitoring have shown that post-prandial glucose excursion may occur because of fat, protein, and GI [71,72]. CGM and increasing focus on the daily lives of patients highlight the limitations of the traditional CC method, used to calculate the meal-time insulin dose. From the new insights about the effect of dietary macronutrients on post-prandial glucose control, it appears that, to improve the calculation of the insulin bolus, CC should be integrated with the counts of fats and proteins. On the other hand, it has been demonstrated that bolus calculation for high fat feeding prevents late rises in postprandial triglycerides and tumour necrosis factor alpha, thus improving cardiovascular risk profile [73]. Therefore, the development of suitable and usable algorithms is necessary, without forgetting the importance of educational therapy for a successful translation of fat/protein counting in real life [74].

4. Conclusions

Current guidelines recommend that the algorithms for prandial insulin dose be based on the carbohydrate amount taken with a meal. CC and intensive insulin therapy enable patients to have greater freedom in the management of the meals or snacks and activities of daily living, without forgetting the principles of healthy eating. A paediatric interdisciplinary T1D care team is fundamental. It has to provide education, monitoring, and support to the children and their caregivers, bearing in mind crucial aspects of children and adolescents with T1D: physical and psychological development and T1D complications.

CC may improve metabolic control and reduce HbA_{1c} concentration. Moreover, with developments in medical technology and with the new insights into the effect of dietary macronutrients on post-prandial glucose control, it appears that, to improve the calculation of the insulin bolus, the CC should be integrated with the counts of fats and proteins. Research into suitable and usable algorithms is necessary. Overall, CC may have a positive effect on metabolic control, reduce hypoglycaemia events, improve quality of life, and not influence BMI. However, more high-quality clinical trials are needed to confirm this positive impact.

Acknowledgments: This review, including the costs to publish in open access, was supported by a grant from the World Association of Infectious Diseases (WAidid).

Author Contributions: Giorgia Tascini wrote the first draft of the manuscript; Maria Giulia Berioli and Laura Cerquiglini revised the text; Elisa Santi, Giulia Mancini, Francesco Rogari and Giada Toni gave a support in the literature review; Susanna Esposito critically revised the text and made substantial scientific contributions. All the authors approved the final version of the manuscript.

References

1. Switzer, S.M.; Moser, E.G.; Rockler, B.E.; Garg, S.K. Intensive insulin therapy in patients with type 1 diabetes mellitus. *Endocrinol. Metab. Clin. N. Am.* **2012**, *41*, 89–104. [CrossRef] [PubMed]
2. Tamborlane, W.V.; Sikes, K.A. Insulin therapy in children and adolescents. *Endocrinol. Metab. Clin. N. Am.* **2012**, *41*, 145–160. [CrossRef] [PubMed]
3. Malik, F.S.; Taplin, C.E. Insulin therapy in children and adolescents with type 1 diabetes. *Pediatr. Drugs* **2014**, *16*, 141–150. [CrossRef] [PubMed]
4. Golicki, D.T.; Golicka, D.; Groele, L.; Pankowska, E. Continuous glucose monitoring system in children with type 1 diabetes mellitus: A systematic review and meta-analysis. *Diabetologia* **2008**, *51*, 233–240. [CrossRef] [PubMed]

5. Smart, C.E.; Aslander-van de Vliet, E.; Waldron, S. ISPAD Clinical Practice Consensus Guidelines 2009 Compendium: Nutritional management in children and adolescents with diabetes. *Pediatr. Diabetes* **2009**, *10*, 100–117. [CrossRef] [PubMed]
6. Smart, C.E.; Annan, F.; Bruno, L.P.C.; Higgins, L.A.; Acerini, C.L. ISPAD Clinical Practice Consensus Guidelines 2014 Compendium: Nutritional management in children and adolescents with diabetes. *Pediatr. Diabetes* **2014**, *15*, 135–153. [CrossRef] [PubMed]
7. Gillespie, S.J.; Kulkarni, K.D.; Daly, A.E. Using carbohydrate counting in diabetes clinical practice. *J. Am. Diet. Assoc.* **1998**, *98*, 897–905. [CrossRef]
8. Kawamura, T. The importance of carbohydrate counting in the treatment of children with diabetes. *Pediatr. Diabetes* **2007**, *8*, 57–62. [CrossRef] [PubMed]
9. Sheard, N.F.; Clark, N.G.; Brand-Miller, J.C.; Franz, M.J.; Pi-Sunyer, F.X.; Mayer-Davis, E.; Kulkarni, K.; Geil, P. Dietary carbohydrate (amount and type) in the prevention and management of diabetes: A statement by the American diabetes association. *Diabetes Care* **2004**, *27*, 2266–2271. [CrossRef] [PubMed]
10. THE DCCT Research Group. Nutrition interventions for intensive therapy in the Diabetes Control and Complications Trial. *J. Am. Diet. Assoc.* **1993**, *93*, 768–772.
11. Rabbone, I.; Canova, A.; Tuli, G.; Gioia, E.; Sicignano, S.; Cerutti, F. The calculation of carbohydrates in type 1 diabetes in children. *G. Ital. Diabetol. Metab.* **2011**, *31*, 150–154. (In Italian)
12. Deeb, A.; Al Hajeri, A.; Alhmoudi, I.; Nagelkerke, N. Accurate carbohydrate counting is an important determinant of postprandial glycemia in children and adolescents with type 1 diabetes on insulin pump therapy. *J. Diabetes Sci. Technol.* **2017**, *11*, 753–758. [CrossRef] [PubMed]
13. Wolever, T.M.; Hamad, S.; Chiasson, J.L.; Josse, R.G.; Leiter, L.A.; Rodger, N.W.; Ross, S.A.; Ryan, E.A. Day-to-day consistency in amount and source of carbohydrate associated with improved blood glucose control in type 1 diabetes. *J. Am. Coll. Nutr.* **1999**, *18*, 242–247. [CrossRef] [PubMed]
14. Slama, G.; Klein, J.C.; Delage, A.; Ardila, E.; Lemaignen, H.; Papoz, L.; Tchobroutsky, G. Correlation between the nature and amount of carbohy- drate in meal intake and insulin delivery by the artificial pancreas in 24 insulin-dependent diabetics. *Diabetes* **1981**, *30*, 101–105. [CrossRef] [PubMed]
15. Halfon, P.; Belkhadir, J.; Slama, G. Correlation between amount of carbohydrate in mixed meals and insulin delivery by artificial pancreas in seven IDDM subjects. *Diabetes Care* **1989**, *12*, 427–429. [CrossRef] [PubMed]
16. Walsh, J.; Roberts, R.; Bayle, T.; Varma, C.B. *Using Insulin, Everything You Need for Success with Insulin*; Torrey Pines Press: San Diego, CA, USA, 2003.
17. Walsh, J.; Roberts, R. *Pumping Insulin*, 4th ed.; Torrey Pines Press: San Diego, CA, USA, 2000.
18. Danne, T. Current practice of insulin pump therapy in children and adolescents-the Hannover recipe. *Pediatr. Diabetes* **2006**, *7*, 25–31. [CrossRef] [PubMed]
19. Hanas, R.; Adolfsson, P. Bolus calculator settings in well-controlled prepubertal children using insulin pumps are characterized by low insulin to carbohydrate ratios and short duration of insulin action time. *J. Diabetes Sci. Technol.* **2017**, *11*, 247–252. [CrossRef] [PubMed]
20. Barclay, A.W.; Petocz, P.; McMillan-Price, J.; Flood, V.M.; Prvan, T.; Mitchell, P.; Brand-Miller, J.C. Glycemic index, glycemic load, and chronic disease risk—A meta-analysis of observational studies. *Am. J. Clin. Nutr.* **2008**, *87*, 627–637. [PubMed]
21. Craig, M.E.; Twigg, S.M.; Donaghue, K.C. National Evidence-Based Clinical Care Guidelines for Type 1 Diabetes in Children, Adolescents and Adults. Available online: https://www.google.com.hk/url?sa=t&rct=j&q=&esrc=s&source=web&cd=1&ved=0ahUKEwjkvJndgOHYAhVItpQKHSCHAj0QFgglMAA&url=https%3A%2F%2Fdiabetessociety.com.au%2Fdownloads%2FType1guidelines(7Feb11).pdf&usg=AOvVaw1sAlGP3LfMJDEqvaxMzrbE (accessed on 19 December 2017).
22. Gupta, L.; Khandelwal, D.; Kalra, S. Applied carbohydrate counting. *J. Pak. Med. Assoc.* **2017**, *67*, 1456–1457. [PubMed]
23. Gilbertson, H.R.; Brand-Miller, J.C.; Thorburn, A.W.; Evans, S.; Chondros, P.; Werther, G.A. The effect of flexible low glycemic index dietary advice versus measured carbohydrate exchange diets on glycemic control in children with type 1 diabetes. *Diabetes Care* **2001**, *24*, 1137–1143. [CrossRef] [PubMed]
24. Goksen, D.; Altinok, Y.A.; Ozen, S.; Demir, G.; Darcan, S. Effects of carbohydrate counting method on metabolic control in children with type 1 diabetes mellitus. *J. Clin. Res. Pediatr. Endocrinol.* **2014**, *1*, 74–78. [CrossRef] [PubMed]

25. De Albuquerque, I.Z. Carbohydrate counting, nutritional status and metabolic profile of adolescents with type 1 diabetes mellitus. *Sci. Med.* **2014**, *24*, 21–24.
26. Enander, R.; Gundevall, C.; Strömgren, A.; Chaplin, J.; Hanas, R. Carbohydrate counting with a bolus calculator improves post-prandial blood glucose levels in children and adolescents with type 1 diabetes using insulin pumps. *Pediatr. Diabetes* **2012**, *13*, 545–551. [CrossRef] [PubMed]
27. Kalergis, M.; Pacaud, D.; Strychar, I.; Meltzer, S.; Jones, P.J.; Yale, J.F. Optimizing insulin delivery: Assessment of three strategies in intensive diabetes management. *Diabetes Obes. Metab.* **2000**, *2*, 299–305. [CrossRef] [PubMed]
28. Bell, K.J.; Barclay, A.W.; Petocz, P.; Colagiuri, S.; Brand-Miller, J.C. Efficacy of carbohydrate counting in type 1 diabetes: A systematic review and meta-analysis. *Lancet Diabetes Endocrinol.* **2014**, *2*, 133–140. [CrossRef]
29. Trento, M.; Trinetta, A.; Kucich, C.; Grassi, G.; Passera, P.; Gennari, S.; Paganin, V.; Tedesco, S.; Charrier, L.; Cavallo, F.; et al. Carbohydrate counting improves coping ability and metabolic control in patients with type 1 diabetes managed by group care. *J. Endocrinol. Investig.* **2011**, *34*, 101–105. [CrossRef] [PubMed]
30. Schmidt, S.; Meldgaard, M.; Serifovski, N.; Storm, C.; Christensen, T.M.; Gade-Rasmussen, B.; Nørgaard, K. Use of an automated bolus calculator in MDI-treated type 1 diabetes: The BolusCal Study, a randomized controlled pilot study. *Diabetes Care* **2012**, *35*, 984–990. [CrossRef] [PubMed]
31. Scavone, G.; Manto, A.; Pitocco, D.; Gagliardi, L.; Caputo, S.; Mancini, L.; Zaccardi, F.; Ghirlanda, G. Effect of carbohydrate counting and medical nutritional therapy on glycemic control in Type 1 diabetic subjects: A pilot study. *Diabet. Med.* **2010**, *27*, 477–479. [CrossRef] [PubMed]
32. DAFNE Study Group. Training in flexible, intensive insulin management to enable dietary freedom in people with type 1 diabetes: Dose adjustment for normal eating (DAFNE) randomised controlled trial. *BMJ* **2002**, *325*, 746.
33. Fu, S.; Li, L.; Deng, S.; Zan, L.; Liu, Z. Effectiveness of advanced carbohydrate counting in type 1 diabetes mellitus: A systematic review and meta-analysis. *Sci. Rep.* **2016**, *6*, 37067. [CrossRef] [PubMed]
34. Schmidt, S.; Schelde, B.; Nørgaard, K. Effects of advanced carbohydrate counting in patients with type 1 diabetes: A systematic review. *Diabet. Med.* **2014**, *31*, 886–896. [CrossRef] [PubMed]
35. Abaci, A.; Atas, A.; Unuvar, T.; Bober, E.; Buyukgebiz, A. The effect of carbohydrate counting on metabolic control in patients with type 1 diabetes mellitus. *Gulhane Med. J.* **2009**, *51*, 1–5.
36. Alemzadeh, R.; Palma-Sisto, P.; Parton, E.; Totka, J.; Kirby, M. Beneficial effects of flexible insulin therapy in children and adolescents with type 1 diabetes mellitus. *Acta Diabetol.* **2003**, *40*, 137–142. [CrossRef] [PubMed]
37. Alemzadeh, R.; Berhe, T.; Wyatt, D.T. Flexible insulin therapy with glargine insulin improved glycemic control and reduced severe hypoglycemia among preschool-aged children with type 1 diabetes mellitus. *Pediatrics* **2005**, *115*, 1320–1324. [CrossRef] [PubMed]
38. Hayes, R.L.; Garnett, S.P.; Clarke, S.L.; Harkin, N.M.; Chan, A.K.; Ambler, G.R. A flexible diet using an insulin to carbohydrate ratio for adolescents with type 1 diabetes—A pilot study. *Clin. Nutr.* **2012**, *31*, 705–709. [CrossRef] [PubMed]
39. Gupta, L.; Khandelwal, D.; Kalra, S. Carbohydrate counting-1: South Asian framework. *J. Pak. Med. Assoc.* **2017**, *67*, 1296–1298. [PubMed]
40. Bishop, F.; Maahs, D.; Spiegel, G. The carbohydrate counting in adolescents with type 1 diabetes (CCAT) study. *Diabetes Spectr.* **2009**, *22*, 56–62. [CrossRef]
41. Smart, C.E.; Ross, K.; Edge, J.A.; King, B.R.; McElduff, P.; Collins, C.E. Can children with Type 1 diabetes and their caregivers estimate the carbohydrate content of meals and snacks? *Diabet. Med.* **2010**, *27*, 348–353. [CrossRef] [PubMed]
42. Rabasa-Lhoret, R.; Garon, J.; Langelier, H.; Poisson, D.; Chiasson, J.L. Effects of meal carbohydrate content on insulin requirements in type 1 diabetic patients treated intensively with the basal-bolus (ultralente-regular) insulin regimen. *Diabetes Care* **1999**, *22*, 667–673. [CrossRef] [PubMed]
43. Mehta, S.N.; Quinn, N.; Volkening, L.K.; Laffel, L.M. Impact of carbo- hydrate counting on glycemic control in children with type 1 diabetes. *Diabetes Care* **2009**, *32*, 1014–1016. [CrossRef] [PubMed]
44. Nebel, I.T.; Bluher, M.; Starcke, U.; Muller, U.A.; Haak, T.; Paschke, R. Evaluation of a computer based interactive diabetes education program designed to train the estimation of the energy or carbohydrate contents of foods. *Patient Educ. Couns.* **2002**, *46*, 55–59. [CrossRef]

45. Ahola, A.J.; Makimattila, S.; Saraheimo, M.; Mikkilä, V.; Forsblom, C.; Freese, R.; Groop, P.H. FinnDIANE Study Group. Many patients with type 1 diabetes estimate their prandial insulin need inappropriately. *J. Diabetes* **2010**, *2*, 194–202. [CrossRef] [PubMed]
46. Funnell, M.M.; Brown, T.L.; Childs, B.P.; Haas, L.B.; Hosey, G.M.; Jensen, B.; Maryniuk, M.; Peyrot, M.; Piette, J.D.; Reader, D.; et al. National standards for diabetes self-management education. *Diabetes Care* **2012**, *35*, S101–S108. [CrossRef] [PubMed]
47. Norris, S.L.; Lau, J.; Smith, S.J.; Schmid, C.H.; Engelgau, M.M. Self-management education for adults with type 2 diabetes: A meta-analysis of the effect on glycemic control. *Diabetes Care* **2002**, *25*, 1159–1171. [CrossRef] [PubMed]
48. Plank, J.; Kohler, G.; Rakovac, I.; Semlitsch, B.M.; Horvath, K.; Bock, G.; Kraly, B.; Pieber, T.R. Long-term evaluation of a structured outpatient education programme for intensified insulin therapy in patients with type 1 diabetes: A 12-year follow-up. *Diabetologia* **2004**, *47*, 1370–1375. [CrossRef] [PubMed]
49. Smart, C.E.; Ross, K.; Edge, J.A.; Collins, C.E.; Colyvas, K.; King, B.R. Children and adolescents on intensive insulin therapy maintain postprandial glycaemic control without precise carbohydrate counting. *Diabet. Med.* **2009**, *26*, 279–285. [CrossRef] [PubMed]
50. Salardi, S.; Tonioli, S.; Tassoni, R.; Tellarini, M.; Mazzanti, I.; Caccianti, E. Growth and growth factors in diabetes mellitus. *Arch. Dis. Child.* **1987**, *62*, 57–62. [CrossRef] [PubMed]
51. Chiarelli, F.; Giannini, C.; Mohn, A. Growth, growth factors and diabetes. *Eur. J. Endocrinol.* **2004**, *151*, U109–U117. [CrossRef] [PubMed]
52. Dias, V.M.; Pandini, J.A.; Nunes, R.R.; Sperandei, S.L.; Portella, E.S.; Cobas, R.A.; Gomes, M.B. Effect of the carbohydrate counting method on glycemic control in patients with type 1 diabetes. *Diabetol. Metab. Syndr.* **2010**, *2*, 54. [CrossRef] [PubMed]
53. Pitocco, D.; Rizzi, A.; Scavone, G.; Tanese, L.; Zaccardi, F.; Manto, A.; Ghirlanda, G. Fields of application of continuous subcutaneous insulin infusion in the treatment of diabetes and implications in the use of rapid-acting insulin analogues. *Minerva Endocrinol.* **2013**, *38*, 321–328. [PubMed]
54. Laurenzi, A.; Bolla, A.M.; Panigoni, G.; Doria, V.; Uccellatore, A.; Peretti, E.; Saibene, A.; Galimberti, G.; Bosi, E.; Scavini, M. Effects of carbohydrate counting on glucose control and quality of life over 24 weeks in adult patients with type 1 diabetes on continuous subcutaneous insulin infusion: A randomized, prospective clinical trial (GIOCAR). *Diabetes Care* **2011**, *34*, 823–827. [CrossRef] [PubMed]
55. Marigliano, M.; Morandi, A.; Maschio, M.; Sabbion, A.; Contreas, G.; Tomasselli, F.; Tommasi, M.; Maffeis, C. Nutritional education and carbohydrate counting in children with type 1 diabetes treated with continuous subcutaneous insulin infusion: The effects on dietary habits, body composition and glycometabolic control. *Acta Diabetol.* **2013**, *50*, 959–964. [CrossRef] [PubMed]
56. Rydall, A.C.; Rodin, G.M.; Olmested, M.P.; Devenyi, R.G.; Daneman, D. Disordered eating behavior and microvascu-lar complications in young women with insulin-dependent diabetes mellitus. *N. Engl. J. Med.* **1997**, *336*, 1905–1906. [CrossRef] [PubMed]
57. Colton, P.; Olmested, M.; Daneman, D.; Rydall, A.; Rodin, G. Disturbed eating behavior and eating disorders in preteen and early teenage girls with type 1 diabetes: A case-controlled study. *Diabetes Care* **2004**, *27*, 1654–1659. [CrossRef] [PubMed]
58. Cooke, D.; O'Hara, M.C.; Beinart, N.; Heller, S.; La Marca, R.; Byrne, M.; Mansell, P.; Dinneen, S.F.; Clark, M.; Bond, R.; et al. NIHR DAFNE Study Group. Linguistic and psychometric validation of the Diabetes-Specific Quality-of-Life Scale in U.K. English for adults with type 1 diabetes. *Diabetes Care* **2013**, *36*, 1117–1125. [CrossRef] [PubMed]
59. Kime, N.H.; Waldron, S.; Webster, E.; Lange, K.; Zinken, K.; Danne, T.; Aschemeier, B.; Sumnik, Z.; Cinek, O.; Raposo, J.F.; et al. Pediatric diabetes training for healthcare professionals in Europe: Time for change. *Pediatr. Diabetes* **2017**. [CrossRef] [PubMed]
60. Coates, V.E.; Horigan, G.; Davies, M.; Davies, M.T. Exploring why young people with Type 1 diabetes decline structured education with a view to overcoming barriers. *Diabet. Med.* **2017**, *34*, 1092–1099. [CrossRef] [PubMed]
61. Bruttomesso, D.; Cipponeri, E. The binomial cho counting and home glycemic self-control: Is it applied? *Il Giornale di AMD* **2013**, *16*, 144–149. (In Italian)
62. Colin, I.M.; Paris, I. Glucose meters with built-in automated bolus calculator: Gadget or real value for insulin-treated diabetic patients? *Diabetes Ther.* **2013**, *4*, 1–11. [CrossRef] [PubMed]

63. Vallejo Mora, M.D.R.; Carreira, M.; Anarte, M.T.; Linares, F.; Olveira, G.; González Romero, S. Bolus calculator reduces hypoglycemia in the short term and fear of hypoglycemia in the long term in subjects with type 1 diabetes (CBMDI Study). *Diabetes Technol. Ther.* **2017**, *19*, 402–409. [CrossRef] [PubMed]
64. Pankowska, E.; Blazik, M. Bolus calculator with nutrition database software, a new concept of prandial insulin programming for pump users. *J. Diabetes Sci. Technol.* **2010**, *4*, 571–576. [CrossRef] [PubMed]
65. Shashaj, B.; Busetto, E.; Sulli, N. Benefits of a bolus calculator in pre- and postprandial glycaemic control and meal flexibility of paediatric patients using continuous subcutaneous insulin infusion (CSII). *Diabet. Med.* **2008**, *25*, 1036–1042. [CrossRef] [PubMed]
66. Pańkowska, E.; Szypowska, A.; Lipka, M.; Szpotańska, M.; Błazik, M.; Groele, L. Application of novel dual wave meal bolus and its impact on glycated hemoglobin A1c level in children with type 1 diabetes. *Pediatr. Diabetes* **2009**, *10*, 298–303. [CrossRef] [PubMed]
67. Rabbone, I.; Scaramuzza, A.E.; Ignaccolo, M.G.; Tinti, D.; Sicignano, S.; Redaelli, F.; De Angelis, L.; Bosetti, A.; Zuccotti, G.V.; Cerutti, F. Carbohydrate counting with an automated bolus calculator helps to improve glycaemic control in children with type 1 diabetes using multiple daily injection therapy: An 18-month observational study. *Diabetes Res. Clin. Pract.* **2014**, *103*, 388–394. [CrossRef] [PubMed]
68. Krebs, J.D.; Parry Strong, A.; Cresswell, P.; Reynolds, A.N.; Hanna, A.; Haeusler, S. A randomised trial of the feasibility of a low carbohydrate diet vs standard carbohydrate counting in adults with type 1 diabetes taking body weight into account. *Asia Pac. J. Clin. Nutr.* **2016**, *25*, 78–84. [PubMed]
69. De Bock, M.; Lobley, K.; Anderson, D.; Davis, E.; Donaghue, K.; Pappas, M.; Siafarikas, A.; Cho, Y.H.; Jones, T.; Smart, C. Endocrine and metabolic consequences due to restrictive carbohydrate diets in children with type 1 diabetes: An illustrative case series. *Pediatr. Diabetes* **2017**. [CrossRef] [PubMed]
70. Ahern, J.A.; Gatcomb, P.M.; Held, N.A.; Petit, W.A., Jr.; Tamborlane, W.V. Exaggerated hyperglycemia after a pizza meal in well-controlled diabetes. *Diabetes Care* **1993**, *16*, 578–580. [CrossRef] [PubMed]
71. Herman, W.H. Approaches to glycemic treatment Sec. 7: In standards of medical care in diabetes. *Diabetes Care* **2015**, *38*, S41–S48.
72. Bell, K.J.; Smart, C.E.; Steil, G.M.; Brand-Miller, J.C.; King, B.; Wolpert, H.A.; Kirstine, J. Impact of fat, protein, and glycemic index on postprandial glucose control in type 1 diabetes: Implications for intensive diabetes management in the continuous glucose monitoring era. *Diabetes Care* **2015**, *38*, 1008–1015. [CrossRef] [PubMed]
73. Campbell, M.D.; Walker, M.; Ajjan, R.A.; Birch, K.M.; Gonzalez, J.T.; West, D.J. An additional bolus of rapid-acting insulin to normalise postprandial cardiovascular risk factors following a high-carbohydrate high-fat meal in patients with type 1 diabetes: A randomised controlled trial. *Diabetes Vasc. Dis. Res.* **2017**, *14*, 336–344. [CrossRef] [PubMed]
74. Kordonouri, O.; Hartmann, R.; Remus, K.; Bläsig, S.; Sadeghian, E.; Danne, T. Benefit of supplementary fat plus protein counting as compared with conventional carbohydrate counting for insulin bolus calculation in children with pump therapy. *Pediatr. Diabetes* **2012**, *13*, 540–544. [CrossRef] [PubMed]

15

Interstitial Glucose and Physical Exercise in Type 1 Diabetes: Integrative Physiology, Technology and the Gap In-Between

Othmar Moser [1,2], Jane E. Yardley [3] and Richard M. Bracken [1,2,*]

[1] Diabetes Research Group, Medical School, Swansea University, Swansea SA2 8PP, UK; othmar.moser@swansea.ac.uk
[2] Applied Sport, Technology, Exercise and Medicine Research Centre (A-STEM), College of Engineering, Swansea University, Swansea SA1 8EN, UK
[3] Kinesiology, Sport and Recreation, Social Sciences, University of Alberta, Edmonton, AB T4V 2R3, Canada; jane.yardley@ualberta.ca
* Correspondence: r.m.bracken@swansea.ac.uk

Abstract: Continuous and flash glucose monitoring systems measure interstitial fluid glucose concentrations within a body compartment that is dramatically altered by posture and is responsive to the physiological and metabolic changes that enable exercise performance in individuals with type 1 diabetes. Body fluid redistribution within the interstitial compartment, alterations in interstitial fluid volume, changes in rate and direction of fluid flow between the vasculature, interstitium and lymphatics, as well as alterations in the rate of glucose production and uptake by exercising tissues, make for caution when interpreting device read-outs in a rapidly changing internal environment during acute exercise. We present an understanding of the physiological and metabolic changes taking place with acute exercise and detail the blood and interstitial glucose responses with different forms of exercise, namely sustained endurance, high-intensity, and strength exercises in individuals with type 1 diabetes. Further, we detail novel technical information on currently available patient devices. As more health services and insurance companies advocate their use, understanding continuous and flash glucose monitoring for its strengths and limitations may offer more confidence for patients aiming to manage glycemia around exercise.

Keywords: continuous glucose monitoring; flash glucose monitoring; exercise; interstitium

---

1. Introduction

Type 1 diabetes is characterized by the autoimmune destruction of pancreatic β-cells within the islets of Langerhans and loss of endogenous insulin production. Most diagnoses are made early in life and result in a life-long dependency on pharmacological insulin, carbohydrate counting, and frequent blood glucose measurements to manage blood glucose levels [1]. In the United Kingdom, over a quarter of a million people have type 1 diabetes and this number is rising. The cost to the National Health Service (NHS) for treatment and care is approximately £1.8+ billion a year [2]. Low levels of physical activity are evident in people with type 1 diabetes [3] and large cohort studies demonstrate an increased risk of cardiovascular disease [4,5]; however, regular physical activity is advocated [6,7] and conveys important health benefits [8]. Nevertheless, the increased risk of developing hypoglycemia and the loss of glucose control around exercise are major concerns for people with type 1 diabetes, contributing to the failure to initiate or maintain regular physical activity [9].

Frequent finger prick blood sampling and adjustments in exogenous basal and/or bolus insulin and carbohydrate intake are necessary to minimize glycemic disturbances with physical exercise [6,7].

However, mimicking the natural secretory pattern of endogenous insulin in individuals without diabetes whilst maintaining glycemia within a normal physiological range is challenging around exercise [6,10]. In the Diabetes Control and Complications Trial, intensive treatment to maintain euglycemia between 4 and 7 mmol/L with either an external insulin pump or three or more daily insulin injections and frequent blood glucose measurements delayed the onset and slowed the progression of retinopathy, nephropathy, and neuropathy compared with conventional therapy of one or two daily insulin injections over a 6.5-year period [11–14]. However, an increased occurrence of severe hypoglycemia was evident with intensive treatment compared to the conventional arm [15]. Thus, more frequent finger prick sampling is inconvenient for patients, increases cost to healthcare providers, and might still not stabilize glycemic control.

In recent years, devices that monitor glucose levels continuously offer opportunities for painless observations of glucose that may guide better glucose management in the daily life of people with type 1 diabetes [16]. Emerging work now demonstrates longitudinal improvements in glucose management with the use of continuous glucose monitoring systems in the daily life of people with type 1 diabetes [17]. Flash glucose monitoring systems, similar to continuous glucose monitoring systems, are now available on prescription in the UK NHS for patients with type 1 diabetes. Current devices monitor dynamic interstitial glucose information for up to two weeks without the need for confirmatory finger prick blood glucose measures. However, whilst mean absolute relative differences demonstrate strong similarity to reference blood values [18], these data are generally reported during rest and not during dynamic exercise.

Performing an acute bout of exercise evokes rapid changes in many physiological systems and demands constant adjustment to facilitate glucose provision to the exercising tissues in both healthy individuals and people with type 1 diabetes [10,19]. The net exercise-induced glucose response in the circulation results from changes in carbohydrate ingestion, hepatic release and uptake, skeletal muscle and adipose tissue uptake (amongst other organs), or hepatic gluconeogenesis, and is dependent on the exercise characteristics: type, mode, intensity, and duration [20–23]. Importantly, (and often overlooked) acute exercise also causes significant redistribution in body fluid between the interstitium, lymphatics, and bloodstream [24]. Changes in posture, sweating, muscle contraction, and hydration dramatically impact interstitial fluid volume and result in altered concentrations of glucose due to fluid redistribution within this compartment.

This review does not seek to revise the historical development of interstitial glucose monitoring technology or its inclusion around physical activity *per se* but rather seeks to focus on our current understanding of acute physiological changes around exercise involving the interstitium and device performance around acute physical exercise in individuals with type 1 diabetes. A firm understanding of the complex physiological adaptations to acute exercise may inform the reader of the strengths and limitations in tracking glucose using continuous and flash monitoring systems in a dynamic metabolic environment such as exercise and offer more confidence for people with type 1 diabetes to better manage glycemia around exercise.

2. Physiological Adjustments to Increased Blood Flow and Glucose Provision during Physical Exercise

2.1. Initiation of Physical Exercise

Complex physiological adaptations dictate the ability of skeletal muscle to generate and maintain power in healthy individuals and people with type 1 diabetes [25,26]. The cardiorespiratory system plays a critical role in facilitating increased provision of glucose and oxygen (alongside the removal of carbon dioxide and other metabolic by-products) to exercising muscle. Yet, physical exercise begins with mental activity! In the brain, increased nerve impulses from the cerebral cortex act on the medulla oblongata and suppress vagal tone to stimulate an increase in cardiac output (i.e., heart rate × stroke volume) from ~5 L/min at rest to over 25 L/min in individuals with type 1 diabetes [27]. Central brain areas also raise the baroreflex level to allow blood pressure regulation at a higher set-point, which facilitates higher sympathoadrenal activity and allows further increases in cardiac output. Skeletal muscle arterioles dilate via the actions of increased circulating catecholamines and sympathetic nerve activity on vascular β-adrenoceptors [20]. In non-active splanchnic and renal beds, a greater vascular constriction occurs to allow more blood to flow to exercising areas [27].

2.2. Continuation of Physical Exercise

As exercise continues, cardiovascular and respiratory systems continuously adjust to the exercise workload to ensure glucose- and oxygen (O_2)-rich blood reaches working muscles at the required rate. Elevated cerebral motor center activity and skeletal muscle afferent fiber mechanical (tension) and metabolic (e.g., H^+, K^+, and local ischemia) signals stimulate sympathetic nervous system activity and causes increases in circulating catecholamines that act on adrenoceptors on vessels and skeletal muscle cells and consequently vasodilation in healthy individuals [28]. Local to the exercising muscle and heart, metabolites cause vasodilation of skeletal muscle and coronary arterioles. This exercise-induced hyperemia or 'exercise pressor reflex' decreases vascular resistance and increases blood flow concomitant with increased capillary recruitment [29]. In high-intensity activities such as sprinting or strength exercises that involve a Valsalva-type maneuver, vascular compression and decreased blood flow induce the buildup of metabolites that activate chemoreceptors, resulting in a greater exercise pressor reflex than dynamic activities, and cause increased cardiac output, total peripheral resistance, and tachycardia that alters blood flow rate in healthy individuals [29]. Increased sympathoadrenal activity constricts arterioles in the non-exercising areas. Also, exercise-induced sympathoadrenal activity increases suppression of vagal activity proportional to the exercise intensity and vasoconstriction of the smooth muscle arterioles. Cutaneous blood flow is initially reduced via vasoconstriction but then increases as vasodilatation occurs due to a rise in body temperature to promote cooling [20]. However, with long duration high-intensity exercise, cutaneous perfusion may again fall as vasoconstriction re-diverts blood flow to muscle. Brain blood flow tends to remain largely constant. During inspiration, pressure in the thoracic cavity falls. With diaphragm contraction during inspiration, there is an increased abdominal pressure that compresses veins and venous blood flow in the abdomen and drives blood back to the heart [30]. The thoracoabdominal pump is also appreciable during heavy exercise as tidal volume and breath frequency increase ventilation rates to over 150 L/min, which was observed in healthy and diseased individuals.

2.3. Blood Flow Distribution to Skeletal Muscle during Exercise

At rest, around two-thirds of the blood volume is present in veins and most capillaries are closed; blood flow rates to skeletal muscle is approximately 20–30 $mL \cdot min^{-1} \cdot kg\ muscle^{-1}$ at an open capillary density of ~100 capillaries per mm^2 in healthy individuals [31]. During exercise, open capillaries increase five-fold due to vasodilation from sympathoadrenal activity and locally from factors emanating from skeletal muscle metabolism (decrease in pO_2, rise in pCO_2, decreased pH, temperature, adenosine, NO, P_i, K^+). Thus, increased cardiac output and localized vasodilation together account for up to a 100-fold increase in blood flow to working tissues (2–3 $L \cdot min^{-1} \cdot kg\ muscle^{-1}$ during heavy exercise). Further, to facilitate this increased rate of blood flow, a rapid shunting of venous blood to the arterial circuit occurs by vasoconstriction of major veins.

Notwithstanding rapid blood redistribution within the circulation, plasma volume may fall ~20% (1 L) with intense exercise over 15 min due to fluid movement towards active muscle [28]. Alterations in the osmolarity of skeletal myocyte cytoplasm and interstitial fluid due to local release of metabolic factors from skeletal muscle increase solutes in the interstitial fluid [28]. Also, an increased perfusion of capillary beds in active muscle increases capillary hydrostatic pressure, which drives more fluid from the plasma to the interstitium [20]. The extent of plasma volume reduction can be magnified by the ambient temperature and humidity and offset by oral consumption of fluids. The overall effect of a net loss in plasma volume is an apparent increase in red blood cell count and hemoglobin concentration, which increases the O_2-carrying capacity per liter of blood, but at the expense of a reduction in total blood volume and an increase in viscosity. The movement of fluid from the plasma to the interstitium is offset to a certain extent by fluid movement back into the circulation from tissues that undergo vasoconstriction (gut, kidneys) [32].

3. The Interstitial Compartment and Factors Influencing Movement of Interstitial Fluid during Exercise

The interstitial space lies between the circulatory system and organs such as skeletal muscle, myocardium, and liver and contains approximately three-quarters of the body's total extracellular fluid (e.g., ~10–12 L in a 70-kg person) [33]. Plasma and lymph fluid represent most of the remaining quarter (~3 L) of extracellular fluid. Interstitial fluid represents a quarter of total body water mixing with plasma, lymph fluid, and sweat [33].

The factors that determine the speed and magnitude of movement of fluid between capillaries and interstitium are determined by Starling forces [34]. The net filtration pressure (NFP) is determined by two pressure differentials that determine the net drive for directional fluid movement between the capillary and interstitial space, namely:

(i) Colloid osmotic pressure between capillary (P_c) and interstitial space (P_{if})

Capillary colloidal pressure is exerted by proteins such as albumin, which causes fluid to be pulled back into the capillary at the venous end due to a higher solute concentration [35]. The remaining fluid left in the interstitial space is drained by the lymphatic capillaries and returned to the circulation. The interstitial colloidal pressure is regulated by the interstitial fluid concentration and the permeability of the capillary to different proteins. As plasma contains more protein than the interstitial fluid, capillary colloidal pressure tends to dominate all the way along the capillary wall [35].

(ii) Hydrostatic pressures from capillary (π_c) to interstitial space (π_{if})

Colloidal hydrostatic pressure is exerted by the plasma fluid against the capillary wall, moving the fluid into the interstitium through filtration and is greater at the arterial end of a capillary due to the higher blood pressure [36]. The interstitial hydrostatic pressure is determined by the interstitial fluid volume and the surrounding tissues' compliance with changes in volume and pressure; skin and skeletal muscle have higher compliance to changes in volume and pressure with more soft tissue surrounding them than the brain [37].

Thus, net filtration pressure (NFP) = $P_c + \pi_{if} - P_{if} - \pi_c$ and the transendothelial fluid filtration rate (cm^3/s) is represented by Equation (1):

$$J_v = L_p S\,[(P_c - P_{if}) - \sigma(\pi_c - \pi_{if})] \quad (1)$$

where

- L_p is the hydraulic conductivity (which provides a measure of water permeability; $m^2{\cdot}s{\cdot}kg^{-1}$ or $m{\cdot}s^{-1}{\cdot}mmHg^{-1}$);
- S is the surface area available for fluid exchange in m^2;
- σ is the osmotic reflection coefficient (dimensionless unit) where σ close to 1.0 indicates the capillary is fully effective in allowing fluid and smaller solutes to filter to the interstitial space while larger protein molecules such as albumin are retained. Where σ is <1.0, capillary filter function is reduced.

Acute physical exercise does not alter the characteristics of the microvascular exchange vessels [38–40]. Thus, S (the surface area available for fluid exchange) contributes most to the enhanced filtration rates with acute exercise but alterations in hydraulic conductivity (L_p) and/or the osmotic reflection coefficient (σ) do not.

Although most pressure fluctuations are absorbed at the level of precapillary resistance vessels, even modest increases in capillary filtration drive lead to fluid accumulation in the interstitial compartment and can increase from 0.008–0.015 mL/min/mmHg for resting skeletal muscle to greater than 4-fold during exercise in healthy individuals [24]. Thus, the rate of fluid filtration from the blood to the tissue interstitial space can reach 1.5 mL·min^{-1}·100 g muscle^{-1} during intense rhythmic contraction [39–42]. This rapid rate of fluid movement with exercise initially exceeds the drainage capacity of the lymphatic system and, converse to the loss of plasma fluid, is a gain in interstitial fluid volume of ~15–20% in exercising tissue [43]. This is due to several factors: (i) exercise-induced capillary hydrostatic pressure increasing with arteriolar vasodilation [43]; (ii) relaxation of vascular smooth muscle in arterioles increasing capillary surface area by recruiting capillaries that were previously closed [41]; and (iii) a muscular contraction-induced increase in interstitial fluid osmolarity due to released metabolites (e.g., K^+, lactate, H^+, adenosine, ammonia) from active skeletal muscle cells that transiently raises interstitial fluid osmolarity by ~20–30 mmol/L or 7–10% [41]. Also, an expanded interstitial fluid volume increases the diffusion distance for glucose molecules and may hinder cellular metabolism in swollen tissues. Interstitial (or cellular) edema can also impair glucose tissue perfusion by collapsing capillaries in swollen tissue [44].

The initial rate of hypervolemia in the interstitium slows as exercise continues due to (i) a compensatory absorption of interstitial fluid by vasoconstricted vascular beds where capillary pressure is lower in non-exercising tissues; and (ii) the subsequent reduction in flow rate allows better lymphatic drainage [43] with one-way flow [44] and flow-induced lymphatic dilation. Muscle contraction increases interstitial fluid pressure and reduces the transcapillary hydrostatic gradient, further reducing fluid accumulation with sustained exercise [45].

4. Interstitial Glucose Metabolism during Exercise

The small amount of glucose in the interstitium of an adult individual with type 1 diabetes (e.g., 10 mmol/L = 1.8 g/L = 18 g with an interstitial fluid volume of 10 L) represents the point measurement of glucose changes at that measured site. Patients in a fasted, resting state produce small rate changes in the disappearance and/or appearance of glucose. However, acute exercise dramatically increases carbohydrate combustion and the metabolic turnover [46] of glucose increases 40 to 50-fold in exercising tissues (Table 1) [33,47]. The magnitude of change in interstitial glucose with acute physical exercise in people with type 1 diabetes is dependent on the type, mode, intensity, and duration of exercise, as well as the time of day, circulating insulin levels, and whether the individual is fasted or fed.

Table 1. Glucose transport from blood to skeletal muscle (per 110/g) [33,47].

	Rest	Heavy Exercise	Fractional Δ (Exercise/Rest)
Skeletal muscle glucose consumption (J_s), μmol/min	1.4	60	×43
Arterial glucose concentration (C_a), mM	5.0	5.0	-
Venous concentration (C_v), mM	4.4	4.0	×0.9
Extraction E, %	11.2	20	×1.8
Blood flow, mL/min	2.5	60	×24
Perfused capillary density, per mm^2	250	1000	×4
Diffusion capacity (PS), cm^3/min	5	20	×4
Mean concentration difference across capillary wall ($\Delta C = J_s/PS$), mM	0.3	3.0	×10
Mean pericapillary concentration (Ci), mM	4.7	2.0	×0.4
Krogh Cylinder radius, μm	36	18	×0.5

4.1. Glucose Transport to Exercising Muscle

Capillary recruitment shortens the diffusion distance and increases the surface area, with the diffusional capacity increased further by an effect of blood flow on permeability. A fall in tissue glucose concentrations raises the gradient across the capillary wall and the increase in diffusional flux raises the fractional extraction and arteriovenous concentration difference (C_a-C_v) [48]. An increased blood flow delivers glucose faster to the capillary and prevents a major fall in the mean intra-capillary plasma concentration, thereby avoiding a flow-limitation of exchange. The new trans-capillary glucose flux is, thus, determined from the Fick principle equaling blood flow × increased arteriovenous concentration difference (Table 1) [48].

4.2. Exercising Skeletal Muscle Tissue Is a Glucose Consumer; Inactive Tissue Acts as a Glucose Store

Glucose entry into muscle occurs across the cell membrane via the glucose transporter type-4 (GLUT-4) [49]. Once inside the muscle, glucose is irreversibly converted to glucose 6-phosphate via the enzyme hexokinase to prevent loss of this valuable nutrient from muscle and is either utilized via glycolysis or stored as glycogen until needed [49]. Skeletal muscle glycogen stores are about 300–350 g and can be manipulated with low carbohydrate diets to reduce estimated whole-body stores from 300 to 50 mmol·glucosyl units per kg^{-1} wet weight in healthy individuals [50]. Conversely, short-term high carbohydrate diets markedly increase muscle glycogen stores to more than 500 mmol·glucosyl units per kg^{-1} wet weight. Carbohydrate combustion in the absence of oxygen is important for releasing energy during high-intensity exercises such as sprinting or strength exercises. For example, a 6 second cycle sprint reduces quadriceps muscle glycogen concentration by 14% from 316 ± 75 to 273 ± 80 mmol·glucosyl units per kg^{-1} wet weight [51] and by 32% after a 30 second sprint [21]. Consequently, blood lactate and H+ concentrations increase from ~1.0 to over 20 mmol/L and 7.4 to <7 pH units and alters osmolarity in the interstitial space [21,51]. The net glucose uptake into tissues during exercise depends on the exercise characteristics; moderate intensity exercise causes similar whole-body rates of glucose appearance and disappearance. In contrast, high-intensity exercise causes a disproportionate rate of increase in glucose appearance compared to disappearance [52].

4.3. Hepatocytes Take Up and Release Glucose

The liver glycogen content is approximately 80–110 g for a 70-kg person and similar to muscle is easily manipulated with low carbohydrate diets, reducing hepatic stores from 232 to 24–55 mmol·glucosyl units per kg^{-1} wet weight within 24 h in healthy people [53]. Conversely, high carbohydrate diets markedly increase hepatic glycogen stores to supernormal values of 424–624 mmol·glucosyl units per kg^{-1} wet weight [53], especially if preceded by glycogen-depleting exercise, a concept known as glycogen supercompensation [50]. In contrast to skeletal myocytes, hepatocytes contain a phosphatase enzyme that catalyzes stored glucose, allowing the glucose to leave the liver cell and enter the interstitial space prior to appearing in the circulation. A strong counter-regulatory hormone response elicited by high-intensity exercise acts on hepatocytes to promote hepatic glucose release and consequent exercise-induced hyperglycemia in people with type 1 diabetes [54]. Carbohydrate combustion in the presence of oxygen can increase from resting values of ~0.25 g/min to over 3.0 g/min and the liver plays an important role in the later stages of endurance exercise to support exercise metabolism beyond that of lipid [20]. On the other hand, one day of starvation and/or prolonged exercise might almost deplete endogenous carbohydrate stores, excepting for the body's ability to minimize this loss through the manufacture of new glucose from amino acids, ketoacids, or lactate in the liver; the contribution of gluconeogenesis to exercise is important [20,22].

4.4. Exogenous 'On-Board' Insulin Concentrations Differ When Compared with Endogenous Insulin

In people that do not have diabetes, plasma insulin falls with exercise duration and/or intensity due to exercise-induced catecholamine inhibition on pancreatic ß-cell function [55]. However, no such reductions on exogenous insulin are seen in individuals with type 1 diabetes. Indeed, there is evidence of increased circulating insulin with exercise [56]. Insulin stimulates vasodilation around subcutaneous depots where injected insulin may be flushed into the extracellular space and increase glucose uptake and hepatic glucose inhibition [57].

4.5. *Ingested Carbohydrate from the Gastrointestinal Tract*

Ingested carbohydrates (e.g., a mixture of glucose and fructose) can be assimilated from the small intestine at an upper limit of ~1.8 g/min [58]. Interestingly, glucose alone can be absorbed and utilized at rates of ~1.0–1.1 g/min, due to rate limits in the capacities of the glucose transporter type-2 (GLUT-2), glucose transporter type-5 (GLUT-5), and/or sodium–glucose linked transporter-1 (SGLT-1) carriers in the intestinal membrane [59]. In people with type 1 diabetes, carbohydrate ingestion in readiness for exercise increases blood glucose with the overall magnitude dependent on factors such as amount, digestibility, and glycemic index [6]. This new glucose appearance into body fluid compartments alters body fluid osmolarity.

5. Interstitial Glucose Responses to Different Forms of Exercise

Continuous glucose monitoring systems use an enzymatic technique that reacts with circulating glucose in the interstitium [60]. This reaction releases one electron for each glucose molecule and transmits it to an electrode. Within this electrode, an electric current is generated that is passed from a transmitter (attached or incorporated) to a reader (e.g., mobile phone) to reflect the interstitial glucose levels [60].

Data on head-to-head comparisons between continuous and flash glucose monitoring systems remain rare. Aberer et al. [61] have shown that the Abbott FreeStyle Libre (Abbott, Alameda, CA, USA) flash glucose monitoring system was the most accurate (median absolute relative differences (MARD) 8.7 ± 5.9%, n = 13), followed by Dexcom G4 Platinum (Dexcom, San Diego, CA, USA) (MARD 15.7 ± 14.6%, n = 24), and Medtronic MiniMed 640 G (Medtronic MiniMed, Inc., Northridge, CA, USA) (MARD 19.4 ± 13.5%, n = 22) during 30 min (2 × 15 with a 5 min rest) of low-intensity continuous exercise. However, it must be mentioned that only thirteen comparison points between blood glucose and interstitial glucose concentrations were available for the flash glucose monitoring system. Unfortunately, in this trial, glucose concentrations were not classified for hypo-, eu-, and hyperglycemia during exercise. Disagreements in absolute glucose values during exercise between different compartments were found in healthy individuals [62] and in patients with type 1 diabetes [63–65]. Interstitial glucose concentrations measured via the SEVEN® PLUS CGM (Dexcom, San Diego, CA, USA) system during exercise under euglycemic conditions are higher compared to capillary (finger sticks) and venous blood, and the capillary blood levels seem to be higher than the venous blood levels [62]. In patients with type 1 diabetes performing high-intensity interval exercise and continuous exercise, no clear trend was found in comparing the capillary blood glucose concentration (earlobe) and interstitial glucose concentration when using the Guardian REAL-time system and the Enlite sensor (Medtronic MiniMed, Inc., Northridge, CA, USA) (no classification for glycemic ranges was performed) [63]. However, in a different study comparing the interstitial glucose (G4 Platinum, Dexcom, San Diego, CA, USA) and venous blood glucose concentration, a trend towards lower levels were found in venous blood when exercising within a euglycemic range (blood glucose during high-intensity interval exercise: 7.56 ± 0.21; blood glucose during continuous exercise: 6.71 ± 0.23) [64]. Interestingly, significantly lower glucose concentrations were found in the interstitium compared to the venous system for continuous exercise and for resistance exercise under a euglycemic range when using the CGMS® System Gold® (Medtronic MiniMed, Inc., Northridge, CA, USA) [65].

The duration of exercise seems not to influence the differences in glucose levels in different compartments [63–65]. However, it might be that longer-duration exercise and the potential for dehydration could decrease the glucose supply within the interstitium, resulting in lower glucose levels compared to the capillary and venous systems. Furthermore, the lag time in interstitium could be influenced by the intensity of exercise and the amount of circulating insulin. Low insulin reductions combined with high exercise intensities could increase the lag time between the blood and the interstitium, resulting in severe impairments for continuous and flash glucose monitoring systems. The type and mode of exercise seem not to influence continuous glucose monitoring accuracy [63–65]. During high-intensity interval exercise and continuous exercise, continuous glucose monitoring technology shows sufficient potential to trace changes in glucose concentrations [63,64]. During resistance exercise, a mean difference of −0.71 mmol/L was found [65]. However, it should be considered that during resistance exercise the site of sensor placement might directly influence its performance. Therefore, it is prudent to place the sensor away from working muscles.

Only a single study assessed continuous glucose monitoring accuracy during exercise under hypoglycemic conditions [66]. When a hypoglycemic alarm was set at 5.5 mmol/L, the system overestimated the interstitial glucose by 1.6 mmol/L. Therefore, a higher alarm level setting is recommended to avoid exercise-induced hypoglycemia.

Future research should clearly evaluate sensor performance under hypo-, eu-, and hyperglycemic ranges during exercise. Additionally, reported sensor performance during exercise needs to be adjusted for any treatments (e.g., carbohydrate ingestion, bolus insulin correction).

6. Continuous and Flash Glucose Monitor Performance

Twenty years of intensive research reveal marked improvements in continuous glucose monitoring performance in the reflection of accuracy, precision, and reliability. Since the start of the millennium, MARDs have been halved from 20% to 10% [67,68]. The Dexcom G5™ Mobile continuous glucose monitoring system, which is approved for patients aged two years and older, shows a MARD of 9% for adults and 10% for pediatric patients [68]. Sensor lifetime is 7 days accompanied with 2 calibrations to capillary blood glucose concentration per day. Its predecessor model, the Dexcom G4® system (Dexcom, San Diego, CA, USA), was found to be less accurate with MARDs of 13% for adults and 15% for pediatric patients [69–72]. Sensor lifetime is also 7 days, accompanied with 2 calibrations to capillary blood glucose concentration per day.

Medtronic's (Medtronic MiniMed, Inc., Northridge, CA, USA) flagships are the MiniMed 670 G hybrid closed-loop system and 640 G with SmartGuard® (predictive low glucose), as well as the Medtronic Paradigm Minimed Veo® (530 G) with low glucose suspend. Recently, the MARD for the Medtronic 640 G system was found at 9.6%, using the Guardian™ sensor 3 [73]. Predecessor models using Enlite™ sensor technologies resulted in MARDs of 13.6–14.2% for adults and of about 21% for children from 4–14 years for blood glucose levels below 6.7 mmol/L [72,74]. Sensors need to be changed after 6 days, requiring 2 calibrations per day.

A slightly different technology, Abbotts FreeStyle® Libre FGM system (Abbott, Alameda, CA, USA), was also found to track changes in interstitial glucose accurately with a MARD of 10–11.4% [18,72]. This device shows a sensor lifetime of 14 days and is factory-calibrated. The FreeStyle® Navigator II CGM system has a MARD of 12.3% with a sensor lifetime of up to 5 days and needs to be calibrated 3–4 times per day [72].

Notable, a novel analytical framework that enables spectroscopy-based longitudinal tracking of blood glucose without extensive a priori information was investigated by Spegazzini et al. [75]. Using blood glucose monitoring by Raman spectroscopy as an example, it was found that the efficacy of this approach was comparable to conventional calibration methods (35% reduction in error over partial least squares regression when applied to glucose tolerance tests).

7. Continuous and Flash Glucose Monitoring Systems' (Dis) Advantages and Exercise

These commonly used devices reveal different advantages and disadvantages for daily life; furthermore, accuracy during exercise might be divergent to general MARDs (Table 2).

Table 2. Advantages, disadvantages, and exercise performance in continuous and flash glucose monitoring systems.

	Advantage	Disadvantage	Exercise Performance
Dexcom G5™	Hypo- and hyperglycemia alerts; rise and fall (rate of change) alerts; compatible with mobile devices; online live monitoring with different mobile devices (e.g., for parents), CE [1] mark (European Union). Approved for non-adjuvant use; compatible with Apple iPhone 4S and subsequent iOS models	Requires calibration to blood glucose; no integrated bolus wizard	N/A for Dexcom G5™
Dexcom G4™	Hypo- and hyperglycemia alerts; rise and fall (rate of change) alerts; available integrated with the Animas Vibe pump	Requires calibration to blood glucose; no integrated bolus wizard	Continuous exercise: MARD [2] 13.6–18.6%; interval exercise: MARD 13.3–17.7% [61,64,76] (interstitial glucose compared to venous plasma glucose)
Medtronic 670 G with SmartGuard®	Hybrid closed-loop system when combined with insulin pump (automatic insulin delivery when glucose is high); predictive low glucose-suspend when combined with insulin pump; predictive low glucose alert; hypo- and hyperglycemia alerts; rise and fall (rate of change) alerts; Bluetooth connected to glucometer (CONTOUR, NEXT LINK 2.4); bolus wizard	Requires calibration to blood glucose	N/A [3] for this specific system
Medtronic 640 G with SmartGuard®	Predictive low glucose-suspend when combined with insulin pump; predictive low glucose alert; hypo- and hyperglycemia alerts; rise and fall (rate of change) alerts; Bluetooth connected to glucometer (CONTOUR, NEXT LINK 2.4); bolus wizard	Requires calibration to blood glucose	Continuous exercise: MARD 19.4% [61] (interstitial glucose compared to venous plasma glucose)
Medtronic Paradigm Minimed® Veo (530 G)	Low-glucose-suspend when combined with insulin pump; hypo- and hyperglycemia alerts; rise and fall (rate of change) alerts; Bluetooth connected to glucometer (CONTOUR, NEXT LINK 2.4); bolus wizard;	Requires calibration to blood glucose	Continuous exercise: MARD 12.8–23.7%; interval exercise: MARD 15.5–26.5% [63] (interstitial glucose compared to capillary blood glucose)
FreeStyle® Libre Flash glucose monitoring	Factory-calibrated; long sensor lifetime (14 days); integrated glucometer; integrated blood ketone measurement; cheap sensor costs; integrated bolus wizard	No automatic hypo- or hyperglycemia alerts; not combinable with pump	Continuous exercise: MARD 8.7% [61] (interstitial glucose compared to venous plasma glucose)
FreeStyle® Navigator II CGM system	30 m transmission range; new result every minute; hypo- and hyperglycemia alerts; early warning alarms; integrated glucometer	Fixed time points for calibration: 1, 2, 10, 24, and 72 h after sensor insertion	N/A for the second generation

[1] CE (Conformité Européenne) marking is a certification mark that indicates conformity with health, safety, and environmental protection standards for products sold within the European Economic Area. [2] MARD: Median Absolute Relative Difference. [3] N/A: Not Applicable.

8. Continuous and Flash Glucose Monitor Algorithms

As continuous and flash glucose monitoring systems measure glucose within the interstitial fluid, a certain lag time is present for the glucose to diffuse from the blood into the interstitium. To overcome this lag time and to reduce the risk of inadequate therapy decisions (e.g., overdose in bolus insulin correction), several algorithms are incorporated in continuous and flash glucose monitoring systems. Generally, so-called algorithmically "smart sensors" incorporate three software modules that need to work in real time [77,78]:

- denoising the random noise component
- enhancing the accuracy
- predicting the future glucose concentration

As used by Facchinetti et al. [77], an adaptive self-tunable Bayesian smoother is able to automatically estimate the signal-to-noise ratio present in the continuous glucose monitoringdata [79]. For the enhancement of accuracy, a stochastic deconvolution-based re-calibration algorithm is applied, which re-scales the interstitial glucose data using a simple linear regressor whose parameters are re-calculated for each self-measured blood glucose value [78,80]. Especially this or a similar denoising and enhancement algorithm is inwrought in the Dexcom (Dexcom, San Diego, CA, USA) G4 and G5 sensor technology (505 algorithm).

Predicting future glucose concentrations is based on an autoregressive model of order, one based on the findings of Sparacino et al. [81]. For example, the Medtronic 640 G with SmartGuard® (Medtronic MiniMed, Inc., Northridge, CA, USA) uses an algorithm that predicts the decrease of 20 mg/dL within the next 30 min above the pre-defined "low-threshold". When combined with an insulin pump, it suspends the infusion of insulin before reaching this value and automatically restarts when it predicts that glucose levels will increase by 20 mg$\cdot$dL^{-1} above the pre-defined low glucose threshold [78].

9. Future Directions

9.1. *Artificial Pancreas*

In line with a recent review, a threshold low-glucose suspend of insulin infusion might be the first step towards an artificial pancreas [72]. The future of artificial pancreas devices promises a more accurate mimicking of endogenous responses to glucose fluctuations; achieved via dual hormone closed-loop systems using insulin and glucagon [82,83]. This system is able to reduce significantly hypoglycemic episodes. Intriguingly, the beneficial effects of dual- compared to single hormone closed-loop systems were observed during continuous and interval exercises [84]. In this study, glucagon was given a microboluses to avoid drastic increases in blood glucose concentrations. Glucagon delivery was based on logical rules considering glucose concentration estimates and their trends. Importantly, the insulin delivery algorithm took account of the injected glucagon onboard via the dual-hormone artificial pancreas. During continuous exercise, a total glucagon dose of 0.126 ± 0.057 mg was administered and during interval exercise 0.093 ± 0.068 mg. The split total glucagon dose was delivered every 10 min during the 60 min exercise sessions. Mini-doses of glucagon were found to be efficacious and safe to treat mild hypoglycemia in adults with type 1 diabetes [85]. Successful hypoglycemia-treatment criteria were met for 94% when using a mini-dose of glucagon in comparison to 95% when giving oral glucose tablets.

Instead of glucagon selective antagonism of somatostatin receptor type 2 (SSTR2) might also be reasonable (within the artificial pancreas) [86]. SSTR2 antagonism after recurrent hypoglycemia ameliorates the glucagon and corticosterone responses, as well as decreases the risk of insulin-induced hypoglycemia in rats with type 1 diabetes. However, a safety profile of SSTR2 antagonism will need to be established. Potential adverse effects might be increased gastric acid secretion and effects on pituitary and adrenal hormone secretion [87].

In real life, the only commercially available system (FDA approved), which is similar to an artificial pancreas, is the hybrid closed-loop system from Medtronic (670 G with SmartGuard®) (Medtronic MiniMed, Inc., Northridge, CA, USA). However, from the authors' point of view, the fundamental problem in the development of a "real" artificial pancreas might be the sensor inaccuracy and sensor/interstitial glucose lag time to blood glucose concentration. For example, the Abbott FreeStyle Libre (Abbott, Alameda, CA, USA) flash glucose monitoring system shows an average lag time of 4.5–4.8 min (for both clinic and home-phases) [18]. In a rapidly changing internal environment during acute exercise combined with low doses of circulating bolus insulin this lag time could potentially rise by 200%, as observed in our lab in two ongoing clinical trials (U1111-1174-6676; DRKS00013477). Furthermore, if the artificial pancreas is designated to work autonomously, the use of detectors of physical activity (e.g., heart rate monitor, accelerometer, small spirometry devices) needs to be incorporated from the very early stages of development.

9.2. Implantable Sensors

In a recent pivotal study, the MARD of the Eversense implantable continuous glucose monitoring sensor (Senseonics Inc., Germantown, MD, USA) was found at 11.1% against reference glucose values above 4.2 mmol/L [88]. Implantable continuous glucose monitoring systems may provide advantages since frequent sensor insertions are not needed and the transmitter can be removed without sensor replacement. However, the implantation and removal are a minor surgical procedure and accompanied by some discomfort.

10. Conclusions

As more health services and insurance companies advocate their use, understanding continuous and flash glucose monitoring systems for its strengths and limitations around exercise may offer more confidence for patients aiming to better manage glycemia. This review detailed the complexities of acute physical exercise and offers an integrated understanding of the efficacy of glucose monitoring with current technology around a heightened metabolic state such as exercise.

Author Contributions: O.M., J.E.Y. and R.M.B. wrote the paper.

References

1. Chiang, J.L.; Kirkman, M.S.; Laffel, L.M.B.; Peters, A.L. Type 1 diabetes through the life span: A position statement of the American Diabetes Association. *Diabetes Care* **2014**, *37*, 2034–2054. [CrossRef] [PubMed]
2. The Health and Social Care Information Centre National Diabetes Audit 2012–2013, Report 2. Available online: http://content.digital.nhs.uk/catalogue/PUB16496/nati-diab-audi-12-13-rep2.pdf (accessed on 27 November 2017).
3. Plotnikoff, R.C.; Taylor, L.M.; Wilson, P.M.; Courneya, K.S.; Sigal, R.J.; Birkett, N.; Raine, K.; Svenson, L.W. Factors associated with physical activity in Canadian adults with diabetes. *Med. Sci. Sports Exerc.* **2006**, *38*, 1526–1534. [CrossRef] [PubMed]
4. Laing, S.P.; Swerdlow, A.J.; Slater, S.D.; Burden, A.C.; Morris, A.; Waugh, N.R.; Gatling, W.; Bingley, P.J.; Patterson, C.C. Mortality from heart disease in a cohort of 23,000 patients with insulin-treated diabetes. *Diabetologia* **2003**, *46*, 760–765. [CrossRef] [PubMed]
5. Dorman, J.S.; Laporte, R.E.; Kuller, L.H.; Cruickshanks, K.J.; Orchard, T.J.; Wagener, D.K.; Becker, D.J.; Cavender, D.E.; Drash, A.L. The Pittsburgh insulin-dependent diabetes mellitus (IDDM) morbidity and mortality study: Mortality results. *Diabetes* **1984**, *33*, 271–276. [CrossRef] [PubMed]
6. Riddell, M.C.; Gallen, I.W.; Smart, C.E.; Taplin, C.E.; Adolfsson, P.; Lumb, A.N.; Kowalski, A.; Rabasa-Lhoret, R.; McCrimmon, R.J.; Hume, C.; et al. Exercise management in type 1 diabetes: A consensus statement. *Lancet Diabetes Endocrinol.* **2017**, *8587*, 1–14. [CrossRef]
7. Colberg, S.R.; Sigal, R.J.; Yardley, J.E.; Riddell, M.C.; Dunstan, D.W.; Dempsey, P.C.; Horton, E.S.; Castorino, K.; Tate, D.F. Physical activity/exercise and diabetes: A position statement of the American Diabetes Association. *Diabetes Care* **2016**, *39*, 2065–2079. [CrossRef] [PubMed]
8. Chimen, M.; Kennedy, A.; Nirantharakumar, K.; Pang, T.T.; Andrews, R.; Narendran, P. What are the health benefits of physical activity in type 1 diabetes mellitus? A literature review. *Diabetologia* **2012**, *55*, 542–551. [CrossRef] [PubMed]

9. Brazeau, A.-S.; Rabasa-Lhoret, R.; Strychar, I.; Mircescu, H. Barriers to physical activity among patients with type 1 diabetes. *Diabetes Care* **2008**, *31*, 2108–2109. [CrossRef] [PubMed]
10. Galassetti, P.; Riddell, M.C. Exercise and type 1 diabetes (T1DM). *Compr. Physiol.* **2013**, *3*, 1309–1336. [PubMed]
11. The Diabetes Control and Complications Trial Research Group. The effect of intensive treatment of diabetes on the development and progression of long-term complications in insulin-dependent diabetes mellitus. *N. Engl. J. Med.* **1993**, *329*, 977–986.
12. The Diabetes Control and Complications Trial Research Group. The effect of intensive diabetes treatment on the development and progression of long-term complications in adolescents with insulin-dependent diabetes mellitus: Diabetes control and complications trial. *J. Pediatr.* **1994**, *125*, 177–188.
13. The Epidemiology of Diabetes Interventions and Complications Research Group. Intensive diabetes therapy and carotid intima–media thickness in type 1 diabetes mellitus. *N. Engl. J. Med.* **2003**, *348*, 2294–2303.
14. Diabetes Control and Complications Trial/Epidemiology of Diabetes Interventions and Complications (DCCT/EDIC) Study Research Group. Intensive diabetes treatment and cardiovascular disease in patients with type 1 diabetes. *N. Engl. J. Med.* **2005**, *353*, 2643–2653.
15. The DCCT Research Group. Epidemiology of severe hypoglycemia in the diabetes control and complications trial. *Am. J. Med.* **1991**, *90*, 450–459.
16. Rodbard, D. Continuous glucose monitoring: A review of successes, challenges, and opportunities. *Diabetes Technol. Ther.* **2016**, *18*, 3–13. [CrossRef] [PubMed]
17. Parkin, C.G.; Graham, C.; Smolskis, J. Continuous glucose monitoring use in type 1 diabetes: Longitudinal analysis demonstrates meaningful improvements in HbA1c and reductions in health care utilization. *J. Diabetes Sci. Technol.* **2017**, *11*, 522–528. [CrossRef] [PubMed]
18. Bailey, T.; Bode, B.W.; Christiansen, M.P.; Klaff, L.J.; Alva, S. The performance and usability of a factory-calibrated flash glucose monitoring system. *Diabetes Technol. Ther.* **2015**, *17*, 787–794. [CrossRef] [PubMed]
19. Richter, E.A.; Derave, W.; Wojtaszewski, J.F.P. Glucose, exercise and insulin: Emerging concepts. *J. Physiol.* **2001**, *535*, 313–322. [CrossRef] [PubMed]
20. Brooks, G.A.; Fahey, T.D.; Baldwin, K.M. *Exercise Physiology: Human Bioenergetics and Its Applications*, 4th ed.; McGraw-Hill: New York, NY, USA, 2005.
21. Nevill, M.E.; Boobis, L.H.; Brooks, S.; Williams, C. Effect of training on muscle metabolism during treadmill sprinting. *J. Appl. Physiol.* **1989**, *67*, 2376–2382. [CrossRef] [PubMed]
22. Emhoff, C.-A.W.; Messonnier, L.A.; Horning, M.A.; Fattor, J.A.; Carlson, T.J.; Brooks, G.A. Gluconeogenesis and hepatic glycogenolysis during exercise at the lactate threshold. *J. Appl. Physiol.* **2013**, *114*, 297–306. [CrossRef] [PubMed]
23. Bergman, B.C.; Horning, M.A.; Casazza, G.A.; Wolfel, E.E.; Butterfield, G.E.; Brooks, G.A. Endurance training increases gluconeogenesis during rest and exercise in men. *Am. J. Physiol. Endocrinol. Metab.* **2000**, *278*, 244E–251E. [CrossRef] [PubMed]
24. Korthuis, R.J. *Skeletal Muscle Circulation*; Morgan & Claypool Life Sciences: Williston, ND, USA, 2011.
25. Spriet, L.L. New insights into the interaction of carbohydrate and fat metabolism during exercise. *Sports Med.* **2014**, *44*, 87–96. [CrossRef] [PubMed]
26. Jenni, S.; Oetliker, C.; Allemann, S.; Ith, M.; Tappy, L.; Wuerth, S.; Egger, A.; Boesch, C.; Schneiter, P.; Diem, P.; et al. Fuel metabolism during exercise in euglycaemia and hyperglycaemia in patients with type 1 diabetes mellitus—A prospective single-blinded randomised crossover trial. *Diabetologia* **2008**, *51*, 1457–1465. [CrossRef] [PubMed]
27. Rissanen, A.P.E.; Tikkanen, H.O.; Koponen, A.S.; Aho, J.M.; Peltonen, J.E. Central and peripheral cardiovascular impairments limit V O2peak in Type 1 diabetes. *Med. Sci. Sports Exerc.* **2015**, *47*, 223–230. [CrossRef] [PubMed]
28. Astrand, P.-O.; Rodahl, K.; Dahl, H.A.; Stromme, S.B. *Textbook of Work Physiology: Physiological Bases of Exercise*, 3rd ed.; McGraw Hill: New York, NY, USA, 1986.
29. Secher, N.H.; Amann, M. Human investigations into the exercise pressor reflex. *Exp. Physiol.* **2012**, *97*, 59–69. [CrossRef] [PubMed]
30. Saltin, B.; Boushel, R.; Niels, S.; Jere, M. *Exercise and Circulation in Health and Disease*; Human Kinetics: Champaign, IL, USA, 1999.

31. Saltin, B.; Radegran, G.; Koskolou, M.D.; Roach, R.C. Skeletal muscle blood flow in humans and its regulation during exercise. *Acta Physiol. Scand.* **1998**, *1*, 421–436. [CrossRef] [PubMed]
32. Middlekauff, H.R.; Nitzsche, E.U.; Nguyen, A.H.; Hoh, C.K.; Gibbs, G.G. Modulation of renal cortical blood flow during static exercise in humans. *Circ. Res.* **1997**, *80*, 62–68. [CrossRef] [PubMed]
33. Levick, J.R. *An Introduction to Cardiovascular Physiology*, 5th ed.; Taylor & Francis Ltd.: London, UK, 2010.
34. Kvietys, P.R. *The Gastrointestinal Circulation*; Morgan & Claypool Life Sciences: Williston, ND, USA, 2010.
35. Metheny, N.M.; Metheny, N.M. *Fluid and Electrolyte Balance: Nursing Considerations*, 5th ed.; Jones & Bartlett Learning: Burlington, ON, Canada, 2012.
36. Martini, F.H.; Nath, J.L. *Fundamentals of Anatomy and Physiology*; Wiley-Blackwell: Hoboken, NJ, USA, 2009.
37. Klabunde, R.E. *Cardiovascular Physiology Concepts*, 2nd ed.; Lippincott Williams & Wilkins: Philadelphia, PA, USA, 2004.
38. Arturson, G.; Kjellmer, I. Capillary permeability in skeletal muscle during rest and activity. *Acta Physiol. Scand.* **1964**, *62*, 41–45. [CrossRef] [PubMed]
39. Jacobsson, S.; Kjellmer, I. Flow and protein content of lymph in resting and exercising skeletal muscle. *Acta Physiol. Scand.* **1964**, *60*, 278–285. [CrossRef] [PubMed]
40. Jacobsson, S.; Kjellmer, I. Accumulation of fluid in exercising skeletal muscle. *Acta Physiol. Scand.* **1964**, *60*, 286–292. [CrossRef] [PubMed]
41. Lundvall, J. Tissue hyperosmolality as a mediator of vasodilatation and transcapillary fluid flux in exercising skeletal muscle. *Acta Physiol. Scand. Suppl.* **1972**, *379*, 1–142. [PubMed]
42. Lundvall, J.; Mellander, S.; Westling, H.; White, T. Fluid transfer between blood and tissues during exercise. *Acta Physiol. Scand.* **1972**, *85*, 258–269. [CrossRef] [PubMed]
43. Kjellmer, I. Studies on exercise hyperemia. *Acta Physiol. Scand. Suppl.* **1964**, *244*, 1–27.
44. Scallan, J.; Huxley, V.H.; Korthuis, R.J. *Capillary Fluid Exchange: Regulation, Functions, and Pathology*; Morgan & Claypool Life Sciences: Williston, ND, USA, 2010.
45. Stick, C.; Jaeger, H.; Witzleb, E. Measurements of volume changes and venous pressure in the human lower leg during walking and running. *J. Appl. Physiol.* **1992**, *72*, 2063–2068. [CrossRef] [PubMed]
46. Richter, E.A.; Ploug, T.; Galbo, H. Increased muscle glucose uptake after exercise. No need for insulin during exercise. *Diabetes* **1985**, *34*, 1041–1048. [CrossRef] [PubMed]
47. Renkin, E.M.; Michel, C.C. Capillary Permeability to Small Solutes. In *Handbook of Physiology: The Cardiovascular System, Microcirculation*; Crone, C., Levitt, D.G., Eds.; American Physiological Society: Bethesda, MD, USA, 1984.
48. Blomstrand, E.; Saltin, B. Effect of muscle glycogen on glucose, lactate and amino acid metabolism during exercise and recovery in human subjects. *J. Physiol.* **1999**, *514*, 293–302. [CrossRef] [PubMed]
49. Rose, A.J.; Richter, E.A. Skeletal muscle glucose uptake during exercise: How is it regulated? *Physiology (Bethesda)* **2005**, *20*, 260–270. [CrossRef] [PubMed]
50. Hultman, E. Studies on muscle metabolism of glycogen and active phosphate in man with special reference to exercise and diet. *Scand. J. Clin. Lab. Investig. Suppl.* **1967**, *94*, 1–63.
51. Gaitanos, G.; Willians, L.; Boobis, L.; Brooks, S. Human muscle metabolism maximal exercise. *Appl. Physiol.* **1993**, *75*, 712–719. [CrossRef] [PubMed]
52. Marliss, E.B.; Vranic, M. Intense exercise has unique effects on both insulin release and its roles in glucoregulation: Implications for diabetes. *Diabetes* **2002**, *51*, 271S–283S. [CrossRef]
53. Nilsson, L.H.; Hultman, E. Liver glycogen in man—The effect of total starvation or a carbohydrate—Poor diet followed by carbohydrate refeeding. *Scand. J. Clin. Lab. Investig.* **1973**, *32*, 325–330. [CrossRef]
54. Fahey, A.J.; Paramalingam, N.; Davey, R.J.; Davis, E.A.; Jones, T.W.; Fournier, P.A. The effect of a short sprint on postexercise whole-body glucose production and utilization rates in individuals with type 1 diabetes mellitus. *J. Clin. Endocrinol. Metab.* **2012**, *97*, 4193–4200. [CrossRef] [PubMed]
55. Gyntelberg, F.; Rennie, M.J.; Hickson, R.C.; Holloszy, J.O. Effect of training on the response of plasma glucagon to exercise. *J. Appl. Physiol.* **1977**, *43*, 302–305. [CrossRef] [PubMed]
56. West, D.J.; Morton, R.D.; Bain, S.C.; Stephens, J.W.; Bracken, R.M. Blood glucose responses to reductions in pre-exercise rapid-acting insulin for 24 h after running in individuals with type 1 diabetes. *J. Sports Sci.* **2010**, *28*, 781–788. [CrossRef] [PubMed]

57. Clark, M.G.; Wallis, M.G.; Barrett, E.J.; Vincent, M.A.; Richards, S.M.; Clerk, L.H.; Rattigan, S. Blood flow and muscle metabolism: A focus on insulin action. *Am. J. Physiol. Endocrinol. Metab.* **2003**, *284*, 241E–258E. [CrossRef] [PubMed]
58. Gonzalez, J.T.; Fuchs, C.J.; Betts, J.A.; van Loon, L.J. Glucose plus fructose ingestion for post—Exercise recovery—Greater than the sum of its parts? *Nutrients* **2017**, *9*, E344. [CrossRef] [PubMed]
59. Jeukendrup, A.E. Training the gut for athletes. *Sports Med.* **2017**, *47*, 101–110. [CrossRef] [PubMed]
60. Klonoff, D.C.; Ahn, D.; Drincic, A. Continuous glucose monitoring: A review of the technology and clinical use. *Diabetes Res. Clin. Pract.* **2017**, *133*, 178–192. [CrossRef] [PubMed]
61. Aberer, F.; Hajnsek, M.; Rumpler, M.; Zenz, S.; Baumann, P.M.; Elsayed, H.; Puffing, A.; Treiber, G.; Pieber, T.R.; Sourij, H.; et al. Evaluation of subcutaneous glucose monitoring systems under routine environmental conditions in patients with type 1 diabetes. *Diabetes Obes. Metab.* **2017**, *19*, 1051–1055. [CrossRef] [PubMed]
62. Herrington, S.J.; Gee, D.L.; Dow, S.D.; Monosky, K.A.; And, E.D.; Pritchett, K.L. Comparison of glucose monitoring methods during steady-state exercise in women. *Nutrients* **2012**, *4*, 1282–1292. [CrossRef] [PubMed]
63. Moser, O.; Mader, J.; Tschakert, G.; Mueller, A.; Groeschl, W.; Pieber, T.; Koehler, G.; Messerschmidt, J.; Hofmann, P. Accuracy of continuous glucose monitoring (CGM) during continuous and high-Intensity interval exercise in patients with type 1 diabetes mellitus. *Nutrients* **2016**, *8*, 489. [CrossRef] [PubMed]
64. Bally, L.; Zueger, T.; Pasi, N.; Carlos, C.; Paganini, D.; Stettler, C. Accuracy of continuous glucose monitoring during differing exercise conditions. *Diabetes Res. Clin. Pract.* **2016**, *112*, 1–5. [CrossRef] [PubMed]
65. Yardley, J.E.; Sigal, R.J.; Kenny, G.P.; Riddell, M.C.; Lovblom, L.E.; Perkins, B. A Point accuracy of interstitial continuous glucose monitoring during exercise in type 1 diabetes. *Diabetes Technol. Ther.* **2013**, *15*, 46–49. [CrossRef] [PubMed]
66. Iscoe, K.E.; Davey, R.J.; Fournier, P.A. Increasing the low-glucose alarm of a continuous glucose monitoring system prevents exercise-induced hypoglycemia without triggering any false alarms. *Diabetes Care* **2011**, *34*, 109e. [CrossRef] [PubMed]
67. Gross, T.M.; Bode, B.W.; Einhorn, D.; Kayne, D.M.; Reed, J.H.; White, N.H.; Mastrototaro, J.J. Performance evaluation of the MiniMed continuous glucose monitoring system during patient home use. *Diabetes Technol. Ther.* **2000**, *2*, 49–56. [CrossRef] [PubMed]
68. FDA Advisory Panel. FDA advisory panel votes to recommend non-adjunctive use of Dexcom G5 mobile CGM. *Diabetes Technol. Ther.* **2016**, *18*, 512–516.
69. Matuleviciene, V.; Joseph, J.I.; Andelin, M.; Hirsch, I.B.; Attvall, S.; Pivodic, A.; Dahlqvist, S.; Klonoff, D.; Haraldsson, B.; Lind, M. A clinical trial of the accuracy and treatment experience of the Dexcom G4 sensor (Dexcom G4 system) and Enlite sensor (Guardian REAL-time system) tested simultaneously in ambulatory patients with type 1 diabetes. *Diabetes Technol. Ther.* **2014**, *16*, 759–767. [CrossRef] [PubMed]
70. Kropff, J.; Bruttomesso, D.; Doll, W.; Farret, A.; Galasso, S.; Luijf, Y.M.; Mader, J.K.; Place, J.; Boscari, F.; Pieber, T.R.; et al. Accuracy of two continuous glucose monitoring systems: A head-to-head comparison under clinical research centre and daily life conditions. *Diabetes Obes. Metab.* **2014**, *17*, 343–349. [CrossRef] [PubMed]
71. Luijf, Y.M.; Mader, J.K.; Doll, W.; Pieber, T.; Farret, A.; Place, J.; Renard, E.; Bruttomesso, D.; Filippi, A.; Avogaro, A.; et al. Accuracy and reliability of continuous glucose monitoring systems: A head-to-head comparison. *Diabetes Technol. Ther.* **2013**, *15*, 721–726. [CrossRef] [PubMed]
72. Rodbard, D. Continuous glucose monitoring: A review of recent studies demonstrating improved glycemic outcomes. *Diabetes Technol. Ther.* **2017**, *19* (Suppl. 3), 25S–37S. [CrossRef] [PubMed]
73. Christiansen, M.P.; Garg, S.K.; Brazg, R.; Bode, B.W.; Bailey, T.S.; Slover, R.H.; Sullivan, A.; Huang, S.; Shin, J.; Lee, S.W.; et al. Accuracy of a fourth-generation subcutaneous continuous glucose sensor. *Diabetes Technol. Ther.* **2017**, *19*, 446–456. [CrossRef] [PubMed]
74. Lawson, M.L.; Bradley, B.; McAssey, K.; Clarson, C.; Kirsch, S.E.; Mahmud, F.H.; Curtis, J.R.; Richardson, C.; Courtney, J.; Cooper, T.; et al. The JDRF CCTN CGM TIME Trial: Timing of initiation of continuous glucose monitoring in established pediatric type 1 diabetes: Study protocol, recruitment and baseline characteristics. *BMC Pediatr.* **2014**, *14*, 183. [CrossRef] [PubMed]

75. Spegazzini, N.; Barman, I.; Dingari, N.C.; Pandey, R.; Soares, J.S.; Ozaki, Y.; Dasari, R.R. Spectroscopic approach for dynamic bioanalyte tracking with minimal concentration information. *Sci. Rep.* **2014**, *4*, 7013. [CrossRef] [PubMed]
76. Taleb, N.; Emami, A.; Suppere, C.; Messier, V.; Legault, L.; Chiasson, J.-L.; Rabasa-Lhoret, R.; Haidar, A. Comparison of two continuous glucose monitoring systems, Dexcom G4 Platinum and Medtronic Paradigm Veo Enlite system, at rest and during exercise. *Diabetes Technol. Ther.* **2016**, *18*, 561–567. [CrossRef] [PubMed]
77. Facchinetti, A.; Sparacino, G.; Guerra, S.; Luijf, Y.M.; DeVries, J.H.; Mader, J.K.; Ellmerer, M.; Benesch, C.; Heinemann, L.; Bruttomesso, D.; et al. Real-time improvement of continuous glucose monitoring accuracy: The smart sensor concept. *Diabetes Care* **2013**, *36*, 793–800. [CrossRef] [PubMed]
78. Facchinetti, A. Continuous glucose monitoring sensors: Past, present and future algorithmic challenges. *Sensors* **2016**, *16*, 2093. [CrossRef] [PubMed]
79. Facchinetti, A.; Sparacino, G.; Cobelli, C. An online self-tunable method to denoise CGM sensor data. *IEEE Trans. Biomed. Eng.* **2010**, *57*, 634–641. [CrossRef] [PubMed]
80. Guerra, S.; Facchinetti, A.; Sparacino, G.; De Nicolao, G.; Cobelli, C. Enhancing the accuracy of subcutaneous glucose sensors: A real-time deconvolution-based approach. *IEEE Trans. Biomed. Eng.* **2012**, *59*, 1658–1669. [CrossRef] [PubMed]
81. Sparacino, G.; Zanderigo, F.; Corazza, S.; Maran, A.; Facchinetti, A.; Cobelli, C. Glucose Concentration can be Predicted Ahead in Time From Continuous Glucose Monitoring Sensor Time-Series. *IEEE Trans. Biomed. Eng.* **2007**, *54*, 931–937. [CrossRef] [PubMed]
82. Gingras, V.; Rabasa-Lhoret, R.; Messier, V.; Ladouceur, M.; Legault, L.; Haidar, A. Efficacy of dual-hormone artificial pancreas to alleviate the carbohydrate-counting burden of type 1 diabetes: A randomized crossover trial. *Diabetes Metab.* **2016**, *42*, 47–54. [CrossRef] [PubMed]
83. El-Khatib, F.H.; Balliro, C.; Hillard, M.A.; Magyar, K.L.; Ekhlaspour, L.; Sinha, M.; Mondesir, D.; Esmaeili, A.; Hartigan, C.; Thompson, M.J.; et al. Home use of a bihormonal bionic pancreas versus insulin pump therapy in adults with type 1 diabetes: A multicentre randomised crossover trial. *Lancet* **2017**, *389*, 369–380. [CrossRef]
84. Taleb, N.; Emami, A.; Suppere, C.; Messier, V.; Legault, L.; Ladouceur, M.; Chiasson, J.-L.; Haidar, A.; Rabasa-Lhoret, R. Efficacy of single-hormone and dual-hormone artificial pancreas during continuous and interval exercise in adult patients with type 1 diabetes: Randomised controlled crossover trial. *Diabetologia* **2016**, *59*, 2561–2571. [CrossRef] [PubMed]
85. Haymond, M.W.; DuBose, S.N.; Rickels, M.R.; Wolpert, H.; Shah, V.N.; Sherr, J.L.; Weinstock, R.S.; Agarwal, S.; Verdejo, A.S.; Cummins, M.J.; et al. Efficacy and safety of mini-dose glucagon for treatment of non-severe hypoglycemia in adults with type 1 diabetes. *J. Clin. Endocrinol. Metab.* **2017**, *102*, 2994–3001. [CrossRef] [PubMed]
86. Yue, J.T.Y.; Riddell, M.C.; Burdett, E.; Coy, D.H.; Efendic, S.; Vranic, M. Amelioration of hypoglycemia via somatostatin receptor type 2 antagonism in recurrently hypoglycemic diabetic rats. *Diabetes* **2013**, *62*, 2215–2222. [CrossRef] [PubMed]
87. Taleb, N.; Rabasa-Lhoret, R. Can somatostatin antagonism prevent hypoglycaemia during exercise in type 1 diabetes? *Diabetologia* **2016**, *59*, 1632–1635. [CrossRef] [PubMed]
88. Kropff, J.; Choudhary, P.; Neupane, S.; Barnard, K.; Bain, S.C.; Kapitza, C.; Forst, T.; Link, M.; Dehennis, A.; De Vries, J.H. Accuracy and longevity of an implantable continuous glucose sensor in the PRECISE study: A 180-day, prospective, multicenter, pivotal trial. *Diabetes Care* **2017**, *40*, 63–68. [CrossRef] [PubMed]

16

LXRα Regulates Hepatic ChREBPα Activity and Lipogenesis upon Glucose but Not Fructose Feeding in Mice

Qiong Fan [1,*], Rikke C. Nørgaard [1], Christian Bindesbøll [2], Christin Lucas [1], Knut Tomas Dalen [1], Eshrat Babaie [3], Harri M. Itkonen [4], Jason Matthews [1,5], Hilde I. Nebb [1] and Line M. Grønning-Wang [1,*]

1 Department of Nutrition, Institute of Basic Medical Sciences, University of Oslo, 0317 Oslo, Norway; r.c.norgaard@medisin.uio.no (R.C.N.); christin.lucas@medisin.uio.no (C.L.); k.t.dalen@medisin.uio.no (K.T.D.); jason.matthews@medisin.uio.no (J.M.); h.i.nebb@medisin.uio.no (H.I.N.)
2 Department of Molecular Medicine, Institute of Basic Medical Sciences, University of Oslo, 0317 Oslo, Norway; christian.bindesboll@medisin.uio.no
3 Centre for Molecular Medicine Norway, University of Oslo, 0318 Oslo, Norway; eshrat.babaie@ncmm.uio.no
4 Prostate Cancer Research Group, Centre for Molecular Medicine (Norway), University of Oslo and Oslo University Hospitals, 0318 Oslo, Norway; Harri_Itkonen@hms.harvard.edu
5 Department of Pharmacology and Toxicology, University of Toronto, Toronto, ON M5S1A8, Canada
* Correspondence: qiong.fan@medisin.uio.no (Q.F.); l.m.gronning-wang@medisin.uio.no (L.M.G.-W.)

Abstract: Liver X receptors (LXRα/β) and carbohydrate response element-binding proteins (ChREBPα/β) are key players in the transcriptional control of hepatic *de novo* lipogenesis. LXRα/β double knockout (LXR$\alpha^{-/-}/\beta^{-/-}$) mice have reduced feeding-induced nuclear *O*-linked *N*-acetylglucosamine (*O*-GlcNAc) signaling, ChREBPα activity, and lipogenic gene expression in livers, suggesting important roles for LXRs in linking hepatic glucose utilization to lipid synthesis. However, the role of LXRs in fructose-induced ChREBP activation and lipogenesis is currently unknown. In this study, we studied the effects of high fructose or high glucose feeding on hepatic carbohydrate metabolism and lipogenic gene expression in livers from fasted (24 h) and fasted-refed (12 h) wild type and LXRα knockout (LXR$\alpha^{-/-}$) mice. Hepatic lipogenic gene expression was reduced in glucose fed, but not fructose fed LXR$\alpha^{-/-}$ mice. This was associated with lower expression of liver pyruvate-kinase (*L-pk*) and *Chrebpβ*, indicating reduced ChREBPα activity in glucose fed, but not fructose fed mice. Interestingly, ChREBP binding to the *L-pk* promoter was increased in fructose fed LXR$\alpha^{-/-}$ mice, concomitant with increased glucose-6-phosphatase (*G6pc*) expression and *O*-GlcNAc modified LXRβ, suggesting a role for LXRβ in regulating ChREBPα activity upon fructose feeding. In conclusion, we propose that LXRα is an important regulator of hepatic lipogenesis and ChREBPα activity upon glucose, but not fructose feeding in mice.

Keywords: LXR; ChREBP; *de novo* lipogenesis (DNL); *O*-GlcNAc

---

1. Introduction

Diets rich in the simple sugars glucose and fructose stimulate hepatic *de novo* lipogenesis (DNL) and increase circulating triglycerides in humans and rodents [1–4]. Many of the enzymes involved in DNL and triglyceride synthesis are primarily regulated at the transcriptional level in a coordinate manner through multiple transcription factors in response to glucose and insulin [5]. Three transcription factors have been identified as particularly important for regulation of lipogenesis: the liver X receptors (LXRα; Nuclear Receptor Subfamily 1 Group H Member 3 (NR1H3) and LXRβ;

Nuclear Receptor Subfamily 1 Group H Member 2 (NR1H2)), sterol regulatory element-binding protein 1c (SREBP-1c), and carbohydrate response element-binding protein-α (ChREBPα) [5].

The LXRs are classically known as oxysterol-activated nuclear transcription factors and members of the nuclear receptor family. LXRs heterodimerize with retinoic X receptor (RXR; Nuclear Receptor Subfamily 2 Group B (NR2B)) family members to regulate the expression of genes involved in cholesterol homeostasis, lipogenesis, glucose metabolism, and inflammation [6]. LXRα is the predominantly expressed isoform in lipogenic tissues such as liver and adipose, whereas LXRβ is ubiquitously expressed [7]. In response to dietary cholesterol, glucose, and insulin, hepatic LXRs, in particular LXRα, activate transcription of the two other lipogenic transcription factors SREBP-1c and ChREBPα, which alone or in concert with LXRs induce expression of glycolytic and lipogenic enzymes in hepatic DNL, such as glucokinase (*Gk*), liver pyruvate kinase (*L-pk*), ATP citrate lyase (*Acl*), acetyl-CoA carboxylase (*Acc*), fatty acid synthase (*Fasn*), and stearoyl-CoA desaturase-1 (*Scd1*) [6,8]. In addition, LXRs improve glucose tolerance by negatively regulating hepatic glucose-6-phosphate (*G6pc*) expression and glucose production [9–11].

We and others have shown that LXRs and ChREBPα are post-translationally modified by *O*-linked *N*-acetylglucosamine (*O*-GlcNAc) in response to high glucose by *O*-GlcNAc transferase (OGT), which increases their lipogenic potential [12,13]. OGT uses UDP-*N*-acetylglucosamine (UDP-GlcNAc), the high energy product of the hexosamine biosynthetic pathway (HBP), as a substrate for reversible *O*-linked GlcNAcylation of nuclear, cytoplasmic, and mitochondrial target proteins affecting transcription, metabolism, apoptosis, organelle biogenesis, and transport [14]. The HBP is a branch of the glycolytic pathway that couples nutrient sensing to cellular metabolism and signaling via activation of OGT [15]. *O*-GlcNAcylation regulates transcription through OGT-associated chromatin-modifying complexes [16]. In this way, glucose not only serves as an energy source and substrate for lipogenesis, but also acts as a signaling molecule in the regulation of glycolytic and lipogenic gene expression [17]. In line with this notion, *O*-GlcNAc signaling is associated with increased ChREBPα activity, enhanced glycogenic and lipogenic gene expression, and hepatic steatosis [13]. We recently reported that insulin-independent glucose-*O*-GlcNAc signaling potentiates LXR-mediated transactivation of the SREBP-1c and ChREBPα promoters, linking glucose metabolism to LXR activation and lipogenesis [12,18]. Furthermore, we reported that LXRs are important for nuclear *O*-GlcNAc signaling, ChREBPα *O*-GlcNAcylation and *L-pk* promoter binding activity, and glycogenic and lipogenic gene expression, including expression of the newly discovered *Chrebpβ* isoform in mouse livers. Collectively, these data suggest that LXRs connect hepatic glucose utilization to lipogenesis via regulation of nuclear OGT and ChREBPα activity [18,19]. However, the specific roles of LXRα and LXRβ in this process are currently unknown.

ChREBPβ is derived from an alternative promoter within exon 1b of the ChREBP gene, resulting in a shorter constitutively nuclear protein lacking most of the low glucose inhibitory domain (LID) in *N*-terminus [20]. *Chrebpβ* expression is low during prolonged fasting and strongly induced following high carbohydrate refeeding in mice [21]. ChREBPα mediates this response in a tissue-specific manner via transactivation of carbohydrate response elements (ChoREs) upstream of and in exon 1b [21]. Interestingly, ChREBPβ conferred a higher transcriptional activity than ChREBPα under both low and high glucose conditions and appears to be the major regulator of lipogenesis in response to dietary carbohydrates [20,22]. Recently, a role for ChREBP and in particular ChREBPβ, in fructose-induced *de novo* lipogenesis was suggested [21,23]. ChREBP null mice are intolerant to high fructose diet, in part by blunted gene expression of fructose-metabolizing enzyme genes, suggesting also a crucial role for ChREBP in fructose metabolism [24]. Interestingly, a recent study showed that ChREBP induces hepatic *G6pc* expression and glucose production by short-term fructose feeding in mice [25], suggesting a role for ChREBP in contributing to selective hepatic insulin resistance.

The objectives of the present study were to investigate the LXRα dependent effect of dietary fructose and glucose on hepatic ChREBPα activity, glycogenic and lipogenic gene expression, intermediate carbohydrate metabolism, and *O*-GlcNAc levels by using wild type and LXRα deficient mice. The results from this study indicate that LXRα is important in hepatic DNL and ChREBPα activity upon glucose, but not fructose feeding in mice.

2. Materials and Methods

2.1. Materials

Formaldehyde (F1635) and UDP-GlcNAc (U4375) were purchased from Sigma Aldrich (St. Louis, MO, USA). UltraPure™ Phenol: Chloroform:Isoamyl Alcohol (15593-031) was from Invitrogen Aldrich (Thermo Fisher Scientific, Waltham, MA, USA). All other chemicals were of the highest quality available from commercial vendors.

2.2. Animals and Treatment

Wildtype ($LXR\alpha^{+/+}$) and LXRα deficient ($LXR\alpha^{-/-}$) mice were housed in a temperature-controlled (22 °C) facility with a strict 12 h light/dark cycle. Mice had free access to standard chow diet (SDS diets, RM3, #801190, consisting of 12% calories from fat, 27% from protein, and 61% from carbohydrate) and water at all times prior to experiments. The generation of the $LXR\alpha^{-/-}$ mice has been described previously [26]. The $LXR\alpha^{+/+}$ and $LXR\alpha^{-/-}$ mice used were of mixed genetic background (129/Sv/C57BL/6) backcrossed into the C57BL/6N strain for six generations. Twelve-week-old male mice (n = 5) were fasted for 24 h or fasted for 24 h and subsequently refed for 12 h on an isocaloric diet (3.99 kcal/g) containing 60.8% calories from fructose (5BN7) or glucose (5BN8) (TestDiet), 22.6% fat, and 16.7% protein. The mice were sacrificed in a mixed order between fasted and refed groups by cervical dislocation at 7–9 a.m., and tissues were weighed and snap frozen in liquid nitrogen and stored at −80 °C until further analysis. All use of animals was registered and approved by the local veterinary and the Norwegian Animal Research authority (FOTS #5457 and #6378).

2.3. Blood Chemistries

Plasma was separated from blood by centrifugation. Plasma insulin was measured using the Ultrasensitive Insulin Kit from Mercodia (Mercodia AB, Uppsala, Sweden) according to the manufacturer's instructions. Plasma triglycerides (TGs) were determined with a Triglycerides Enzymatic PAP 150 kit (TGPAP 150; BioMérieux, Marcy-l'Étoile, France).

2.4. Metabolomics

Liver tissues (n = 5 mice for each group) were sent to Metabolon, Inc. (Research Triangle Park, Durham, NC, USA) for metabolomics analysis as described [27]. The metabolomics data is included in Supplementary Table S1.

2.5. RNA Extraction, cDNA Synthesis and Real-Time Quantitative PCR (RT-qPCR)

RNA was isolated by phenol chloroform extraction followed by high salt precipitation (0.8 M sodium acetate, 1.5 M NaCl) to avoid contaminating polysaccharides to co-precipitate with RNA. Extracted RNA was further purified using RNeasy spin columns (#74104; QIAGEN, Hilden, Germany). Isolated RNA (500 ng) was reverse transcribed into cDNA using SuperScript III Reverse Transcriptase (Invitrogen, Thermo Fisher Scientific, Waltham, MA, USA) and random hexamer primers. qPCR was performed with 1 μL of the cDNA synthesis reaction using Kapa SYBR FAST qPCR Master Mix (KapaBiosystems, Roche, Basel, Switzerland) on a Bio-Rad CFX96 Touch™ Real-Time PCR Detection System. Gene expression was normalized against the expression of TATA-binding protein (*Tbp*). Assay primers were designed with Primer-BLAST software (NCBI, Bethesda, MD, USA) [28]. Sequences are listed in Supplementary Table S1.

2.6. Liver Extracts and Immunoblot Analysis

Nuclear and cytoplasmic proteins were prepared using NE-PER™ Nuclear and Cytoplasmic Extraction kit (Pierce Biotechnology, Thermo Fisher Scientific, Waltham, MA, USA), with the following inhibitors added to the buffers: 1 mM NaF, 1 mM Na_3VO_4, 1 mM β-glycerophosphate, 1 μM *O*-GlcNAcase inhibitor GlcNAc-thiazoline, and Complete™ protease inhibitors (Roche Applied Science, Penzberg, Germany). Proteins were separated by Sodium Dodecyl Sulfate Polyacrylamide Gel Electrophoresis (SDS-PAGE) (Bio-Rad, Hercules, CA, USA) and blotted onto Polyvinylidene fluoride (PVDF) membrane (Merck Millipore, Billerica, MA, USA). Primary antibodies used were rabbit anti-mouse LXR (1:500) [19], ChREBP (1:1000; #NB400-135; Novus Biologicals, Littleton, CO, USA), FASN (1:500; #sc-55580; Santa Cruz Biotechnology, Dallas, TX, USA), SCD1 (1:2000; #sc-14719; Santa Cruz Biotechnology, Dallas, TX, USA), α-Tubulin (1:20,000; #T5168; Sigma-Aldrich, St. Louis, MO, USA), Lamin A (1:1000; #L1293; Sigma-Aldrich, St. Louis, MO, USA), OGT (1:1000; #AL25) [29], RL2 (1:1000, #MA1-072, Invitrogen, Thermo Fisher Scientific, Waltham, MA, USA), SREBP-1 (1:1000) [30], and L-PK (1:2000; #MABS148; Merck Millipore, Billerica, MA, USA). Secondary horseradish peroxidase-conjugated anti-mouse (#115-035-174) and anti-rabbit (#211-032-171; Jackson ImmunoResearch Laboratories, West Grove, PA, USA); anti-goat (#605-4302; Rockland, Limerick, PA, USA) antibodies were used at 1:10,000 dilutions. Anti-mouse IgM (#A8786; Sigma-Aldrich, St. Louis, MO, USA) was used at 1:5000 dilutions. Blots were quantified from five mice for each experimental group, using the ImageJ software (NIH, Bethesda, Maryland). All lanes were normalized to loading controls as indicated in figure text (α-tubulin or Lamin A).

2.7. Chromatin Immunoprecipitation (ChIP)

ChIP experiments were performed as described previously with modest changes [19]. Briefly, liver tissue was homogenized and crosslinked with 1% formaldehyde/Phosphate-buffered saline (PBS) for 10 min at room temperature. Crosslinking was stopped by 3 min incubation with 125 mM glycine. Samples were washed twice in cold PBS and resuspended in lysis buffer (0.1% SDS, 1% Triton X-100, 0.15 M NaCl, 1 mM Ethylenediaminetetraacetic acid (EDTA), and 20 mM Tris (pH 8.0). Lysed tissue was sonicated to an average size of 200–500 bp fragments using a bioruptor (Diagenode, Seraing, Belgium). Chromatin was immunoprecipitated with 2 μg antibody against ChREBP (NB400-135; Novus Biologicals, Littleton, CO, USA) or rabbit IgG (011-000-002; Jackson ImmunoResearch Laboratory, West Grove, PA, USA) over night at 4 °C. Dynabeads Protein A (Invitrogen) were washed four times in lysis buffer, and then added to the chromatin and rotated at 4 °C for 2 h. Dynabeads were then washed three times with wash buffer 1 (0.1% SDS, 1% Triton X-100, 0.15 M NaCl, 1 mM EDTA, 20 mM Tris (pH 8)); followed by washing once in wash buffer 2 (0.1% SDS, 1% Triton X-100, 0.5 M NaCl, 1 mM EDTA, 20 mM Tris (pH 8)), and then once in wash buffer 3 (0.25 M LiCl, 1% NaDOC, 1% NP-40, 1 mM EDTA, 20 mM Tris (pH 8)), and then once in wash buffer 1. All washing steps were done for five minutes at room temperature. DNA-protein complexes were eluted with 1% SDS and reverse cross-linked overnight at 65 °C. DNA was purified by using the QIAquick PCR Purification Kit (#28104; QIAGEN, Hilden, Germany). DNA enrichment was quantified by quantitative RT-PCR. The binding of ChREBP to the carbohydrate response element (ChoRE) in the promoter-proximal enhancer of *L-pk* has been described previously [13] and the ChIP primers used were as follows: *L-pk* ChoRE (5′-GTCCCACACTTTGGAAGCAT, 5′-CCCAACACTGATTCTACCC). The negative control primers located 2.2 kp downstream from the ChoRE were as follows: 5′-TGCAACTGGGGAACTAGCCA, 5′-AGCTTTGTGTGATGGCTGAAG.

2.8. Wheat Germ Agglutinin (WGA) Pulldown

Nuclear extracts (100 μg) were incubated with protein A/G-agarose beads (sc-2003; Santa Cruz Biotechnology) for 1 h at 4 °C. Cleared extracts were transferred to new tubes and incubated with 30 μL of WGA-agarose (Vector Lab, Burlingame, CA, USA) overnight at 4 °C. After four washes (PBS,

0.2% NP-40), proteins were eluted from the beads in 2× Laemmli buffer and separated by SDS-PAGE. The captured proteins were analyzed by immunoblotting.

2.9. UDP-GlcNAc Measurements

UDP-GlcNAc in liver tissue was extracted and analyzed using described methods [31] with minor changes. Liver tissue (20 μg) was homogenized in liquid nitrogen-chilled CryoGrinder (OPS Diagnostics, Lebanon, NJ, USA), and resuspended in 0.15 mL cold PBS. Ice-cold ethanol (0.45 mL) was added to the samples, followed by sonication in Diagenode Bioruptor to lyse the cells. The lysate was centrifuged at 16,000× *g* for 10 min at 4 °C, and a third of the supernatant was used for determination of protein concentration using the bicinchoninic acid (BCA) assay kit (Pierce, Thermo Fisher Scientific, Waltham, MA, USA), and the rest was vacuum dried in a Savant DNA100 SpeedVac to measure levels of nucleotide sugars with ion-pair reversed phase High-performance liquid chromatography (HPLC). The preparatory columns for HPLC were done as previously reported [32], while the run-time in HPLC was extended up to 2 h. A standard UDP-GlcNAc (100 μM) was spiked into samples to verify the accurate peak.

2.10. Statistical Analysis

Statistical analyses were performed using GraphPad Prims 6 (GraphPad Software Inc., San Diego, CA, USA). All data were presented as means and standard error of the mean (SEM), and error bars for all results were derived from biological replicates rather than technical replicates. Statistical differences between groups were determined by two-way analysis of variance (ANOVA) followed by Tukey's multiple comparison tests. For all statistical tests $p < 0.05$ was considered statistically significant. For metabolomics data, statistical differences between groups were determined by repeated measures two-way ANOVA.

3. Results

3.1. Regulation of Genes Involved in Carbohydrate Metabolism by Dietary Fructose and Glucose-Role of LXRα

To examine LXRα-dependent regulation of genes encoding for glucose and fructose metabolizing enzymes in response to fructose and glucose feeding, wild type and LXRα$^{-/-}$ mice were divided into three groups: fasted (24 h), fasted-refed with 60% fructose, or fasted-refed with 60% glucose for 12 h. No statistically significant differences in food intake or body weight were found among the fructose and glucose fed wild type and LXRα$^{-/-}$ mice (Table 1). A schematic representation of the enzymes involved in carbohydrate metabolism (glycolysis, fructolysis, and gluconeogenesis) is presented in Figure 1A. The majority of the analyzed genes were similarly regulated in wild type and LXRα$^{-/-}$ mice. Both diets upregulated glycolytic *Gk* mRNA to a similar degree, and fructose feeding upregulated the ChREBP target gene *L-pk* mRNA more strongly than glucose feeding, which is in agreement with previous observations [33,34] (Figure 1B). Interestingly, glucose-, but not fructose-mediated induction of *L-pk* was significantly attenuated in LXRα$^{-/-}$ mice. Figure 1C shows genes in the fructolysis pathway, fructokinase (*Fk*) and aldolase B (*AldoB*). Only fructose feeding upregulated Fk and AldoB, as previously reported [33]. We observed increased expression of gluconeogenic genes *G6pc* and glucose transporter 2 (*Glut2*) with fructose feeding in the LXRα$^{-/-}$ mice (Figure 1B,D). These observations were concomitant with an approximately 2-fold increase in plasma insulin levels in fructose fed LXRα$^{-/-}$ mice compared to wild type mice on the same diet (Table 1). These data suggest increased glucose production and glucose output in fructose fed mice lacking LXRα.

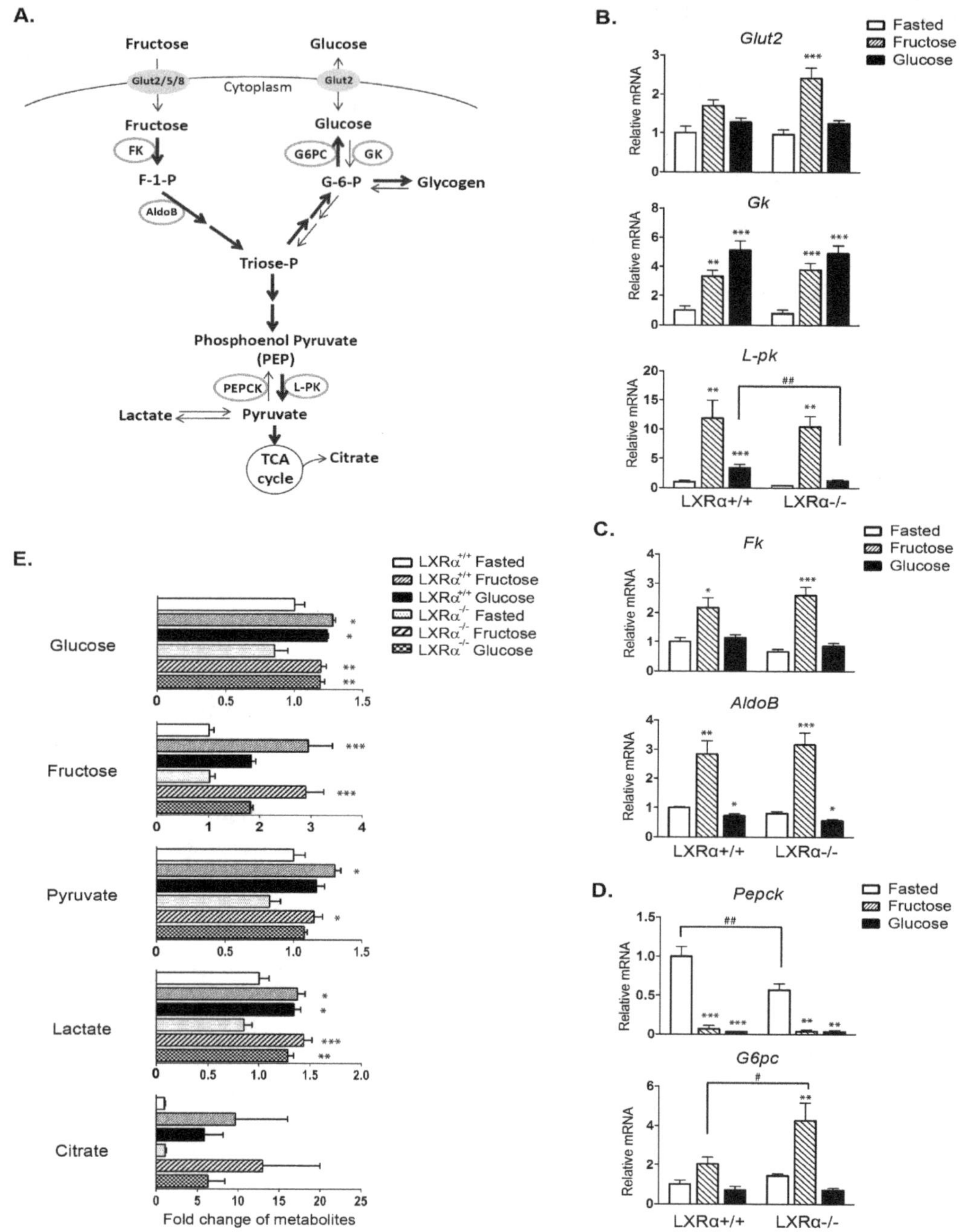

Figure 1. Hepatic liver pyruvate-kinase (*L-pk*) expression by dietary glucose is reduced in LXRα knockout (LXRα$^{-/-}$) mice. The male mice of inbred strain C57 Black 6 (C57BL/6) were fasted 24 h (white bars) or fasted-refed for 12 h on a 60% fructose diet (gray bars) or 60% glucose diet (black bars) as described in Materials and Methods. (**A**) Simplified schematic overview of the genes involved in glycolysis, fructolysis, and gluconeogenesis. F-1-P: fructose-1-phosphate; G-1-P: glucose-1-phosphate; Triose-P: triose phosphate. TCA: tricarboxylic acid; (**B**) Hepatic gene expression of the glycolytic genes glucose transporter 2 (*Glut2*), glucokinase (*Gk*) and *L-pk*; (**C**) Hepatic gene expression of the fructolytic genes fructokinase (*Fk*) and aldolase B (*AldoB*); (**D**) Hepatic gene expression of the gluconeogenic genes phosphoenolpyruvate carboxykinase (*Pepck*) and glucose-6-phosphatase (*G6pc*). Expression of above genes (B-D) were analyzed by real-time quantitative PCR (RT-qPCR) and normalized to TATA-binding protein (*Tbp*); (**E**) Relative metabolite expression levels of hepatic glucose, fructose, pyruvate, lactate, and citrate in response to fructose and glucose feeding in wild type and LXRα$^{-/-}$ mice. Data represent the mean ± standard error of the mean (SEM) (n = 5). Significant differences were found using two-way analysis of variance (ANOVA) followed by Tukey's multiple comparison test (fasted vs. fructose fed and fasted vs. glucose fed were analyzed separately). * $p < 0.05$, ** $p < 0.01$, *** $p < 0.001$ compared to fasted. # $p < 0.05$, ## $p < 0.01$, compared to LXRα$^{+/+}$ mice.

Table 1. Body weight, food intake, and plasma insulin of fasted and refed mice.

Genotype	Treatment	Body Weight (g)	Food Intake (g)	Plasma Insulin (μg/dL)
$LXR\alpha^{+/+}$	Fasted	30.8 ± 2.0		0.7 ± 0.1
	Refed-Fructose	28.4 ± 1.7	2.4 ± 0.4	2.0 ± 0.7
	Refed-Glucose	29.6 ± 2.3	3.3 ± 0.2	7.0 ± 1.0 ***
$LXR\alpha^{-/-}$	Fasted	32.7 ± 1.5		0.7 ± 0.1
	Refed-Fructose	31.1 ± 2.9	2.8 ± 0.2	5.0 ± 1.5 *
	Refed-Glucose	32.1 ± 3.5	2.7 ± 0.4	7.1 ± 0.8 ***

Wild type ($LXR\alpha^{+/+}$) and LXRα knockout ($LXR\alpha^{-/-}$) mice were treated as explained in Materials and Methods. Values are mean ± standard error of the mean (SEM) (n = 5). Significant differences were calculated by two-way analysis of variance (ANOVA) followed by Tukey's multiple comparisons test. * $p < 0.05$, *** $p < 0.001$ compared to fasted within same genotype.

Metabolite analysis showed significantly increased hepatic levels of glucose and also increased hepatic fructose levels in high glucose fed mice (Figure 1E), suggesting increased activity of aldose reductase upon high glucose consumption, as previously reported [35]. Hepatic glucose levels were also higher in fructose fed mice, in agreement with increased glycogen synthesis and turnover [36,37]. We observed elevated hepatic levels of glycogenic metabolites upon both fructose and glucose feeding, likely derived from the continuous production and turnover of glycogen (Supplementary Table S2). Hepatic pyruvate, lactate, and citrate levels were increased in wild type and $LXR\alpha^{-/-}$ mice upon fructose and glucose feeding (Figure 1E), which correspond with increased carbohydrate oxidation after digestion of these carbohydrate rich diets.

3.2. *Expression of Hepatic de novo Lipogenic Genes Mediated by Dietary Glucose Is Reduced in $LXR\alpha^{-/-}$ Compared to Wild Type Mice*

We next addressed the gene expression of central lipogenic enzymes in fasted and refed mice. A schematic representation of DNL and the enzymes involved is presented in Figure 2A. All lipogenic genes assessed, except for *Scd1*, were more strongly upregulated by fructose compared to glucose feeding (Figure 2B), in agreement with previous reports [21,38,39]. Glucose-induced lipogenic gene expression was reduced in $LXR\alpha^{-/-}$ mice (Figure 2B). In line with previous observations in our laboratory [19], *Scd1* expression was not upregulated after high sugar feeding. SCD1 mRNA and protein expression were almost completely abolished in $LXR\alpha^{-/-}$ fasted mice (Figure 2B,C), consistent with a previous study reporting that LXR directly regulate SCD1 expression [40]. Although lipogenic gene expression was significantly induced by both diets in wild type mice, plasma triglyceride levels were not significantly elevated after 12 h refeeding (Figure 2D).

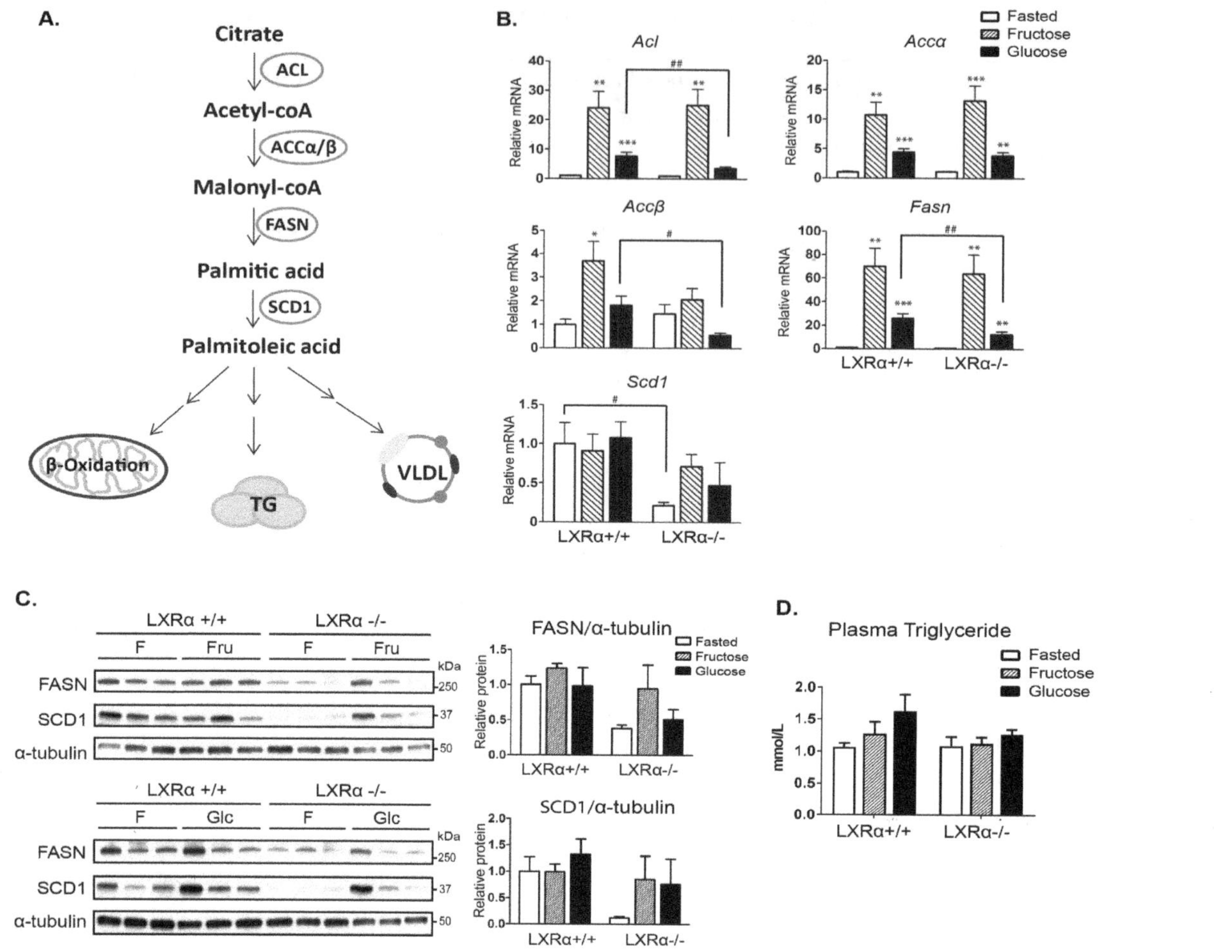

Figure 2. Hepatic *de novo* lipogenic gene expression is dependent on LXRα in response to dietary glucose. (**A**) Simplified schematic overview of genes involved in hepatic *de novo* lipogenesis. VLDL: very low-density lipoprotein; (**B**) Hepatic gene expression of lipogenic genes ATP citrate lyase (*Acl*), acetyl-CoA carboxylase (*Acc*), fatty acid synthase (*Fasn*), and stearoyl-CoA desaturase-1 (*Scd1*) were analyzed by quantitative RT-PCR and normalized to *Tbp*; (**C**) Cytosolic lysates were immunoblotted with antibodies against FASN and SCD1 with α-Tubulin as loading control. Each lane represents independent mice from each experimental group. One representative western blot is shown ($n = 3$). Quantification of cytosolic FASN and SCD1 proteins was analyzed by ImageJ ($n = 5$). F: fasted mice; Fru: fructose-fed mice; Glc: glucose-fed mice; (**D**) Plasma triglycerides (TG). Data represent the mean ± SEM ($n = 5$). Significant differences were found using two-way ANOVA followed by Tukey's multiple comparison test (fasted vs. fructose fed and fasted vs. glucose fed RNA data were analyzed separately). * $p < 0.05$, ** $p < 0.01$, *** $p < 0.001$ compared to fasted. # $p < 0.05$, ## $p < 0.01$, compared to LXR$\alpha^{+/+}$ mice.

3.3. Regulation of *Srebp-1* and *Chrebpβ* Expression Mediated by Dietary Glucose Is Dependent of LXRα

LXRs, and particularly LXRα, are known as upstream regulators of SREBP-1c and CHREBPα expression in response to glucose and insulin, and all three transcription factors are involved in the regulation of hepatic lipogenic enzyme genes described above [6,19]. Recent investigations have shown that ChREBPα is activated by dietary fructose, which in turn induces the expression of *Chrebpβ* [21,23]. We did not observe significant changes in *Chrebpα* mRNA levels by both diets in wild type mice, while high fructose feeding more potently induced *Chrebpβ* mRNA expression as compared to glucose (Figure 3A). Compared to wild type mice, *Chrebpβ* mRNA expression was significantly reduced in glucose fed, but not in fructose fed LXR$\alpha^{-/-}$ mice, concomitant with reduced nuclear LXRβ protein expression in glucose-fed LXRα$^{-/-}$ mice (Figure 3B, quantification is shown in Supplementary Figure S1B). This supports our previous observations that both LXR isoforms are necessary to maintain hepatic ChREBPα activity in response to glucose [19], and suggests that LXRβ is able to compensate for the lack of LXRα in regulation of ChREBPα in fructose fed mice. SREBP-1 mRNA and protein (proform) expression were significantly reduced in glucose fed LXRα$^{-/-}$ mice (Figure 3A,B, quantification in Supplementary Figure S1A), supporting the role of LXRα as a central regulator of hepatic *Srebp-1*expression. Notably, we could only detect the ChREBPα protein but not ChREBPβ in our in vivo liver samples, suggestive of a high turnover (rapid degradation) of the constitutively active nuclear ChREBPβ protein.

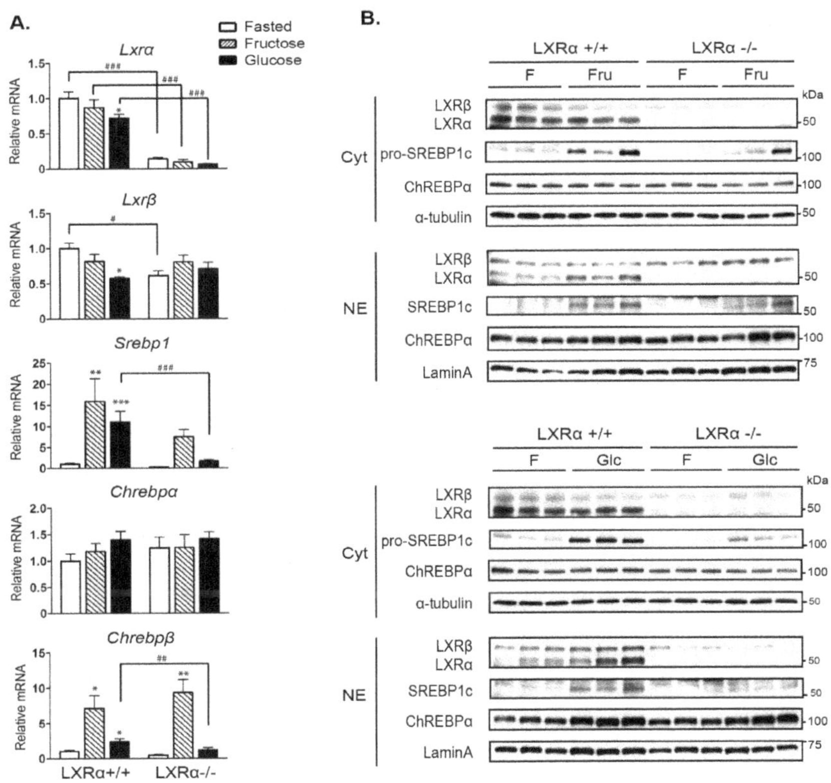

Figure 3. Induction of hepatic *Srebp-1* and carbohydrate response element-binding protein (*Chrebp*)*β* expression by dietary glucose is reduced in LXRα$^{-/-}$ mice. (**A**) Hepatic gene expression of *Lxrα/β*, *Srebp-1*, and *Chrebpα/β* was analyzed by quantitative RT-PCR and normalized to *Tbp*; (**B**) Cytosolic and nuclear lysates were immunoblotted with antibodies against LXR, SREBP-1, and ChREBP with α-Tubulin and Lamin A as loading controls. Each lane represents independent mice from each group. One representative western blot is shown ($n = 3$). Data represent the mean ± SEM ($n = 5$). Significant differences were found using two-way ANOVA followed by Tukey's multiple comparison test (fasted vs. fructose fed and fasted vs. glucose fed RNA data were analyzed separately). * $p < 0.05$, ** $p < 0.01$, *** $p < 0.001$ compared to fasted. # $p < 0.05$, ## $p < 0.01$, ### $p < 0.001$ compared to LXRα$^{+/+}$ mice.

3.4. Dietary Fructose Induces Nuclear O-GlcNAc Signaling

O-GlcNAcylation of ChREBPα has been shown to potentiate its activity, stability, and binding to the *L-pk* promoter in response to refeeding in normal mice and more so in hyperglycemic diabetic mice [13]. The hexosamine biosynthetic pathway (HBP) involving activation of OGT is depicted in Figure 4A. Metabolomics analysis revealed lower levels of *N*-acetylglucosamine-1-P (GlcNAc-1-P) in refed mice with both diets compared to fasting (Supplementary Table S2), suggesting high glutamine-fructose-6-phosphate amidotransferase 2 (GFAT2) activity during fasting, possibly via glucagon-PKA-mediated activation [41]. Although HPLC analysis showed no significant increase in total liver UDP-GlcNAc levels in refed compared to fasted mice (Figure 4B), the fraction of UDP-GlcNAc that is utilized for *O*-GlcNAc modification may be increased towards the nuclear pool after refeeding. Ogt mRNA levels were strongly downregulated upon refeeding (Figure 4C), which is suggestive of a negative feedback regulation due to high OGT activity, as reported previously [42]. We observed increased nuclear protein *O*-GlcNAcylation levels upon fructose refeeding in wild type mice (Figure 4D, quantification in Supplementary Figure S2B). Notably, the *O*-GlcNAcylation of LXRβ was significantly increased in fructose-fed LXRα$^{-/-}$ mice (representative western blots in Figure 4E, quantification (n = 4) in Supplementary Figure S2C).

Because ChREBP binding to its cognate DNA-binding site in the *L-pk* promoter is affected by high glucose feeding, *O*-GlcNAc and LXRα/β signaling in rat and mice livers [13,19,43], we next investigated ChREBP recruitment to the *L-pk* promoter in chromatin immunoprecipitation (ChIP) assays. We did not observe a significant increase in ChREBP recruitment after refeeding in wild type mice, but observed a significant increase after fructose feeding in LXRα$^{-/-}$ mice (Figure 4F). This observation, together with increased *O*-GlcNAcylation of LXRβ, suggests that LXRβ may compensate for the lack of LXRα in regulating ChREBPα activity upon fructose feeding.

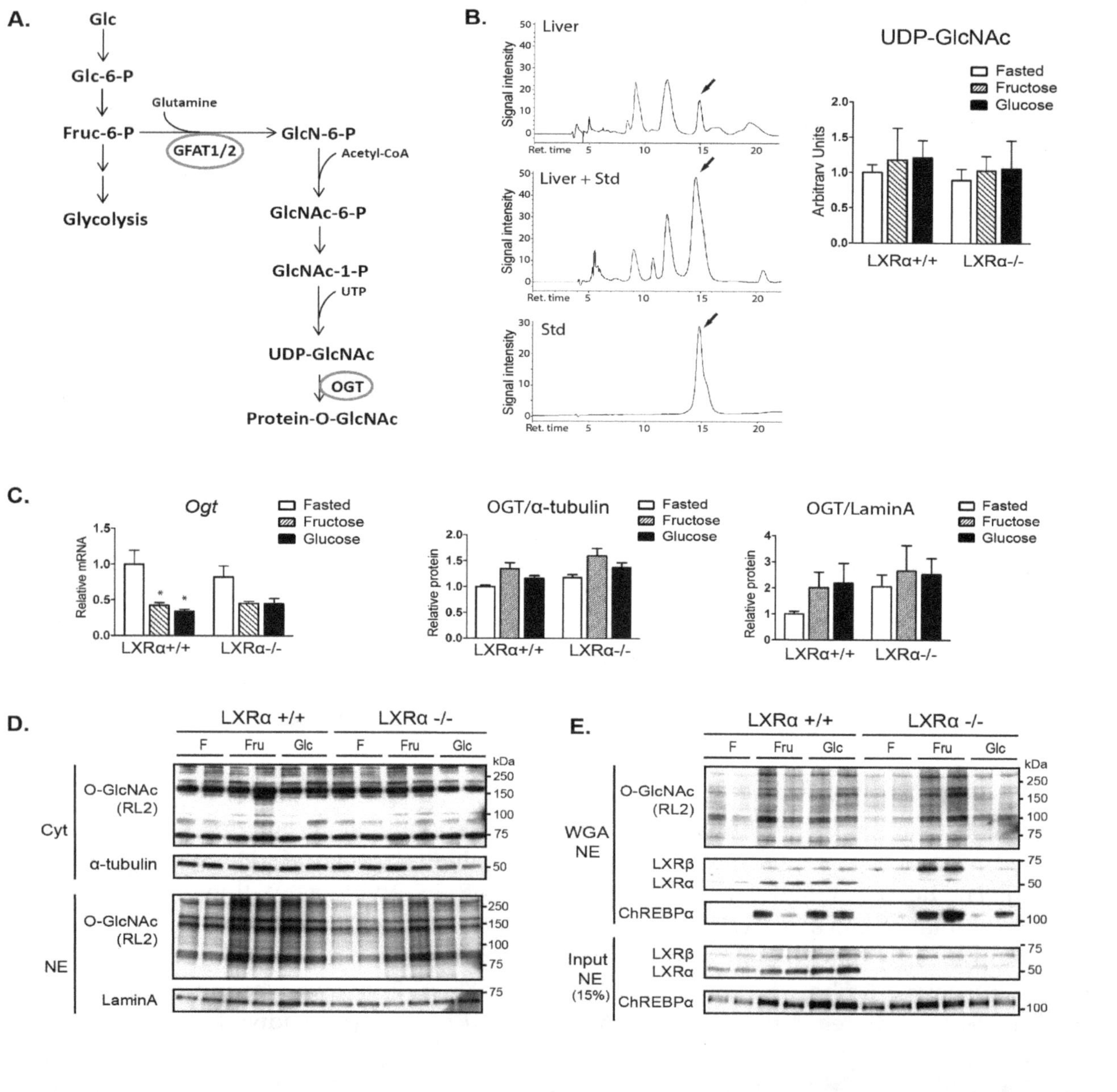

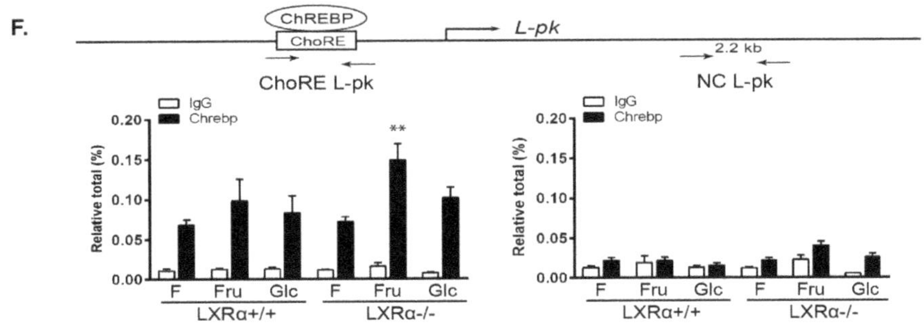

Figure 4. Dietary fructose induces nuclear *O*-GlcNAc signaling. (**A**) Simplified schematic overview of the hexosamine signaling pathway including the rate limiting enzyme GFAT and *O*-GlcNAc transferase (OGT); (**B**) High-performance liquid chromatography (HPLC) analysis of hepatic UDP-GlcNAc levels. Left panel: Example of a typical running profile with or without injection of UDP-GlcNAc standard (Std.) is shown. Right panel: Quantification of the HPLC data normalized to protein concentration; (**C**) Hepatic expression of the *Ogt* gene and cytosolic and nuclear OGT protein were analyzed by quantitative RT-PCR and western blotting/Image J and normalized to *Tbp*, α-tubulin, and Lamin A, respectively. Data represent the mean ± SEM (n = 5); (**D**) Cytosolic and nuclear lysates were immunoblotted with anti-*O*-GlcNAc antibody (RL2) with α-Tubulin and Lamin A as loading controls. Each lane represents independent mice from each group. One representative western blot is shown (n = 2); (**E**) Nuclear lysates were subjected to wheat germ agglutinin (WGA) beads to precipitate *O*-GlcNAcylated proteins. WGA enriched samples (upper panel) and input lysates (bottom panel) were immunoblotted with antibodies detecting *O*-GlcNAcylated proteins (RL2), LXR and ChREBP. Each lane represents independent mice from experimental groups. Representative western blots are shown (n = 2); (**F**) ChREBP binding to the carbohydrate response element (ChoRE) containing region of the *L-pk* promoter and negative control sequence (NC) 2216–2288 bp into the *L-pk* gene after ChoRE sequence was detected by chromatin immunoprecipitation (ChIP) using antibodies against ChREBP or IgG as a control. Data represent the mean ± SEM (n = 5). Significant differences were found using two-way ANOVA followed by Tukey's multiple comparison test. ** $p < 0.01$ compared to fasted.

4. Discussion and Conclusions

The results of this study show that LXRα is important for ChREBPα activity upon glucose, but not fructose feeding in the livers of mice, as visualized by lower expression of ChREBPα specific target genes *L-pk* and *Chrebpβ* in LXRα$^{-/-}$ compared to wild type mice. LXRα is also important for the transcriptional control of classical hepatic DNL genes upon glucose feeding, including *Fasn* and *Accβ*. This suggests that LXRα is important in integrating nutritional cues upon glucose feeding upstream of ChREBPα.

In the human diet, fructose and glucose are rarely consumed in isolation. Studies comparing more commonly consumed sucrose and high fructose corn syrup have yielded different results compared to studies with pure fructose or glucose [37]. However, long-term feeding studies (12 h or more) in rat and mice have shown similar fold induction of hepatic lipogenic genes by high fructose compared to sucrose and always above levels in mice fed high glucose [21,33,34,38]. This is likely due to most of the dietary fructose being taken up by the liver whereas only 30% of dietary glucose is metabolized by the liver; the remaining glucose is metabolized in muscle, adipose tissues, brain, kidney, and red blood cells [44]. However, approximately 30–50% of fructose taken up by the liver is converted to glucose and 15% to lactate in part as a fuel source for extrahepatic tissues [37,45]. This suggests additive effects of hepatic glucose and fructose metabolism and signaling in the control of DNL in response to dietary fructose, at least in the late refed phase. This is supported by a study by Matsuzaka et al. [34] that showed the expression of SREBP-1 and FASN above glucose-induced levels after 9 h fructose feeding concomitant with increased plasma glucose and insulin levels. At 6 h refeeding, however, glucose, but not fructose, strongly induced SREBP-1 and FASN expression. Stamatikos et al. reported increased fructose-induced *Accα* and *Fasn* gene expression following inhibition of Fructose-1,6-biphosphatase (FBPase) in human hepatocyte carcinoma (HepG2) cells, suggesting that dietary fructose induces DNL gene expression independently of its ability to generate glucose [21]. However, these results were not verified in primary hepatocytes, suggesting that this effect may be specific for hepatoma cells.

In the present study, we observed similar hepatic glucose levels in fructose and glucose fed mice, but significantly higher pyruvate levels after fructose feeding. This observation is concomitant with more strongly induced expression of the ChREBP target gene *L-pk* upon fructose feeding than glucose feeding, in agreement with previous observations [34]. This supports the notion that fructose activates ChREBP and *L-pk* expression to a higher degree than glucose, thus generating more substrate to DNL [39,46,47]. Notably, *L-pk* expression was almost back to fasting levels in LXRα depleted glucose fed mice, but not in fructose fed mice, suggesting differential roles of LXRα and ChREBP in response to early phase of glucose and fructose metabolism.

We have recently shown that LXR$\alpha^{-/-}/\beta^{-/-}$ mice have reduced nuclear *O*-GlcNAc levels, ChREBPα activity, and lipogenic gene expression in livers as compared wild type mice upon refeeding with a chow diet [19]. Herein, we provide evidence that LXRα is important for ChREBPα activity upon glucose feeding. The effects on hepatic DNL is less striking when depleting LXRα alone, and LXRα was dispensable in fructose fed, but not glucose fed mice, which were also low in LXRβ protein levels. Levels of nuclear LXRβ protein were maintained in fructose fed but surprisingly strongly reduced in glucose fed LXR$\alpha^{-/-}$ mice, suggesting compensation by LXRβ in regulating SREBP-1c and lipogenic gene expression in fructose fed mice. This may be explained, at least in part, by redundancy between the LXRs [48]. Notably, increased WGA-recovery of LXRβ and ChREBPα, which is indicative of increased *O*-GlcNAc modifications of these proteins, was observed in fructose fed LXR$\alpha^{-/-}$ mice along with increased ChREBP binding to the *L-pk* promoter in these mice. It is thus possible that LXRα, LXRβ, and ChREBPα collectively integrate different sugar metabolites with lipogenesis in a wild type context. Acetyl-CoA generated by the ACL enzyme, which was strongly upregulated by fructose feeding (Figure 1B), also acts as a substrate for protein acetylation [49]. Metabolic sensing by LXRs and ChREBP involves modification by *O*-GlcNAcylation and acetylation [50,51] and there seems to be interplay between OGT and the acetylating p300 transcriptional coregulator [52], which is likely to impact LXR and ChREBP activity [53].

We did not observe reduced levels of nuclear *O*-GlcNAcylated proteins when knocking out LXRα, suggesting that both LXRα and β must be depleted for this phenotype. Because *O*-GlcNAc modification of ChREBPα is important for its activity and because ChREBPα was more modified in fructose fed LXR$\alpha^{-/-}$ mice, it would be interesting to study if the dietary effects of fructose on DNL gene expression and ChREBPα activity would have been more pronounced in an animal model where both LXR isoforms were depleted.

In summary, we provide evidence that hepatic expression of *de novo* lipogenic genes require LXRα activity in response to dietary glucose and that LXRβ may compensate for the lack of LXRα in fructose fed mice. As aberrant *O*-GlcNAc signaling during nutrient stress and diabetes leads to excessive glucose production and lipid accumulation in the liver [54], studies including mutated O-GlcNAc residues in LXRs and ChREBPα will provide a better understanding of the relevance of coordinated *O*-GlcNAcylation of these transcriptional regulators under physiological and pathophysiological conditions.

Supplementary Materials: Figure S1: Quantification of cytosolic and nuclear proteins LXRα/β, SREBP-1 and ChREBPα. Western blot quantification of cytosolic (A) and nuclear (B) proteins was analyzed by ImageJ. Data represent the mean ± SEM (n = 3–4). Significant differences were found using two-way ANOVA followed by Tukey's multiple comparison test. ** $p < 0.01$, *** $p < 0.001$ compared to fasted. # $p < 0.05$, ## $p < 0.01$, ### $p < 0.001$ compared to LXR$\alpha^{+/+}$ mice. Figure S2: Quantification of nuclear lysates input and WGA enriched proteins LXRα/β, ChREBPα and *O*-GlcNAcylation levels (RL2). Western blot quantification of cytosolic lysates (A), nuclear lysates input (B), and WGA enriched (C) proteins were analyzed by ImageJ. Data represent the mean ± SEM (n = 4). Significant differences were found using two-way ANOVA followed by Tukey's multiple comparison test. * $p < 0.05$ compared to fasted. # $p < 0.05$,

$p < 0.01$, ### $p < 0.001$ compared to LXR$\alpha^{+/+}$ mice. Table S1: Mouse SYBR Green Primers sequences. Table S2: Metabolomics analysis of liver tissues of wild type and LXR$\alpha^{-/-}$ mice.

Acknowledgments: This work was supported by grants from the University of Oslo, the Research Council of Norway, the Johan Throne Holst Foundation, the Novo Nordic Foundation, and the Anders Jahre Foundation. The authors thank Timothy F. Osborne (University of California) for providing the SREBP-1 antibody and Gerald Hart (Johns Hopkins University) for providing the OGT AL25 antibody.

Author Contributions: L.M.G., H.I.N., K.T.D. and C.B. conceived and designed the experiments; Q.F., R.C.N., C.L., C.B., K.T.D. and E.B. performed experiments; Q.F., R.C.N., C.L., H.M.I. and J.M. analyzed data; Q.F., H.M.I., L.M.G. and J.M. interpreted results of experiments; Q.F. and L.M.G. prepared figures; Q.F. and L.M.G. drafted manuscript; Q.F. and L.M.G. edited and revised the manuscript; all co-authors approved the final version of manuscript.

References

1. Bantle, J.P.; Raatz, S.K.; Thomas, W.; Georgopoulos, A. Effects of dietary fructose on plasma lipids in healthy subjects. *Am. J. Clin. Nutr.* **2000**, *72*, 1128–1134. [PubMed]
2. Parks, E.J.; Hellerstein, M.K. Carbohydrate-induced hypertriacylglycerolemia: Historical perspective and review of biological mechanisms. *Am. J. Clin. Nutr.* **2000**, *71*, 412–433. [PubMed]
3. Faeh, D.; Minehira, K.; Schwarz, J.M.; Periasamy, R.; Park, S.; Tappy, L. Effect of fructose overfeeding and fish oil administration on hepatic de novo lipogenesis and insulin sensitivity in healthy men. *Diabetes* **2005**, *54*, 1907–1913. [CrossRef] [PubMed]
4. Caton, P.W.; Nayuni, N.K.; Khan, N.Q.; Wood, E.G.; Corder, R. Fructose induces gluconeogenesis and lipogenesis through a SIRT1-dependent mechanism. *J. Endocrinol.* **2011**, *208*, 273–283. [CrossRef] [PubMed]
5. Strable, M.S.; Ntambi, J.M. Genetic control of de novo lipogenesis: Role in diet-induced obesity. *Crit. Rev. Biochem. Mol. Biol.* **2010**, *45*, 199–214. [CrossRef] [PubMed]
6. Grønning-Wang, L.M.; Bindesbøll, C.; Nebb, H.I. *The Role of Liver X Receptor in Hepatic de novo Lipogenesis and Cross-Talk with Insulin and Glucose Signaling*; INTECH Open Access Publisher: Rijeka, Croatia, 2013.
7. Repa, J.J.; Mangelsdorf, D.J. The role of orphan nuclear receptors in the regulation of cholesterol homeostasis. *Annu. Rev. Cell Dev. Biol.* **2000**, *16*, 459–481. [CrossRef] [PubMed]
8. Filhoulaud, G.; Guilmeau, S.; Dentin, R.; Girard, J.; Postic, C. Novel insights into ChREBP regulation and function. *Trends Endocrinol. Metab.* **2013**, *24*, 257–268. [CrossRef] [PubMed]
9. Laffitte, B.A.; Chao, L.C.; Li, J.; Walczak, R.; Hummasti, S.; Joseph, S.B.; Castrillo, A.; Wilpitz, D.C.; Mangelsdorf, D.J.; Collins, J.L.; et al. Activation of liver X receptor improves glucose tolerance through coordinate regulation of glucose metabolism in liver and adipose tissue. *Proc. Natl. Acad. Sci. USA* **2003**, *100*, 5419–5424. [CrossRef] [PubMed]
10. Cao, G.; Liang, Y.; Broderick, C.L.; Oldham, B.A.; Beyer, T.P.; Schmidt, R.J.; Zhang, Y.; Stayrook, K.R.; Suen, C.; Otto, K.A.; et al. Antidiabetic action of a liver x receptor agonist mediated by inhibition of hepatic gluconeogenesis. *J. Boil. Chem.* **2003**, *278*, 1131–1136. [CrossRef] [PubMed]
11. Grempler, R.; Gunther, S.; Steffensen, K.R.; Nilsson, M.; Barthel, A.; Schmoll, D.; Walther, R. Evidence for an indirect transcriptional regulation of glucose-6-phosphatase gene expression by liver X receptors. *Biochem. Biophys. Res. Commun.* **2005**, *338*, 981–986. [CrossRef] [PubMed]
12. Anthonisen, E.H.; Berven, L.; Holm, S.; Nygard, M.; Nebb, H.I.; Gronning-Wang, L.M. Nuclear Receptor Liver X Receptor Is *O*-GlcNAc-modified in Response to Glucose. *J. Biol. Chem.* **2010**, *285*, 1607–1615. [CrossRef] [PubMed]
13. Guinez, C.; Filhoulaud, G.; Rayah-Benhamed, F.; Marmier, S.; Dubuquoy, C.; Dentin, R.; Moldes, M.; Burnol, A.F.; Yang, X.; Lefebvre, T.; et al. *O*-GlcNAcylation increases ChREBP protein content and transcriptional activity in the liver. *Diabetes* **2011**, *60*, 1399–1413. [CrossRef] [PubMed]
14. Bond, M.R.; Hanover, J.A. A little sugar goes a long way: The cell biology of *O*-GlcNAc. *J. Cell Biol.* **2015**, *208*, 869–880. [CrossRef] [PubMed]
15. Hart, G.W.; Slawson, C.; Ramirez-Correa, G.; Lagerlof, O. Cross talk between *O*-GlcNAcylation and phosphorylation: Roles in signaling, transcription, and chronic disease. *Annu. Rev. Biochem.* **2011**, *80*, 825–858. [CrossRef] [PubMed]
16. Gambetta, M.C.; Muller, J. A critical perspective of the diverse roles of *O*-GlcNAc transferase in chromatin. *Chromosoma* **2015**, *124*, 429–442. [CrossRef] [PubMed]

17. Rumberger, J.M.; Wu, T.; Hering, M.A.; Marshall, S. Role of hexosamine biosynthesis in glucose-mediated up-regulation of lipogenic enzyme mRNA levels: Effects of glucose, glutamine, and glucosamine on glycerophosphate dehydrogenase, fatty acid synthase, and acetyl-CoA carboxylase mRNA levels. *J. Biol. Chem.* **2003**, *278*, 28547–28552. [CrossRef] [PubMed]
18. Bindesbøll, C.; Grønning-Wang, L.M. Liver X receptors connect nuclear *O*-GlcNAc signaling to hepatic glucose utilization and lipogenesis. *Recept. Clin. Investig.* **2015**. [CrossRef]
19. Bindesboll, C.; Fan, Q.; Norgaard, R.C.; MacPherson, L.; Ruan, H.B.; Wu, J.; Pedersen, T.A.; Steffensen, K.R.; Yang, X.; Matthews, J.; et al. Liver X receptor regulates hepatic nuclear *O*-GlcNAc signaling and carbohydrate responsive element-binding protein activity. *J. Lipid Res.* **2015**, *56*, 771–785. [CrossRef] [PubMed]
20. Herman, M.A.; Peroni, O.D.; Villoria, J.; Schon, M.R.; Abumrad, N.A.; Bluher, M.; Klein, S.; Kahn, B.B. A novel ChREBP isoform in adipose tissue regulates systemic glucose metabolism. *Nature* **2012**, *484*, 333–338. [CrossRef] [PubMed]
21. Stamatikos, A.D.; da Silva, R.P.; Lewis, J.T.; Douglas, D.N.; Kneteman, N.M.; Jacobs, R.L.; Paton, C.M. Tissue Specific Effects of Dietary Carbohydrates and Obesity on ChREBPα and ChREBPβ Expression. *Lipids* **2016**, *51*, 95–104. [CrossRef] [PubMed]
22. Zhang, P.; Kumar, A.; Katz, L.S.; Li, L.; Paulynice, M.; Herman, M.A.; Scott, D.K. Induction of the ChREBPβ Isoform Is Essential for Glucose-Stimulated β-Cell Proliferation. *Diabetes* **2015**, *64*, 4158–4170. [CrossRef] [PubMed]
23. Erion, D.M.; Popov, V.; Hsiao, J.J.; Vatner, D.; Mitchell, K.; Yonemitsu, S.; Nagai, Y.; Kahn, M.; Gillum, M. P.; Dong, J.; et al. The role of the carbohydrate response element-binding protein in male fructose-fed rats. *Endocrinology* **2013**, *154*, 36–44. [CrossRef] [PubMed]
24. Iizuka, K.; Bruick, R.K.; Liang, G.; Horton, J.D.; Uyeda, K. Deficiency of carbohydrate response element-binding protein (ChREBP) reduces lipogenesis as well as glycolysis. *Proc. Natl. Acad. Sci. USA* **2004**, *101*, 7281–7286. [CrossRef] [PubMed]
25. Kim, M.S.; Krawczyk, S.A.; Doridot, L.; Fowler, A.J.; Wang, J.X.; Trauger, S.A.; Noh, H.L.; Kang, H.J.; Meissen, J.K.; Blatnik, M.; et al. ChREBP regulates fructose-induced glucose production independently of insulin signaling. *J. Clin. Investig.* **2016**, *126*, 4372–4386. [CrossRef] [PubMed]
26. Hessvik, N.P.; Boekschoten, M.V.; Baltzersen, M.A.; Kersten, S.; Xu, X.; Andersen, H.; Rustan, A.C.; Thoresen, G.H. LXRβ is the dominant LXR subtype in skeletal muscle regulating lipogenesis and cholesterol efflux. *Am. J. Physiol. Endocrinol. Metab.* **2010**, *298*, E602–E613. [CrossRef] [PubMed]
27. Rull, A.; Geeraert, B.; Aragones, G.; Beltran-Debon, R.; Rodriguez-Gallego, E.; Garcia-Heredia, A.; Pedro-Botet, J.; Joven, J.; Holvoet, P.; Camps, J. Rosiglitazone and fenofibrate exacerbate liver steatosis in a mouse model of obesity and hyperlipidemia. A transcriptomic and metabolomic study. *J. Proteome Res.* **2014**, *13*, 1731–1743. [CrossRef] [PubMed]
28. Ye, J.; Coulouris, G.; Zaretskaya, I.; Cutcutache, I.; Rozen, S.; Madden, T.L. Primer-BLAST: A tool to design target-specific primers for polymerase chain reaction. *BMC Bioinform.* **2012**, *13*, 134. [CrossRef] [PubMed]
29. Iyer, S.P.; Akimoto, Y.; Hart, G.W. Identification and cloning of a novel family of coiled-coil domain proteins that interact with *O*-GlcNAc transferase. *J. Biol. Chem.* **2003**, *278*, 5399–5409. [CrossRef] [PubMed]
30. Seo, Y.K.; Chong, H.K.; Infante, A.M.; Im, S.S.; Xie, X.; Osborne, T.F. Genome-wide analysis of SREBP-1 binding in mouse liver chromatin reveals a preference for promoter proximal binding to a new motif. *Proc. Natl. Acad. Sci. USA* **2009**, *106*, 13765–13769. [CrossRef] [PubMed]
31. Itkonen, H.M.; Engedal, N.; Babaie, E.; Luhr, M.; Guldvik, I.J.; Minner, S.; Hohloch, J.; Tsourlakis, M.C.; Schlomm, T.; Mills, I.G. UAP1 is overexpressed in prostate cancer and is protective against inhibitors of *N*-linked glycosylation. *Oncogene* **2015**, *34*, 3744–3750. [CrossRef] [PubMed]
32. Nakajima, K.; Kitazume, S.; Angata, T.; Fujinawa, R.; Ohtsubo, K.; Miyoshi, E.; Taniguchi, N. Simultaneous determination of nucleotide sugars with ion-pair reversed-phase HPLC. *Glycobiology* **2010**, *20*, 865–871. [CrossRef] [PubMed]
33. Koo, H.Y.; Wallig, M.A.; Chung, B.H.; Nara, T.Y.; Cho, B.H.; Nakamura, M.T. Dietary fructose induces a wide range of genes with distinct shift in carbohydrate and lipid metabolism in fed and fasted rat liver. *Biochim. Biophys. Acta* **2008**, *1782*, 341–348. [CrossRef] [PubMed]
34. Matsuzaka, T.; Shimano, H.; Yahagi, N.; Amemiya-Kudo, M.; Okazaki, H.; Tamura, Y.; Iizuka, Y.; Ohashi, K.; Tomita, S.; Sekiya, M.; et al. Insulin-independent induction of sterol regulatory element-binding protein-1c expression in the livers of streptozotocin-treated mice. *Diabetes* **2004**, *53*, 560–569. [CrossRef] [PubMed]

35. Lanaspa, M.A.; Ishimoto, T.; Li, N.; Cicerchi, C.; Orlicky, D.J.; Ruzycki, P.; Rivard, C.; Inaba, S.; Roncal-Jimenez, C.A.; Bales, E.S.; et al. Endogenous fructose production and metabolism in the liver contributes to the development of metabolic syndrome. *Nat. Commun.* **2013**, *4*, 2434. [CrossRef] [PubMed]
36. Tounian, P.; Schneiter, P.; Henry, S.; Jequier, E.; Tappy, L. Effects of infused fructose on endogenous glucose production, gluconeogenesis, and glycogen metabolism. *Am. J. Physiol.* **1994**, *267*, E710–E717. [CrossRef]
37. Rippe, J.M.; Angelopoulos, T.J. Sucrose, high-fructose corn syrup, and fructose, their metabolism and potential health effects: What do we really know? *Adv. Nutr. Int. Rev. J.* **2013**, *4*, 236–245. [CrossRef] [PubMed]
38. Janevski, M.; Ratnayake, S.; Siljanovski, S.; McGlynn, M.A.; Cameron-Smith, D.; Lewandowski, P. Fructose containing sugars modulate mRNA of lipogenic genes ACC and FAS and protein levels of transcription factors ChREBP and SREBP1c with no effect on body weight or liver fat. *Food Funct.* **2012**, *3*, 141–149. [CrossRef] [PubMed]
39. Koo, H.Y.; Miyashita, M.; Cho, B.H.; Nakamura, M.T. Replacing dietary glucose with fructose increases ChREBP activity and SREBP-1 protein in rat liver nucleus. *Biochem. Biophys. Res. Commun.* **2009**, *390*, 285–289. [CrossRef] [PubMed]
40. Chu, K.; Miyazaki, M.; Man, W.C.; Ntambi, J.M. Stearoyl-coenzyme A desaturase 1 deficiency protects against hypertriglyceridemia and increases plasma high-density lipoprotein cholesterol induced by liver X receptor activation. *Mol. Cell. Biol.* **2006**, *26*, 6786–6798. [CrossRef] [PubMed]
41. Hu, Y.; Riesland, L.; Paterson, A.J.; Kudlow, J.E. Phosphorylation of mouse glutamine-fructose-6-phosphate amidotransferase 2 (GFAT2) by cAMP-dependent protein kinase increases the enzyme activity. *J. Biol. Chem.* **2004**, *279*, 29988–29993. [CrossRef] [PubMed]
42. Taylor, R.P.; Geisler, T.S.; Chambers, J.H.; McClain, D.A. Up-regulation of *O*-GlcNAc transferase with glucose deprivation in HepG2 cells is mediated by decreased hexosamine pathway flux. *J. Boil. Chem.* **2009**, *284*, 3425–3432. [CrossRef] [PubMed]
43. Ishii, S.; Iizuka, K.; Miller, B.C.; Uyeda, K. Carbohydrate response element binding protein directly promotes lipogenic enzyme gene transcription. *Proc. Natl. Acad. Sci. USA* **2004**, *101*, 15597–15602. [CrossRef] [PubMed]
44. Moore, M.C.; Coate, K.C.; Winnick, J.J.; An, Z.; Cherrington, A.D. Regulation of hepatic glucose uptake and storage in vivo. *Adv. Nutr. (Bethesda, Md.)* **2012**, *3*, 286–294. [CrossRef] [PubMed]
45. Sun, S.Z.; Empie, M.W. Fructose metabolism in humans—What isotopic tracer studies tell us. *Nutr. Metab.* **2012**, *9*, 89. [CrossRef] [PubMed]
46. Parks, E.J.; Skokan, L.E.; Timlin, M.T.; Dingfelder, C.S. Dietary sugars stimulate fatty acid synthesis in adults. *J. Nutr.* **2008**, *138*, 1039–1046. [PubMed]
47. Moore, J.B.; Gunn, P.J.; Fielding, B.A. The role of dietary sugars and *de novo* lipogenesis in non-alcoholic fatty liver disease. *Nutrients* **2014**, *6*, 5679–5703. [CrossRef] [PubMed]
48. Quinet, E.M.; Savio, D.A.; Halpern, A.R.; Chen, L.; Schuster, G.U.; Gustafsson, J.A.; et al. Liver X receptor (LXR)-β regulation in LXRα-deficient mice: Implications for therapeutic targeting. *Mol. Pharmacol.* **2006**, *70*, 1340–1349. [CrossRef] [PubMed]
49. Choudhary, C.; Weinert, B.T.; Nishida, Y.; Verdin, E.; Mann, M. The growing landscape of lysine acetylation links metabolism and cell signalling. *Nat. Rev. Mol. Cell Biol.* **2014**, *15*, 536–550. [CrossRef] [PubMed]
50. Li, X.; Zhang, S.; Blander, G.; Tse, J.G.; Krieger, M.; Guarente, L. SIRT1 deacetylates and positively regulates the nuclear receptor LXR. *Mol. Cell* **2007**, *28*, 91–106. [CrossRef] [PubMed]
51. Bricambert, J.; Miranda, J.; Benhamed, F.; Girard, J.; Postic, C.; Dentin, R. Salt-inducible kinase 2 links transcriptional coactivator p300 phosphorylation to the prevention of ChREBP-dependent hepatic steatosis in mice. *J. Clin. Investig.* **2010**, *120*, 4316–4331. [CrossRef] [PubMed]
52. Allison, D.F.; Wamsley, J.J.; Kumar, M.; Li, D.; Gray, L.G.; Hart, G.W.; Jones, D.R.; Mayo, M.W. Modification of RelA by *O*-linked *N*-acetylglucosamine links glucose metabolism to NF-κB acetylation and transcription. *Proc. Natl. Acad. Sci. USA* **2012**, *109*, 16888–16893. [CrossRef] [PubMed]
53. Oosterveer, M.H.; Schoonjans, K. Hepatic glucose sensing and integrative pathways in the liver. *Cell. Mol. Life Sci. CMLS* **2014**, *71*, 1453–1467. [CrossRef] [PubMed]
54. Zhang, K.; Yin, R.; Yang, X. *O*-GlcNAc: A Bittersweet Switch in Liver. *Front. Endocrinol.* **2014**, *5*, 221. [CrossRef] [PubMed]

17

The Influence of Pre-Exercise Glucose versus Fructose Ingestion on Subsequent Postprandial Lipemia

Tsung-Jen Yang [1], Chih-Hui Chiu [2], Mei-Hui Tseng [3], Cheng-Kang Chang [3] and Ching-Lin Wu [4,*]

1 Department of Physical Education, National Taiwan Normal University, Taipei 106, Taiwan; andy32437@yahoo.com.tw
2 Graduate Program in Department of Exercise Health Science, National Taiwan University of Sport, Taichung 404, Taiwan; loveshalom@hotmail.com
3 Sport Science Research Center, National Taiwan University of Sport, Taichung 404, Taiwan; tsengmh2009@gmail.com (M.-H.T.); wspahn@seed.net.tw (C.-K.C.)
4 Graduate Institute of Sports and Health Management, National Chung Hsing University, Taichung 402, Taiwan
* Correspondence: psclw@dragon.nchu.edu.com

Abstract: Ingestion of low glycemic index (LGI) carbohydrate (CHO) before exercise induced less insulin response and higher fat oxidation than that of high GI (HGI) CHO during subsequent exercise. However, the effect on the subsequent postprandial lipid profile is still unclear. Therefore, the aim of this study was to investigate ingestion of CHO drinks with different GI using fructose and glucose before endurance exercise on the subsequent postprandial lipid profile. Eight healthy active males completed two experimental trials in randomized double-blind cross-over design. All participants ingested 500 mL CHO (75 g) solution either fructose (F) or glucose (G) before running on the treadmill at 60% VO_2max for 1 h. Participants were asked to take an oral fat tolerance test (OFTT) immediately after the exercise. Blood samples were obtained for plasma and serum analysis. The F trial was significantly lower than the G trial in TG total area under the curve (AUC; 9.97 $\pm$ 3.64 vs. 10.91 $\pm$ 3.56 mmol $\times$ 6 h/L; $p = 0.033$) and incremental AUC (6.57 $\pm$ 2.46 vs. 7.14 $\pm$ 2.64 mmol/L $\times$ 6 h, $p = 0.004$). The current data suggested that a pre-exercise fructose drink showed a lower postprandial lipemia than a glucose drink after the subsequent high-fat meal.

Keywords: glycemic index; triacylglycerol; high-density lipoprotein; fat oxidation; oral fat tolerance test

1. Introduction

An increase in postprandial plasma triacylglycerol (TG) concentrations was suggested to cause damage on vascular subcutaneous cells and vascular walls [1]. The postprandial lipemia phenomena may last for 6 to 8 h [2], suggesting that a high postprandial TG concentration in the circulation is likely lasting an entire day after breakfast is ingested. A number of studies indicated that an increase in postprandial TG level correlates positively with the mortality rate and risk of cardiovascular disease (CVD) [3–5]. In order to reduce high postprandial TG concentrations, several studies proposed that endurance exercise was effective for lowering postprandial TG concentrations [6–8].

A high-carbohydrate (CHO) diet increases the storage and use of muscle glycogen, and improves exercise performance [9,10]. However, a high CHO diet might cause a rise in very-low-density lipoprotein (VLDL) concentration [11–13] and a reduction in the level of high-density lipoprotein cholesterol (HDL-C) [14], which were considered to increase the risk of CVD. Previous study showed exercise intervention might elevate the level of HDL-C, increase lipoprotein lipase (LPL) activity [15], increase the transportation of blood lipids into the muscle cells for storage or use, and lower postprandial TG concentrations [11,16]. Katsanos and colleagues [17] showed that following moderate-intensity endurance exercise there was significantly lower insulin concentration and TG area under the curve (AUC) over 6 h after ingestion of a high-fat meal when compared to the no exercise trial. Therefore, insulin action may play one of the key factors in influencing postprandial TG levels [18,19].

A rise in insulin concentration by following CHO ingestion results in an increase in the rate of CHO oxidation, and the rate of fat oxidation inhibited [18]. Previous studies examined ingesting CHO meals with a low glycemic index (LGI) and a high glycemic index (HGI) before exercise on substrate utilization during exercise [20–22]. The results suggested that ingestion of the LGI meal induced lower insulin response and showed a significantly higher rate of fat oxidation than that of the HGI meal during subsequent exercise [20,22]. Ingesting CHO with a distinct GI stimulates insulin response, leading to changes in the fat oxidation rate during exercise, which possibly exerts varying degrees of influence on postprandial lipid metabolism when the body is recovering from the exercise. Kaviani and colleagues [23] reported that ingestion of a post-exercise LGI meal induced lower postprandial TG concentrations when compared to that of the HGI meal. However, how the pre-exercise CHO influenced the subsequent postprandial lipid profile is still unclear.

An extant study verified that exercise intervention effectively lowered the increased level of blood lipids due to CHO ingestion [24,25]. We hypothesize that ingestion of an LGI drink prior the exercise may induce higher fat oxidation than ingestion of an HGI drink during exercise and subsequently induces a higher plasma TG clearance rate during the postprandial period after a high fat meal. To date, no studies have been conducted on postprandial lipid profiles immediately after exercise with ingestion of pre-exercise GI CHO. Therefore, the purpose of the present study was to determine the effect of fructose versus glucose pre-exercise drinks and exercise intervention on the subsequent postprandial lipid profile.

2. Materials and Methods

Eight healthy active males voluntary participated in the present study (age 23.1 $\pm$ 0.7 years, weight 68.9 $\pm$ 2.0 kg, and maximal oxygen consumption (VO_2max) 47.7 $\pm$ 1.6 mL/kg/min). This study was conducted in the Sports Science Research Center of National Taiwan University of Sport, with the approval of the Human Subject Committee of National Taiwan University of Sport (NTCPE-95-01). Participants were given their written informed consent after complete understood the study design and possible risks. All participants completed the health history questionnaire before undertaking the experiments.

2.1. Experimental Design

A randomized double-blind cross-over experimental design was adopted and the trial order was counter-balanced for this study. All of the participants underwent two experimental trials separated at least seven days. The participants were asked to ingest CHO-containing either a fructose or glucose drink 30 min before running on the treadmill for 1 h at 60% VO_2max. Immediately after the exercise the participants were asked to take an oral fat tolerance test (OFTT), which asked participants to ingest a high-fat meal to observe postprandial lipemia for 6 h [26]. The participants were asked to record their diet for three days before the first trial and were required to repeat the same diet before the next trial. A standardized lunch and dinner was served for the participants on the day before the main trial. The participants were asked to avoid any heavy physical activity or exercise three days before the main trials. In addition, they were asked to refrain from smoking and ingesting alcohol- and caffeine-containing beverages before the experiment.

2.2. Preliminary Measurements

Two preliminary tests were conducted: running economy (RE) test and VO_2max measurement.

RE test: The RE protocol was a four-stage test running on a treadmill (Medtrack ST65, Quinton, Seattle, Washington, USA) at an initial speed of 7.0–8.0 km/h and increase at 1.0–1.5 km/h every 4 min. The oxygen uptake (VO_2) was measured 1 min before the end of each stage using a gas analyzer (Vmax Series 29C, Sensor Medics, Yorba Linda, CA, USA). The four VO_2 measurements were substituted in a linear regression equation to calculate the relationship between VO_2 and running speed [22].

VO_2max test: The speed of the treadmill was set at a constant pace. The initial slope of the treadmill was set at 3.5% and increased at 2.5% every 3 min. Participants were encouraged to complete every stage of the exercise until volitional fatigue. The VO_2max criteria were a plateau in VO_2, heart rate coming close to the age-predicted maximal heart rate, and respiratory exchange ratio (RER) ≥ 1.15.

2.3. Test Drink, Oral Fat Tolerance Test, and Lunch and Dinner before Experiment Day

Participants ingested different GI carbohydrate drinks that we provided in the present study: (a) a high-GI drink (GI = 100; HGI); and (b) a low-GI drink (GI = 40; LGI). Carbohydrate source: HGI was 75 g glucose (Wako Pure Chemical Industries, Ltd., Osaka, Japan), or LGI was 75 g fructose (Shimakyu's Pure Chemicals, Osaka, Japan) in 500 mL water.

An oral fat tolerance test meal included white bread, whipping cream, nuts, butter, and cereal. The meal provided as based on the body weight of the participants and contained 1.2 g/kg fat, 1.1 g/kg CHO, 0.33 g/kg protein, and 16.5 kcal/kg [26]. All of the foods were purchased from the same supermarket, and the foods were of the same brand. The calorie value of the foods, as well as CHO, protein, and fat contents, were calculated according to the nutritional label by the manufacturer.

The standardized lunch and dinner before the main trial were described in the previous study [26] and were purchased from the same convenience store. The lunch provided 840.0 ± 57.0 kcal, with 50.7 ± 0.3% energy from carbohydrate (106.5 ± 7.4 g), 31.5 ± 0.5% from fat (29.4 ± 1.8 g), and 17.8 ± 0.5% from protein (37.5 ± 3.2 g). The standard dinner offered 692 kcal, with 50% energy from carbohydrate (86.5 g), 32% from fat (24.6 g), and 18% from protein (31.1 g). The calculated GI value was 68.8.

2.4. Protocol

Participants were given the same lunch and dinner one day before the start of the experiment. They were instructed to report to the laboratory after overnight fasting for 12 h. After their height and weight were measured, they were asked to ingest a fructose (F) or glucose (G) drink (500 mL). Following 30 min of a resting period, the participants ran at 60% VO_2max for 1 h on the treadmill. After the exercise was completed, fasting blood specimens were drawn at 0 h from the antecubital vein by a catheter. Subsequently, the participants were asked to ingest an OFTT meal within 20 min, and their blood specimens were collected at 0.5, 1, 2, 3, 4, 5, and 6 h after the meal. The participants were required to sit quietly in the laboratory to avoid any physical activities during the 6 h postprandial period. The environmental temperature was maintained at 22 °C–25 °C and a humidity of 50–60%.

2.5. Blood Sample Collection and Analysis

A catheter (Venflon 20G, Ohmeda, Sweden) was connected to the three-way stopcock (Connecta Ltd., Helsingborg, Sweden) with a 10-cm long tube for collecting 10 mL blood samples at each time point. The 10-cm long blood tube was regularly washed with sterile sodium chloride solution (0.9% *w/v*) to prevent blood coagulation in the tube. A non-heparinized tube was used to collect 2 mL of blood sample, and it was allowed to stand for 1 h to wait for the blood to coagulate. Another tube containing ethylenediaminetetraacetic acid (EDTA) was used to collect 8 mL of blood sample. The collected sample was then centrifuged (Eppendorf 5810, Hamburg, Germany) at 4 °C at 2000 rpm for 20 min. The extracted serum and plasma samples were stored at −70 °C in a freezer before analysis. Plasma glucose (Shino, Tokyo, Japan), TG (Wako, Osaka, Japan), non-esterified fatty acid (NEFA; Wako, Neuss, Germany), glycerol (Randox, Co., Antrim, UK), and HDL-C (Kyowa, Osaka, Japan) were measured using an automated biochemical analyzer (Hitachi 7020, Tokyo, Japan). Electrochemiluminescence (Elecsys 2010, Roche Diagnostics, Basel, Switzerland) immunoassay was used to analyze the serum insulin concentrations (Roche Diagnostics, Mannheim, Germany). The intra-assay coefficients of the variation of the blood sample measurement were: TG: CV(%) = 4.9; insulin: CV(%) = 2.8; NEFA: CV(%) = 4.51; glycerol: CV(%) = 6.42; glucose: CV(%) = 6.9; and HDL-C: CV(%) = 4.9.

2.6. Statistical Analyses

All collected data was presented as mean $\pm$ SD. Changes in blood samples were analyzed by a two-way ANOVA with repeated measures. The Bonferroni post hoc test for comparison with two groups for each time point was used when the ANOVA showed a significant interaction effect (condition $\times$ time). The blood biochemistry concentrations over the time AUCs were analyzed using a paired T-test. The differences between F and G trials were evaluated by Cohen's effect size (ES). The analysis was performed with SPSS 23.0. A p-value less than 0.05 was considered statistically significant.

3. Results

3.1. Plasma Triacylglycerol

Plasma TG IAUC (Figure 1a) was significantly lower in the F than in the G trial (6.57 $\pm$ 2.46 vs. 7.14 $\pm$ 2.64 mmol/L $\times$ 6 h, $p = 0.004$); plasma TG total AUC (Figure 1b) was significantly lower in the F compared with the G trial (9.97 $\pm$ 3.64 vs. 10.91 $\pm$ 3.56 mmol/L $\times$ 6 h, $p = 0.033$). Plasma TG concentration over 6 h (Figure 1c) showed no significant difference between trials by time interaction (condition $\times$ time, $p = 0.628$; condition, $p = 0.342$; time, $p < 0.001$).

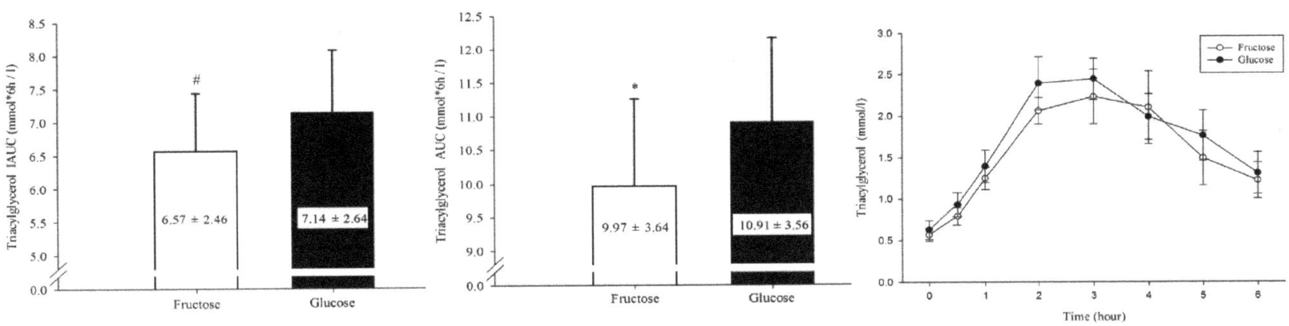

(a) (b) (c)

Figure 1. Triacylglycerol (TG) incremental area under the curve (**a**) and TG area under the curve (**b**) in 6 h and postprandial TG concentration over 6 h (**c**). # F was significantly lower than G ($p = 0.004$). * F was significantly lower than G ($p = 0.033$).

3.2. Serum Insulin and Plasma Glucose

Serum insulin concentration and plasma glucose concentration over the 6 h are displayed in Figure 2. There was no significant difference in serum insulin (condition $\times$ time, $p = 0.557$; condition, $p = 0.893$; Figure 2a). Plasma glucose concentration showed no significant difference between trials (condition $\times$ time, $p = 0.191$; condition, $p = 0.763$; Figure 2b). There were no significant differences between trials in serum insulin AUC and glucose AUC ($p = 0.717$; $p = 0.951$; Table 1).

3.3. Plasma Non-Esterified Fatty Acids (NEFA), Glycerol

Plasma NEFA concentration was significantly higher before OFTT (after exercise) in the F trial than in the G trial (0.39 $\pm$ 0.1 vs. 0.24 $\pm$ 0.06 mmol/L; $p = 0.011$; Table 2). Plasma NEFA concentration over 6 h showed no significant difference between trials (condition × time, $p = 0.052$; condition, $p = 0.563$; time, $p < 0.001$; Figure 3a). There was no difference between trials in plasma NEFA AUC (F: 3.05 ± 0.45; G: 3.06 ± 0.54, $p = 0.962$; Table 1).

Plasma glycerol concentration was significantly higher before OFTT (after exercise) in the F trial than in the G trial (168.75 ± 38.86 vs. 131.75 ± 45.30 μmol/L; $p = 0.015$; Table 2). Plasma glycerol concentration over 6 h showed no significant difference between trials (condition × time, $p = 0.141$; condition, $p = 0.064$; time, $p < 0.001$; Figure 3b). There was no difference between trials in plasma glycerol AUC (F: 395.84 ± 69.55; G: 363.19 ± 64.67, $p = 0.192$; Table 1).

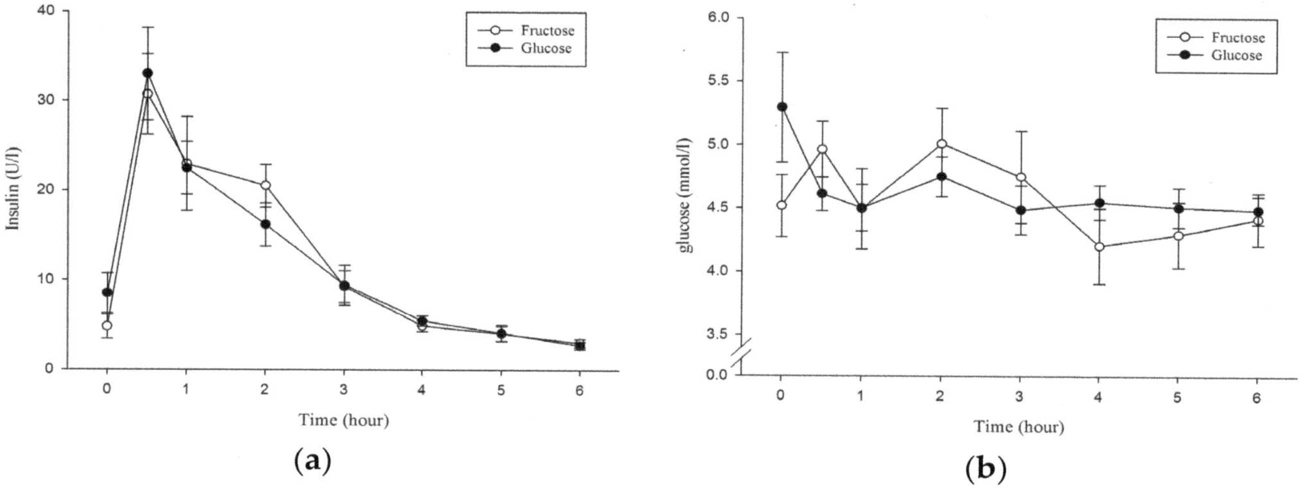

Figure 2. Serum insulin concentrations (**a**) and plasma glucose concentrations (**b**) during the 6 h postprandial period, $p < 0.05$.

Table 1. The plasma and serum sample concentrations area under the curve.

	Fructose	Glucose	p	ES
Insulin (μU/mL × 6 h)	74.06 ± 20.95	71.73 ± 17.88	0.717	0.12
TG (mmol/L × 6 h)	9.97 ± 3.64	10.91 ± 3.56	0.033 *	0.26
TG IAUC (mmol/L × 6 h)	6.57 ± 2.46	7.14 ± 2.64	0.004 *	0.22
Glucose (mmol/L × 6 h)	27.46 ± 3.30	27.56 ± 1.59	0.951	0.04
NEFA (mmol/L × 6 h)	3.05 ± 0.45	3.06 ± 0.54	0.962	0.02
Glycerol (μmol/L × 6 h)	395.84 ± 69.55	363.19 ± 64.67	0.192	0.49
HDL-C (mmol/L × 6 h)	8.02 ± 1.68	7.49 ± 1.52	0.003 *	0.33

* Significant difference between F and G ($p < 0.05$). Values are mean ± SD. TG: triacylglycerol; IAUC: incremental area under the curve; NEFA: non-esterified fatty acids; HDL-C: high density lipoprotein cholesterol.

Table 2. The plasma and serum sample concentrations before OFTT.

	Fructose	Glucose	p	ES
Insulin (μU/mL)	4.78 ± 3.86	8.50 ± 6.31	0.177	0.71
TG (mmol/L)	0.57 ± 0.21	0.63 ± 0.31	0.580	0.23
Glucose (mmol/L)	4.52 ± 0.69	5.29 ± 1.22	0.101	0.78
NEFA (mmol/L)	0.39 ± 0.10	0.24 ± 0.06	0.011 *	1.82
Glycerol (μmol/L)	168.8 ± 38.86	131.7 ± 45.30	0.015 *	0.88
HDL-C (mmol/L)	1.47 ± 0.31	1.33 ± 0.27	0.184	0.48

* Significant difference between F and G ($p < 0.05$). Values are mean ± SD. TG: triacylglycerol; NEFA: non-esterified fatty acids; HDL-C: high density lipoprotein cholesterol.

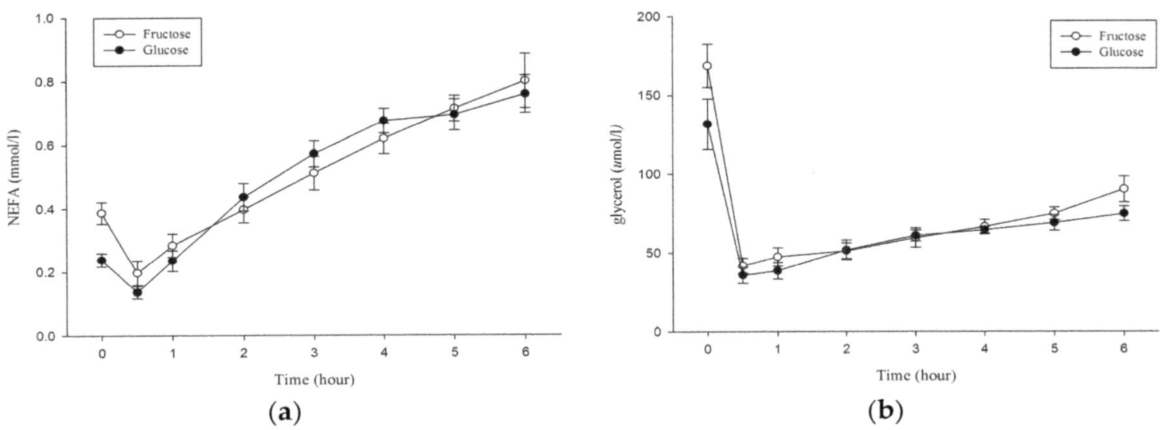

Figure 3. Plasma NEFA concentrations (**a**); and glycerol concentrations (**b**) during the 6 h postprandial period. NEFA: non-esterfied fatty acid.

3.4. *Plasma High-Density Lipoprotein Cholesterol*

Plasma HDL-C concentrations (Figure 4) showed no significant difference between trials by time interaction (condition × time, $p = 0.336$; condition, $p = 0.118$; time, $p = 0.021$). Plasma HDL-C AUC was significantly higher in the F trial compared to the G trial (8.02 ± 1.68 vs. 7.49 ± 1.52 mmol/L × 6 h, $p = 0.003$; Table 1).

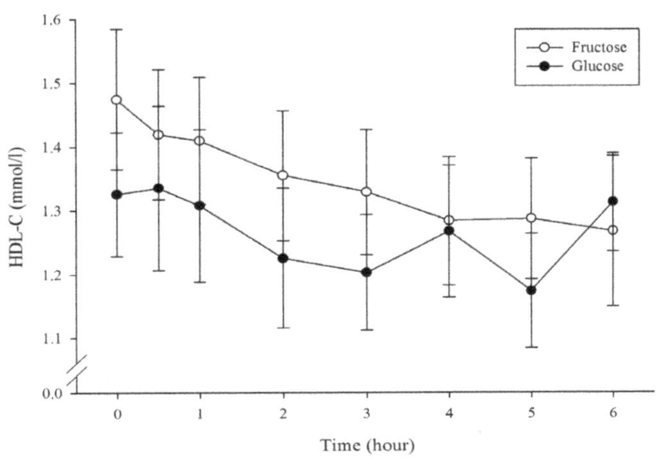

Figure 4. Plasma HDL-C concentrations during the 6 h postprandial period.

4. Discussion

The major finding of this study is that ingestion of fructose before endurance exercise lowered subsequent postprandial plasma TG concentrations compared to that of the glucose drink. Several studies demonstrated that endurance exercise effectively reduced postprandial lipemia [7,8,17,25,27]. To our knowledge, no studies have been conducted on how pre-exercise CHO with different GI and endurance exercises influence the subsequent lipid profile after oral ingestion of a high-fat meal.

A previous study reported that while a lower insulin level was induced by ingesting an LGI meal before exercise, a lower CHO oxidation rate was observed compared with when an HGI meal was ingested during exercise [20,22]. After ingestion of the HGI CHO meal, the rise in insulin level, in turn, decreases the fat oxidation rate during exercise, thereby inhibiting exercise-induced lipid metabolism [22,28]. Although we did not measure the RER to examine the rate of substrate utilization during exercise, the plasma NEFA and glycerol concentrations of the F trial was significantly higher than that of the G trial following 60 min of exercise (Figure 3). The current result is similar to previous studies, which might indicate a higher fat oxidation occurred in the F trial during exercise in the current study [20,22]. Therefore, the current study supported those of previous studies that, after ingesting a CHO diet with different GI and engaging in exercise, the LGI trial showed a significantly higher fat oxidation rate during the exercise than did the HGI trial [20–22]. This result verifies that ingesting an LGI CHO drink before exercise could depress lipid metabolism less during exercise compared with the HGI CHO drink. The higher fat oxidation occurring in the F trial during exercise might result in a higher plasma TG clearance rate during subsequent postprandial period.

Previous study demonstrated that the additional insulin administration after ingestion of high fat meal showed an improvement in postprandial TG disposal in type I diabetes [29]. The study indicated that the insulin concentration played an important role on postprandial TG removal. However, the current study did not find differences in insulin concentration between trials during OFTT. This might be due to the exercise before OFTT diminishing the difference in postprandial insulin response even though we fed different GI CHO before exercise.

In the present study, the postprandial TG AUC and IAUC in the F trial demonstrated significantly lower values than the G trial (Figure 1). An increase in the plasma TG removal rate is possibly the factor causing a reduction in the plasma TG level, including decreasing the release of liver TG and increasing the transport of TG into muscle cells, or storage and utilization [24,30,31]. Ingestion of fructose was thought to increase postprandial lipemia in a sedentary population. Chong and colleagues [32] concluded that ingestion of fructose induced lower insulin secretion and might result in less activation of lipoprotein lipase (LPL), which consequently leads to impairing TG clearance. However, the negative effect may be offset by increasing physical activities [33]. Interestingly, Egli and colleagues [34] reported exercise prevented short-term high-fructose diet induced hypertriglyceridemia and increased lipid oxidation. After exercise, muscle LPL activity is increased, stimulating the transport of TG into the muscle cell for storage and utilization, which may reduce plasma TG concentration [24,35]. A previous study determined that a single session of exercise significantly enhanced the muscle LPL activity [36,37]. Seip and colleagues [38] also found that the expression of LPL genes in fat tissues did not differ significantly after exercise, which further reflects the importance of muscle to blood lipid metabolism after exercise. However, the different insulin responses caused by ingestion of CHO solution with different GI were likely to influence the muscle LPL activity [36,39]. In addition, the levels of glycogen and insulin increased considerably following ingestion of CHO; however, LPL activity was significantly decreased [40,41]. Seip and colleagues [42] demonstrated that the LPL mRNA level was significantly increased after 4 h of exercise, while lower insulin level was observed. This result caused a rise in VLDL concentration and a reduction in HDL-C release [39,43]. Another study reported that glucose ingestion elicits an insulin response that is evidently more apparent than that of fructose ingestion [44,45]. Moreover, the fat oxidation rate during exercise is relatively higher after fructose ingestion [46], which also influences LPL activity, eliciting changes in the postprandial TG level. This probably partially explains why the F trial postprandial TG level was significantly lower than that of the G trial in the current study.

The postprandial HDL-C level is related to the metabolic rate of TG-rich lipoprotein [24], and exercise may promote a rise in HDL-C concentration [47,48]. However, HDL-C concentration could be influenced by the insulin level [49]. The result of the present study indicated that when the participants ingested the F drink before exercise, the significantly higher postprandial HDL-C level was observed compared with when ingesting the G solution (Figure 4). A previous study reported when CHO ingestion was controlled for four weeks, the fasting insulin level increased significantly, and the HDL-C level was significantly lower than the pretest value [50]. Another study compared ingestion of different concentrations of CHO beverages and found that low CHO intervention resulted in higher HDL-C concentration, which was effective for triggering a decrease in the postprandial TG level [51]. Compared with ingesting the F drink, ingesting the G drink induced higher insulin response which, in turn, caused a reduction in the postprandial HDL-C level, thereby weakening the TG removal capability.

Previous studies have largely explored the relationship between exercise intervention and postprandial lipid metabolism. No studies have investigated ingestion of different GI CHO before exercise generating an influence on the postprandial lipemia immediately after exercise. This is the first study to elucidate the interactive effects of different GI drinks and exercise intervention on lipid metabolism following OFTT. We found that intervention might exert a retention effect, suggesting that ingesting a CHO drink with different GI before exercise influences the rate of substrate utilization during exercise, as well as the postprandial lipid level when OFTT is ingested after exercise.

Limitations

One of the major limitation of the present study was that the participants were given 75 g glucose or fructose drinks which were not adjusted by their body weight, although the different body size may have resulted in different magnitudes of glycemia when ingesting of the same amount of CHO. However, the design of the present study was mainly to induce different glycemic and insulinemic responses via different GI carbohydrate prior to exercise in order to influence the subsequent substrate utilization. In addition, the present study design was a with-in subject design. Therefore, we speculate that even if we adjust the amount of pre-exercise CHO by the subject's body weight, the outcome will possibly be similar to the present results.

5. Conclusions

This study found that when fructose was ingested before endurance exercise, the fructose trial significantly lowered TG AUC and IAUC compared with the glucose trial after OFTT. This result is possibly related to the pre-exercise low insulin level that induced higher fat oxidation during exercise. However, the mechanism involved remains elusive and warrants further investigation in the future.

Acknowledgments: The study was funded by National Science Council in Taiwan (NSC 96-2413-H-028-003-MY2). We deeply appreciated Sport Science Research Center of National Taiwan University of Sport provided the technical supported for this study.

Author Contributions: Ching-Lin Wu and Cheng-Kang Chang conceived and designed the experiments; Mei-Hui Tseng and Tsung-Jen Yang performed the experiments; Chih-Hui Chiu and Tsung-Jen Yang analyzed the data; Ching-Lin Wu, Cheng-Kang Chang, and Chih-Hui Chiu contributed reagents/materials/analysis tools; and Ching-Lin Wu and Tsung-Jen Yang wrote the paper.

References

1. Lefebvre, P.J.; Scheen, A.J. The postprandial state and risk of cardiovascular disease. *Diabet. Med.* **1998**, *15*, S63–S68. [CrossRef]
2. Chan, D.C.; Pang, J.; Romic, G.; Watts, G.F. Postprandial hypertriglyceridemia and cardiovascular disease: Current and future therapies. *Curr. Atheroscler. Rep.* **2013**, *15*, 309. [CrossRef] [PubMed]
3. Nordestgaard, B.G.; Benn, M.; Schnohr, P.; Tybjaerg-Hansen, A. Nonfasting triglycerides and risk of myocardial infarction, ischemic heart disease, and death in men and women. *JAMA* **2007**, *298*, 299–308. [CrossRef] [PubMed]
4. Patsch, J.R.; Miesenbock, G.; Hopferwieser, T.; Muhlberger, V.; Knapp, E.; Dunn, J.K.; Gotto, A.M., Jr.; Patsch, W. Relation of triglyceride metabolism and coronary artery disease. Studies in the postprandial state. *Arterioscler. Thromb.* **1992**, *12*, 1336–1345. [CrossRef] [PubMed]
5. Sharrett, A.R.; Chambless, L.E.; Heiss, G.; Paton, C.C.; Patsch, W. Association of postprandial triglyceride and retinyl palmitate responses with asymptomatic carotid artery atherosclerosis in middle-aged men and women. The Atherosclerosis Risk in Communities (ARIC) Study. *Arterioscler. Thromb. Vasc. Biol.* **1995**, *15*, 2122–2129. [CrossRef] [PubMed]

6. Aldred, H.E.; Perry, I.C.; Hardman, A.E. The effect of a single bout of brisk walking on postprandial lipemia in normolipidemic young adults. *Metabolism* **1994**, *43*, 836–841. [CrossRef]
7. Gill, J.M.; Al-Mamari, A.; Ferrell, W.R.; Cleland, S.J.; Sattar, N.; Packard, C.J.; Petrie, J.R.; Caslake, M.J. Effects of a moderate exercise session on postprandial lipoproteins, apolipoproteins and lipoprotein remnants in middle-aged men. *Atherosclerosis* **2006**, *185*, 87–96. [CrossRef] [PubMed]
8. Tsetsonis, N.V.; Hardman, A.E.; Mastana, S.S. Acute effects of exercise on postprandial lipemia: A comparative study in trained and untrained middle-aged women. *Am. J. Clin. Nutr.* **1997**, *65*, 525–533. [CrossRef] [PubMed]
9. Hargreaves, M.; Hawley, J.A.; Jeukendrup, A. Pre-exercise carbohydrate and fat ingestion: Effects on metabolism and performance. *J. Sports Sci.* **2004**, *22*, 31–38. [CrossRef] [PubMed]
10. Wright, D.A.; Sherman, W.M.; Dernbach, A.R. Carbohydrate feedings before, during, or in combination improve cycling endurance performance. *J. Appl. Phys.* **1991**, *71*, 1082–1088. [CrossRef] [PubMed]
11. Parks, E.J. Effect of dietary carbohydrate on triglyceride metabolism in humans. *J. Nutr.* **2001**, *131*, 2772S–2774S. [CrossRef] [PubMed]
12. Shin, Y.; Park, S.; Choue, R. Comparison of time course changes in blood glucose, insulin and lipids between high carbohydrate and high fat meals in healthy young women. *Nutr. Res. Pract.* **2009**, *3*, 128–133. [CrossRef] [PubMed]
13. Siri-Tarino, P.W.; Sun, Q.; Hu, F.B.; Krauss, R.M. Saturated fat, carbohydrate, and cardiovascular disease. *Am. J. Clin. Nutr.* **2010**, *91*, 502–509. [CrossRef] [PubMed]
14. Abbasi, F.; McLaughlin, T.; Lamendola, C.; Kim, H.S.; Tanaka, A.; Wang, T.; Nakajima, K.; Reaven, G.M. High carbohydrate diets, triglyceride-rich lipoproteins, and coronary heart disease risk. *Am. J. Cardiol.* **2000**, *85*, 45–48. [CrossRef]
15. Hamilton, M.T.; Etienne, J.; McClure, W.C.; Pavey, B.S.; Holloway, A.K. Role of local contractile activity and muscle fiber type on LPL regulation during exercise. *Am. J. Physiol.* **1998**, *275*, E1016–E1022. [CrossRef] [PubMed]
16. Zhang, J.Q.; Thomas, T.R.; Ball, S.D. Effect of exercise timing on postprandial lipemia and HDL cholesterol subfractions. *J. Appl. Phys.* **1998**, *85*, 1516–1522. [CrossRef] [PubMed]
17. Katsanos, C.S.; Grandjean, P.W.; Moffatt, R.J. Effects of low and moderate exercise intensity on postprandial lipemia and postheparin plasma lipoprotein lipase activity in physically active men. *J. Appl. Physiol.* **2004**, *96*, 181–188. [CrossRef] [PubMed]
18. McLaughlin, T.; Abbasi, F.; Lamendola, C.; Yeni-Komshian, H.; Reaven, G. Carbohydrate-induced hypertriglyceridemia: An insight into the link between plasma insulin and triglyceride concentrations. *J. Clin. Endocrinol. Metab.* **2000**, *85*, 3085–3088. [CrossRef] [PubMed]
19. Olefsky, J.M.; Farquhar, J.W.; Reaven, G.M. Reappraisal of the role of insulin in hypertriglyceridemia. *Am. J. Med.* **1974**, *57*, 551–560. [CrossRef]
20. Stevenson, E.J.; Williams, C.; Mash, L.E.; Phillips, B.; Nute, M.L. Influence of high-carbohydrate mixed meals with different glycemic indexes on substrate utilization during subsequent exercise in women. *Am. J. Clin. Nutr.* **2006**, *84*, 354–360. [PubMed]
21. Wee, S.L.; Williams, C.; Tsintzas, K.; Boobis, L. Ingestion of a high-glycemic index meal increases muscle glycogen storage at rest but augments its utilization during subsequent exercise. *J. Appl. Physiol.* **2005**, *99*, 707–714. [CrossRef] [PubMed]
22. Wu, C.L.; Nicholas, C.; Williams, C.; Took, A.; Hardy, L. The influence of high-carbohydrate meals with different glycaemic indices on substrate utilisation during subsequent exercise. *Br. J. Nutr.* **2003**, *90*, 1049–1056. [CrossRef] [PubMed]
23. Kaviani, M.; Chilibeck, P.D.; Yee, P.; Zello, G.A. The effect of consuming low-versus high-glycemic index meals after exercise on postprandial blood lipid response following a next-day high-fat meal. *Nutr. Diabetes* **2016**, *6*, e216. [CrossRef] [PubMed]
24. Gill, J.M.; Herd, S.L.; Vora, V.; Hardman, A.E. Effects of a brisk walk on lipoprotein lipase activity and plasma triglyceride concentrations in the fasted and postprandial states. *Eur. J. Appl. Physiol.* **2003**, *89*, 184–190. [CrossRef] [PubMed]
25. Koutsari, C.; Hardman, A.E. Exercise prevents the augmentation of postprandial lipaemia attributable to a low-fat high-carbohydrate diet. *Br. J. Nutr.* **2001**, *86*, 197–205. [PubMed]

26. Chiu, C.H.; Burns, S.F.; Yang, T.J.; Chang, Y.H.; Chen, Y.L.; Chang, C.K.; Wu, C.L. Energy replacement using glucose does not increase postprandial lipemia after moderate intensity exercise. *Lipids Health Dis.* **2014**, *13*, 177. [CrossRef] [PubMed]
27. Wu, C.L.; Williams, C. A low glycemic index meal before exercise improves endurance running capacity in men. *Int. J. Sport Nutr. Exerc. Metab.* **2006**, *16*, 510–527. [CrossRef] [PubMed]
28. Gregory, S.; Wood, R.; Matthews, T.; Vanlangen, D.; Sawyer, J.; Headley, S. Substrate Utilization is Influenced by Acute Dietary Carbohydrate Intake in Active, Healthy Females. *J. Sports Sci. Med.* **2011**, *10*, 59–65. [PubMed]
29. Campbell, M.D.; Walker, M.; Ajjan, R.A.; Birch, K.M.; Gonzalez, J.T.; West, D.J. An additional bolus of rapid-acting insulin to normalise postprandial cardiovascular risk factors following a high-carbohydrate high-fat meal in patients with type 1 diabetes: A randomised controlled trial. *Diabetes Vasc. Dis. Res.* **2017**, *14*, 336–344. [CrossRef] [PubMed]
30. Magkos, F.; Wright, D.C.; Patterson, B.W.; Mohammed, B.S.; Mittendorfer, B. Lipid metabolism response to a single, prolonged bout of endurance exercise in healthy young men. *Am. J. Physiol. Endocrinol. Metab.* **2006**, *290*, E355–E362. [CrossRef] [PubMed]
31. Tsekouras, Y.E.; Yanni, A.E.; Bougatsas, D.; Kavouras, S.A.; Sidossis, L.S. A single bout of brisk walking increases basal very low-density lipoprotein triacylglycerol clearance in young men. *Metabolism* **2007**, *56*, 1037–1043. [PubMed]
32. Chong, M.F.; Fielding, B.A.; Frayn, K.N. Mechanisms for the acute effect of fructose on postprandial lipemia. *Am. J. Clin. Nutr.* **2007**, *85*, 1511–1520. [PubMed]
33. Bidwell, A.J.; Fairchild, T.J.; Redmond, J.; Wang, L.; Keslacy, S.; Kanaley, J.A. Physical activity offsets the negative effects of a high-fructose diet. *Med. Sci. Sports Exerc.* **2014**, *46*, 2091–2098. [CrossRef] [PubMed]
34. Egli, L.; Lecoultre, V.; Theytaz, F.; Campos, V.; Hodson, L.; Schneiter, P.; Mittendorfer, B.; Patterson, B.W.; Fielding, B.A.; Gerber, P.A.; et al. Exercise prevents fructose-induced hypertriglyceridemia in healthy young subjects. *Diabetes* **2013**, *62*, 2259–2265. [CrossRef] [PubMed]
35. Malkova, D.; Evans, R.D.; Frayn, K.N.; Humphreys, S.M.; Jones, P.R.; Hardman, A.E. Prior exercise and postprandial substrate extraction across the human leg. *Am. J. Physiol. Endocrinol. Metab.* **2000**, *279*, E1020–E1028. [CrossRef] [PubMed]
36. Kiens, B.; Lithell, H. Lipoprotein metabolism influenced by training-induced changes in human skeletal muscle. *J. Clin. Investig.* **1989**, *83*, 558–564. [CrossRef] [PubMed]
37. Kiens, B.; Richter, E.A. Utilization of skeletal muscle triacylglycerol during postexercise recovery in humans. *Am. J. Physiol.* **1998**, *275*, E332–E337. [CrossRef] [PubMed]
38. Seip, R.L.; Angelopoulos, T.J.; Semenkovich, C.F. Exercise induces human lipoprotein lipase gene expression in skeletal muscle but not adipose tissue. *Am. J. Physiol.* **1995**, *268*, E229–E236. [CrossRef] [PubMed]
39. Pollare, T.; Vessby, B.; Lithell, H. Lipoprotein lipase activity in skeletal muscle is related to insulin sensitivity. *Arterioscler. Thromb. Vasc. Biol.* **1991**, *11*, 1192–1203. [CrossRef]
40. Jacobs, I.; Lithell, H.; Karlsson, J. Dietary effects on glycogen and lipoprotein lipase activity in skeletal muscle in man. *Acta Physiol. Scand.* **1982**, *115*, 85–90. [CrossRef] [PubMed]
41. Lithell, H.; Jacobs, I.; Vessby, B.; Hellsing, K.; Karlsson, J. Decrease of lipoprotein lipase activity in skeletal muscle in man during a short-term carbohydrate-rich dietary regime. With special reference to HDL-cholesterol, apolipoprotein and insulin concentrations. *Metabolism* **1982**, *31*, 994–998. [CrossRef]
42. Seip, R.L.; Mair, K.; Cole, T.G.; Semenkovich, C.F. Induction of human skeletal muscle lipoprotein lipase gene expression by short-term exercise is transient. *Am. J. Physiol.* **1997**, *272*, E255–E261. [CrossRef] [PubMed]
43. Lithell, H.; Karlstrom, B.; Selinus, I.; Vessby, B.; Fellstrom, B. Is muscle lipoprotein lipase inactivated by ordinary amounts of dietary carbohydrates? *Hum. Nutr. Clin. Nutr.* **1985**, *39*, 289–295. [PubMed]
44. Decombaz, J.; Sartori, D.; Arnaud, M.J.; Thelin, A.L.; Schurch, P.; Howald, H. Oxidation and metabolic effects of fructose or glucose ingested before exercise. *Int. J. Sports Med.* **1985**, *6*, 282–286. [CrossRef] [PubMed]
45. Koivisto, V.A.; Karonen, S.L.; Nikkila, E.A. Carbohydrate ingestion before exercise: Comparison of glucose, fructose, and sweet placebo. *J. Appl. Physiol.* **1981**, *51*, 783–787. [CrossRef] [PubMed]
46. Massicotte, D.; Peronnet, F.; Allah, C.; Hillaire-Marcel, C.; Ledoux, M.; Brisson, G. Metabolic response to [13C]glucose and [13C]fructose ingestion during exercise. *J. Appl. Physiol.* **1986**, *61*, 1180–1184. [CrossRef] [PubMed]

47. Blazek, A.; Rutsky, J.; Osei, K.; Maiseyeu, A.; Rajagopalan, S. Exercise-mediated changes in high-density lipoprotein: Impact on form and function. *Am. Heart J.* **2013**, *166*, 392–400. [CrossRef] [PubMed]
48. Grandjean, P.W.; Crouse, S.F.; Rohack, J.J. Influence of cholesterol status on blood lipid and lipoprotein enzyme responses to aerobic exercise. *J. Appl. Physiol.* **2000**, *89*, 472–480. [CrossRef] [PubMed]
49. Laws, A.; Reaven, G.M. Evidence for an independent relationship between insulin resistance and fasting plasma HDL-cholesterol, triglyceride and insulin concentrations. *J. Intern. Med.* **1992**, *231*, 25–30. [CrossRef] [PubMed]
50. Volek, J.S.; Sharman, M.J.; Gomez, A.L.; DiPasquale, C.; Roti, M.; Pumerantz, A.; Kraemer, W.J. Comparison of a very low-carbohydrate and low-fat diet on fasting lipids, LDL subclasses, insulin resistance, and postprandial lipemic responses in overweight women. *J. Am. Coll. Nutr.* **2004**, *23*, 177–184. [CrossRef] [PubMed]
51. Volek, J.S.; Sharman, M.J.; Gomez, A.L.; Scheett, T.P.; Kraemer, W.J. An isoenergetic very low carbohydrate diet improves serum HDL cholesterol and triacylglycerol concentrations, the total cholesterol to HDL cholesterol ratio and postprandial lipemic responses compared with a low fat diet in normal weight, normolipidemic women. *J. Nutr.* **2003**, *133*, 2756–2761. [PubMed]

Permissions

All chapters in this book were first published by MDPI; hereby published with permission under the Creative Commons Attribution License or equivalent. Every chapter published in this book has been scrutinized by our experts. Their significance has been extensively debated. The topics covered herein carry significant findings which will fuel the growth of the discipline. They may even be implemented as practical applications or may be referred to as a beginning point for another development.

The contributors of this book come from diverse backgrounds, making this book a truly international effort. This book will bring forth new frontiers with its revolutionizing research information and detailed analysis of the nascent developments around the world.

We would like to thank all the contributing authors for lending their expertise to make the book truly unique. They have played a crucial role in the development of this book. Without their invaluable contributions this book wouldn't have been possible. They have made vital efforts to compile up to date information on the varied aspects of this subject to make this book a valuable addition to the collection of many professionals and students.

This book was conceptualized with the vision of imparting up-to-date information and advanced data in this field. To ensure the same, a matchless editorial board was set up. Every individual on the board went through rigorous rounds of assessment to prove their worth. After which they invested a large part of their time researching and compiling the most relevant data for our readers.

The editorial board has been involved in producing this book since its inception. They have spent rigorous hours researching and exploring the diverse topics which have resulted in the successful publishing of this book. They have passed on their knowledge of decades through this book. To expedite this challenging task, the publisher supported the team at every step. A small team of assistant editors was also appointed to further simplify the editing procedure and attain best results for the readers.

Apart from the editorial board, the designing team has also invested a significant amount of their time in understanding the subject and creating the most relevant covers. They scrutinized every image to scout for the most suitable representation of the subject and create an appropriate cover for the book.

The publishing team has been an ardent support to the editorial, designing and production team. Their endless efforts to recruit the best for this project, has resulted in the accomplishment of this book. They are a veteran in the field of academics and their pool of knowledge is as vast as their experience in printing. Their expertise and guidance has proved useful at every step. Their uncompromising quality standards have made this book an exceptional effort. Their encouragement from time to time has been an inspiration for everyone.

The publisher and the editorial board hope that this book will prove to be a valuable piece of knowledge for researchers, students, practitioners and scholars across the globe.

List of Contributors

Ian D. Caterson, Alice Meroni and Melinda Phang
Boden Institute of Obesity, Nutrition, Exercise & Eating Disorders, D17-Charles Perkins Centre, University of Sydney, Camperdown, NSW 2006, Australia

Kirsty M. Mckenzie, Hasthi U. Dissanayake and Michael R. Skilton
Boden Institute of Obesity, Nutrition, Exercise & Eating Disorders, D17-Charles Perkins Centre, University of Sydney, Camperdown, NSW 2006, Australia
Sydney Medical School, D17-Charles Perkins Centre, University of Sydney, Camperdown, NSW 2006, Australia

Jonathan Hyett
Sydney Medical School, D17-Charles Perkins Centre, University of Sydney, Camperdown, NSW 2006, Australia

Rowena McMullan
Boden Institute of Obesity, Nutrition, Exercise & Eating Disorders, D17-Charles Perkins Centre, University of Sydney, Camperdown, NSW 2006, Australia
Sydney Medical School, D17-Charles Perkins Centre, University of Sydney, Camperdown, NSW 2006, Australia
Royal Prince Alfred Hospital, Missenden Road, Camperdown, NSW 2050, Australia

David S. Celermajer and Adrienne Gordon
Sydney Medical School, D17-Charles Perkins Centre, University of Sydney, Camperdown, NSW 2006, Australia
Royal Prince Alfred Hospital, Missenden Road, Camperdown, NSW 2050, Australia

Camille Raynes-Greenow
Sydney School of Public Health, Edward Ford Building, Fisher Road, University of Sydney, Sydney, NSW 2006, Australia

Jaimie W. Polson
Sydney Medical School, D17-Charles Perkins Centre, University of Sydney, Camperdown, NSW 2006, Australia
School of Medical Science & Bosch Institute, Anderson Stuart Building (F13), University of Sydney, Sydney, NSW 2006, Australia

Fabienne Rajas, Amandine Gautier-Stein and Gilles Mithieux
Institut National de la Santé et de la Recherche Médicale, U1213, F-69008 Lyon, France
Université de Lyon, F-69008 Lyon, France
Université Lyon 1, F-69622 Villeurbanne, France

Fabrizio Ferretti and Michele Mariani
Department of Communication and Economics, School of Social Sciences, University of Modena and Reggio Emilia, Palazzo Dossetti—Viale Allegri 9, 42121 Reggio Emilia, Italy

Wesley C. Kephart, Petey W. Mumford, Xuansong Mao, Matthew A. Romero, Hayden W. Hyatt and Christopher B. Mobley
School of Kinesiology, Auburn University, Auburn, AL 36849, USA

Yufeng Zhang
Department of Biological Sciences, Auburn University, Auburn, AL 36849, USA

John C. Quindry
Department of Human Health Performance, University of Montana, Missoula, MT 59812, USA

Kaelin C. Young, Darren T. Beck, Jeffrey S. Martin, Danielle J. McCullough, Andreas N. Kavazis and Michael D. Roberts
School of Kinesiology, Auburn University, Auburn, AL 36849, USA
Department of Cell Biology and Physiology, Edward via College of Osteopathic Medicine—Auburn Campus, Auburn, AL 36849, USA

Dominic P. D'Agostino
Department of Molecular Pharmacology and Physiology, University of South Florida, Tampa, FL 33620, USA

Ryan P. Lowery and Jacob M. Wilson
Applied Sports Performance Institute, Tampa, FL 33607, USA

John Monro and Suman Mishra
New Zealand Institute for Plant & Food Research, Palmerston North 4442, New Zealand

Maria L. Stewart
Global Nutrition R & D, Ingredion Incorporated, 10 Finderne Ave, Bridgewater, NJ 08807, USA

Meredith L. Wilcox, Marjorie Bell, Mary A. Buggia and Kevin C. Maki
Midwest Biomedical Research, Center for Metabolic and Cardiovascular Health, 489 Taft Ave Suite 202, Glen Ellyn, IL 60137, USA

Grace J. Campbell and Kim S. Bell-Anderson
Charles Perkins Centre, School of Life and Environmental Sciences, University of Sydney, Sydney, NSW 2006, Australia

Alistair M. Senior
Charles Perkins Centre, School of Mathematics and Statistics, University of Sydney, Sydney, NSW 2006, Australia

Mariko Sanada, Chinatsu Kabe, Hisa Hata, Junichi Uchida, Gaku Inoue, Yoko Tsukamoto, Shogo Tabata, Mitsuhisa Tabata and Satoru Yamada
Kitasato Institute Hospital, Diabetes Center, 5-9-1 Shirokane, Minato-ku, Tokyo 108-0072, Japan

Yoshifumi Yamada
Boei Ika Daigakko Boei Igagku Kenkyu Center, 3-2 Namiki, Tokorozawa, Saitama 359-0042, Japan

Junichiro Irie
School of Medicine, Keio University, Internal Medicine, 35 Shinanomachi, Shinjuku, Tokyo 160-8582, Japan

Justin L. Carlson, Jennifer M. Erickson, Julie M. Hess and Joanne L. Slavin
Department of Food Science and Nutrition, University of Minnesota, 1334 Eckles Ave, St. Paul, MN 55108, USA

Trevor J. Gould
Informatics Institute, University of Minnesota, 101 Pleasant St., Minneapolis, MN 55455, USA

Harry L. Taylor, Yung-Chih Chen, Javier T. Gonzalez and James A. Betts
Department for Health, University of Bath, Bath BA2 7AY, UK

Ching-Lin Wu and Pin-Ging Wang
Graduate Institute of Sports and Health Management, National Chung Hsing University, Taichung 402, Taiwan

Zhuoshi Zhang and Bernard J. Venn
Department of Human Nutrition, University of Otago, Dunedin 9054, New Zealand

John Monro
New Zealand Institute for Plant & Food Research Ltd., Palmerston North 4442, New Zealand

Michael L. Newell
Department of Life Sciences, Faculty of Science and Technology University of Westminster, London W1W 6UW, UK

Gareth A. Wallis
School of Sport, Exercise and Rehabilitation Sciences, University of Birmingham, Birmingham B15 2TT, UK

Angus M. Hunter, Kevin D. Tipton and Stuart D. R. Galloway
Physiology, Exercise and Nutrition Research Group, Faculty of Health Sciences and Sport, University of Stirling, Stirling FK9 4LA, UK

Kerry Bentley-Hewitt and Suman Mishra
New Zealand Institute for Plant & Food Research, Palmerston North 4442, New Zealand

John Monro
New Zealand Institute for Plant & Food Research, Palmerston North 4442, New Zealand
Riddet Institute, Massey University, Palmerston North 4442, New Zealand

Giorgia Tascini, Maria Giulia Berioli, Laura Cerquiglini, Elisa Santi, Giulia Mancini, Francesco Rogari, Giada Toni and Susanna Esposito
Pediatric Clinic, Department of Surgical and Biomedical Sciences, Università degli Studi di Perugia, 06132 Perugia, Italy

Othmar Moser and Richard M. Bracken
Diabetes Research Group, Medical School, Swansea University, Swansea SA2 8PP, UK
Applied Sport, Technology, Exercise and Medicine Research Centre (A-STEM), College of Engineering, Swansea University, Swansea SA1 8EN, UK

Jane E. Yardley
Kinesiology, Sport and Recreation, Social Sciences, University of Alberta, Edmonton, AB T4V 2R3, Canada

Qiong Fan, Rikke C. Nørgaard, Christin Lucas, Knut Tomas Dalen, Hilde I. Nebb and Line M. Grønning-Wang
Department of Nutrition, Institute of Basic Medical Sciences, University of Oslo, 0317 Oslo, Norway

Christian Bindesbøll
Department of Molecular Medicine, Institute of Basic Medical Sciences, University of Oslo, 0317 Oslo, Norway

Eshrat Babaie
Centre for Molecular Medicine Norway, University of Oslo, 0318 Oslo, Norway

Harri M. Itkonen
Prostate Cancer Research Group, Centre for Molecular Medicine (Norway), University of Oslo and Oslo University Hospitals, 0318 Oslo, Norway

Jason Matthews
Department of Nutrition, Institute of Basic Medical Sciences, University of Oslo, 0317 Oslo, Norway
Department of Pharmacology and Toxicology, University of Toronto, Toronto, ON M5S1A8, Canada

Tsung-Jen Yang
Department of Physical Education, National Taiwan Normal University, Taipei 106, Taiwan

Chih-Hui Chiu
Graduate Program in Department of Exercise Health Science, National Taiwan University of Sport, Taichung 404, Taiwan

Mei-Hui Tseng and Cheng-Kang Chang
Sport Science Research Center, National Taiwan University of Sport, Taichung 404, Taiwan

Ching-LinWu
Graduate Institute of Sports and Health Management, National Chung Hsing University, Taichung 402, Taiwan

Index

M

N

O

P

R

S

U

X

www.ingramcontent.com/pod-product-compliance
Lightning Source LLC
LaVergne TN
LVHW061512220926
848485LV00017B/877